FAMILIAL ALZHEIMER'S DISEASE

Neurological Disease and Therapy

Series Editor
William C. Koller
Department of Neurology
University of Kansas Medical Center
Kansas City, Kansas

Volume 1 Handbook of Parkinson's Disease
Edited by William C. Koller

Volume 2 Medical Therapy of Acute Stroke
Edited by Mark Fisher

Volume 3 Familial Alzheimer's Disease: Molecular Genetics and Clinical Perspectives
Edited by Gary D. Miner, Ralph W. Richter, John P. Blass, Jimmie L. Valentine, and Linda A. Winters-Miner

FAMILIAL ALZHEIMER'S DISEASE

Molecular Genetics and Clinical Perspectives

edited by

GARY D. MINER
Familial Alzheimer's Disease Research Foundation
Tulsa, Oklahoma

RALPH W. RICHTER
University of Oklahoma Tulsa Medical College
Tulsa, Oklahoma

JOHN P. BLASS
Cornell University Medical College
New York, New York

JIMMIE L. VALENTINE
Oral Roberts University School of Medicine
Tulsa, Oklahoma

LINDA A. WINTERS-MINER
Familial Alzheimer's Disease Research Foundation
Tulsa, Oklahoma

MARCEL DEKKER, INC. New York and Basel

Library of Congress Cataloging-in-Publication Data

Familial Alzheimer's disease : molecular genetics and clinical perspectives/ edited by Gary D. Miner .... [et al.] . p. cm. –– (Neurological disease and therapy : v. 3)

Bibliography: p.

Includes index.

ISBN 0–8247–8068–X (alk. paper)

1. Alzheimer's disease––Genetic aspects. I. Miner, Gary.

II. Series.

[DNLM: 1. Alzheimer's Disease––genetics. 2. Alzheimer's Disease––physiopathology WM 220 F198]

RC523.F35 1989
616.8'31042––dc20
DNLM/DLC
for Library of Congress 89-7692
CIP

This book is printed on acid-free paper.

MARCEL DEKKER, INC.
270 Madison Avenue, New York, New York 10016

Current printing (last digit):
10 9 8 7 6 5 4 3 2 1

PRINTED IN THE UNITED STATES OF AMERICA

Preface

The ranks of those interested in treating Alzheimer's disease (AD) have shown encouraging growth. For example, since its inception, many scientists have joined with the Familial Alzheimer's Disease Research Foundation (FADRF) in its mission to facilitate cooperative research around the world with the goal of arriving at a speedy answer to the problem of Alzheimer's disease. Another sign of increasing involvement was the First International Symposium on Familial Alzheimer's Disease, held in Tulsa, Oklahoma, in 1987. This was the first time so many (over 165) leading scientists had convened to discuss familial Alzheimer's disease.

Our own involvement began as an idea—a vision—to do something about the problem of familial Alzheimer's disease (FAD). This vision was presented gradually to us from 1973 to 1982, as we became acquainted gradually with FAD families, who asked us to help. We started researching FAD in 1973 on a part-time basis, but it was not until the summers of 1981-1985 that we devoted our full energies to it. Initially, we conducted a neuropsychological risk factor study with the help of some of the families. We tested at the homes of these families, lived with them during these times, attended their family reunions, and, in reality, became closely involved with these families. During this time most of medical research was not addressing their needs, so our help was greatly appreciated.

This book is divided into four parts and an appendix. Part I provides a background to familial Alzheimer's disease with chapters by Folstein and Powell, Bird and Lampe, and Nee and Polinsky. Nee and Polinsky additionally discuss the clinical spectrum of AD, and Jean-Francois Foncin et al. address the sociological aspects of ascertaining large family pedigrees and methods of dealing with and obtaining the cooperation of large families. Linda Teri and Rebecca Logsdon provide a background for neuropsychological investigations of AD, leading into Chapter 14 in Part III.

Part II presents several chapters on the molecular genetics of Alzheimer's disease, beginning with V. Elving Anderson's chapter on genetic heterogeneity. Vance et al's chapter on genetic linkage in late onset FAD follows, as does St. George-Hyslop et al.'s chapter, which discusses early onset FAD. The remaining chapters in Part II deal primarily with chromosome 21, amyloid protein and its gene, representing laboratories from Boston; Rochester, New York; San Diego, California; Perth, Australia; and Heidelberg, West Germany.

Part III deals with promising new avenues of research. Zubenko writes on blood platelet membrane fluidity as a potential biological marker for AD, a discovery that may prove to be very important. The remaining chapters cover several areas, including clinical and research applications of monospecific antibodies to abnormal proteins in AD, levels of met-enkephalin in plasma and CSF, brain imaging technology, neuropsychological associations, and calcium channel binding site densities in AD brain. The section concludes with Denis Gauvreau et al.'s chapter on the IMAGE Project.

Part IV provides an overview of challenges in AD research for the future. It begins with a chapter by the National Institute on Aging's Director of the Alzheimer Disease Research Centers, Dr. Zaven S. Khachaturian. It also includes an excellent review of AD-related legal issues for general and family physicians, who can provide a very useful service to patients and families by making them aware of the legal issues that they will need to address.

The Appendix provides a reference bibliography on FAD literature.

The book's unique importance is the pulling together of research and professional interests in a holistic fashion, to provide a realistic appraisal of where we are and what needs to be done in facing this problem. The book is aimed at research scientists and physicians who must deal with the questions relating to this illness and also deal with the problems facing AD families who are bravely coping with this most dreadful of diseases.

Gary D. Miner
Linda A. Winters-Miner

Contents

Introduction

Realization of the importance and full impact of Alzheimer's disease on our medical establishment, social fabric, and personal lives has been slow in developing and still has not fully permeated all aspects of our society. Although the disease was first described in 1907 by Alzheimer (1) in a 51-year-old patient, many generations of physicians were taught that this was a rather rare familial form of "pre-senile dementia," which carried the implied assumption that senility was a normal accompaniment of old age.

Full realization of the magnitude of Alzheimer's disease has been realized gradually in the medical profession only during the past decade, largely as a result of the efforts of Katzman and associates (2,3), who marshaled evidence by a number of workers for the identity of Alzheimer's disease with the most prevalent form of senile dementia (4-7). Studies of Larsson et al. showing familial association of the Alzheimer's senile dementia complex with an age-related incidence led to the proposal of a predisposing autosomal dominant gene with an age-related penetrance (8).

Along with recognition of the magnitude of Alzheimer's disease has come a more critical examination of our assumptions about the aging process, with the realization that old age is not necessarily synonymous with disease and disability (9). We now believe that they are separate processes, with the aging process merely setting the stage for the development of degenerative diseases by creating a susceptibility to their development. Furthermore, the detailed pathogenesis of these diseases should be amenable to understanding through biomedical research, which in turn should permit our devising a rational approach to an effective therapeutic intervention and eventually possibly even to their prevention. At the same time, we are seeing the fruits of earlier research as shown by the substantial extension of our mean life expectancy from 47 years in 1900 to around 76 years today so that a greater portion of our population is living into the age when senile dementia will be expressed.

The magnitude of our problem is obvious when we consider the following additional statistics about Alzheimer's disease (10). Alzheimer's disease now affects 2.5 to 3 million individuals in the United States and accounts for fully one-half of the admissions to nursing homes. It produces 120,000 deaths per year and one of three families is its victim. It is the fourth most common cause of death and costs the taxpayers $48 billion per year to provide care for its victims. The cost of care for patients with heart disease is $14.5 billion, for cancer $13.1 billion, and for stroke $5.1 billion—making a combined total of $32.7 billion. Thus the total cost of care of Alzheimer's disease patients is greater than that for the three leading killers combined. For comparison, Alzheimer's disease is 10 to 14 times more frequent than multiple sclerosis, muscular dystrophy, or cystic fibrosis. It is 200 times more frequently found than AIDS, yet the federal dollars for research on Alzheimer's disease are only 1/12 those now given for AIDS research. Most disconcerting for families is that the disease is not covered by Medicare, private insurance, or the Veterans Administration (with rare exceptions).

At the present time, there is no animal model on which to do effective research, and there is no treatment to prevent, stop, or reverse the course of this disease. Thus, it is apparent that the only hope for changing these doleful statistics is to invest more dollars and effort in research.

With more than two decades of experience as Director of Human Biochemical Genetics Programs, I am most impressed with the remarkable amount of information that we can gain from studying "nature's experiments"—the inborn errors of metabolism. Each single gene defect serves as a potential spotlight into the dark recesses of metabolic and physiological processes within the cell. The touchstone for illuminating these processes is the identification of the abnormal gene product that is made defective by the primary genetic mutation. Once it is identified, further detailed studies allow the tracing in detail of the consequences of the abnormality and the physiological and metabolic chain of events that are put in disarray and become manifested as clinical evidence of disease. Once that chain of events is identified, we can, in many cases, circumvent the damaging effects of the abnormal gene and thereby effectively treat or even avoid the disease state. Once the responsible gene is identified, advances made in molecular genetics in the past decade give promise of eventually allowing the correction of the metabolic aberration by insertion of a cloned normal gene.

We have also learned during this time some common denominators of genetic disorders. Virtually all hereditary diseases display genetic heterogeneity at a wide range of levels of complexity. In some disorders a variety of primary biochemical or physiological aberrations of function, even including some of different genetic origin, can lead to the same final common pathway to the disease process, such as the hyperuricemia responsible for development of gouty arthritis (11). In some cases, we find even environmental insults can lead to the same final common pathway leading to disease without the need for an abnormal gene, as in the saturnine gout associated with lead poisoning (11). In other cases, the abnormal gene merely sets the stage for an abnormality of response to an environmental assault, as in the association of HLA antigen W27 with the tendency to develop ankylosing spondylitis (12). At the other extreme, this genetic heterogeneity is found even at the molecular level, defining the site and nature of the mutation. As a result, different loci for mutation sites within the same gene can give rise to a spectrum of severity of impairment of function in the resulting gene product, which in turn is reflected in a spectrum of clinical severity in expression of the disease. The range of clinical expression of Lesch-Nyhan disease is an example of this type of correlation with the amount of residual activity of the mutant enzyme hypoxanthine-guanine phosphoribosyltransferase (HPRT) (11). Consequently, it makes good sense to study initially the most severe clinical expression of the disease where the genetic impairment of metabolic function is also most likely to be most extreme.

In the case of Alzheimer's disease the most severe clinical expression should be in patients who show the earliest onset of pathology and symptoms. Other features found in many other genetic diseases could greatly simplify studies of Alzheimer's disease. One of these is the systemic nature of the metabolic aberration responsible for many such diseases. Thus, if the defect is in a "housekeeping" gene expressed in all body cells, the target organ for development of pathology may be the organ in which the gene product is normally expressed most abundantly as in the high activity of HPRT in the basal ganglia and the clinical signs of basal ganglia dysfunction in patients with Lesch-Nyhan disease (11). However, the ubiquitous presence of the genetic abnormality in all cells allows diagnostic tests to be performed on erythrocyte lysates and more detailed metabolic and genetic studies to be done on cultured lymphoblasts or fibroblasts and on the in vitro selection for the same genetic mutation in neuroblastoma cell lines (13). Other examples of the unexpected systemic nature of metabolic abnormalities originally thought to require study of a relatively inaccessible tissue are known (14). These considerations have suggested a similar strategy for study of the genetic abnormality in this disease. The use of fibroblasts or lymphoblasts cultured from patients with familial Alzheimer's disease has already produced some promising results reported in this volume. More extensive exploration of this approach for identifying the responsible genetic and metabolic defect will undoubtedly be made in future studies.

Once the primary abnormalities of metabolism are deduced and the chain of biochemical abnormalities leading to clinical expression of the disease is unraveled, we will be in a much better position to intervene therapeutically in a rational manner and to even devise methods for prevention of the disease. Thus, the contents of this book are going to be of particular interest to all laboratory investigators in the field of Alzheimer's disease.

J. E. Seegmiller, M.D.
Institute for Research on Aging
University of California, San Diego
San Diego, California

ACKNOWLEDGMENT

Supported by the Clayton Foundation for Research, California Division, PHS grants AM13622, GM 28223, HD20034, GM17702, the Keck Foundation, and the Weingart Foundation.

REFERENCES

1. Alzheimer, A. (1907). Ueber eine eigenartige Erkranking der Hirnrinde. *Allgemerine Zeritschrift für Psychiatire* 64: 146-148.
2. Katzman, R. (1976). The prevalence and malignancy of Alzheimer's disease. A major killer. *Arch. Neurology* 33: 217-218.
3. Katzman, R., Terry, R.D., and Bick, K.L. (1979). (Eds.). *Alzheimer's Disease: Senile Dementia and Related Disorders. Aging*, Vol. 7. Raven Press, New York.
4. Newton, R.D. (1948). The identity of Alzheimer's disease and senile dementia and their relationship to senility. *J. Ment. Sci.* 94: 225-249.
5. Neumann, M.A., Cohn, R. (1963). Incidence of Alzheimer's disease in a large mental hospital. *Arch. Neurol.* 69: 615-636.
6. Blessed, G., Tomlinson, B.E., Roth, M. (1968). The association between quantitative measures of dementia and of senile changes in the cerebral gray matter of elderly subjects. *Br. J. Psychiatry* 114: 797-811.
7. Tomlinson, B.E., Blessed, G., Roth, M. (1970). Observations on the brains of demented old people. *J. Neurol. Sci.* 11: 205-242.
8. Larsson, T., Sjogren, T., Jacoson, G. (1963). Senile dementia. *Acta Psychiatr. Scand.* 39: 3-259.
9. Butler, R.N. (1979). Alzheimer's disease-senile dementia and related disorders: The role of NIA. In: *Alzheimer's Disease: Senile Dementia and Related Disorders* (R. Katzman, R.D. Terry, and Katherine L. Bick, Eds.). Raven Press, New York, pp. 5-9.
10. Losing a Million Minds - Confronting the Tragedy of Alzheimer's Disease and Other Dementias. Congress of the U.S., Office Technical Assessment, Washington, D.C. 1987.
11. Seegmiller, J.E. (1980). Diseases of purine and pyrimidine metabolism. In: *Metabolic Control and Disease*, Eighth Ed. (P.K. Bondy and L.E. Rosenberg, Eds.). W.B. Saunders Co., Philadelphia, pp. 777-937.
12. Schlosstein, L., Terasaki, P.I., Bluestone, R., and Pearson, C.M. (1973). High association of an HL-A antigen W27 with ankylosing spondylitis. *N. Engl. J. Med.* 288: 704-706.
13. Skaper, S.D., and Seegmiller, J.E. (1976). Purine metabolism in thioguanine-resistant glioma cells. *Exp. Cell Res.* 100: 415-417.
14. Lust, G., Faure, G., Netter, P., and Seegmiller, J.E. (1981). Increased pyrophosphate in fibroblasts and lymphoblasts from patients with hereditary diffuse articular chondrocalcinosis. *Science* 214: 809-810.

FAMILIAL ALZHEIMER'S DISEASE

Part I
Background to Familial Alzheimer's Disease and Clinical Perspective

1

In Search of the Alzheimer's Disease Gene

MARSHAL F. FOLSTEIN and DIANE POWELL / *The Johns Hopkins University School of Medicine, Baltimore, Maryland*

INTRODUCTION AND RATIONALE

The conjecture that Alzheimer's disease of early or late onset is a clinical-pathological entity that is not the inevitable consequence of aging is supported by several lines of evidence. Only a minority (10-20%) of the elderly become affected even by age 85 (1). Furthermore, certain families appear to be more vulnerable than others (1-4). Compelling evidence for a genetic component in the causation of Alzheimer's disease (AD) has come from several sources. First of all, a number of pedigrees affected with AD over several generations have been reported (5-9). Also, family studies of the relatives of probands (the affected individuals who first come to attention) reveal an increasing risk with age. Furthermore, persons with a known genetic disorder, Down's syndrome, nearly always develop the pathology of Alzheimer's disease, if they live to or past age 30. Moreover, the plausibility of the genetic model is increased by the presence of other insidious late-onset and progressive neurological disorders such as Huntington's disease and spinocerebellar degeneration, which are known to be hereditary.

Other models of causation have been proposed (e.g., slow virus infection or prions, enzyme deficiency, vascular incompetence, aluminum accumulation, and others). These will not be outlined here, but are described in articles by Shore and Wyatt (10) and Glenner (11). Any of these alternative models would be compatible with the genetic model. For example, a genetic vulnerability may be essential for any environmental agent to be pathogenic, as may be the case in familial Creutzfeldt-Jakob disease (CJD). An enzyme deficiency or vascular incompetence could clearly occur on a genetic basis. However, a single theory to explain the cause of all cases assumes a homogeneity of the AD population, which is likely to be heterogeneous. Sporadic (nonfamilial) cases may be a reflection of this heterogeneity. However, in some cases they may be artifacts of noninformative pedigrees (pedigrees in which relatives died of other causes prior to exceeding the age of risk) or be secondary to new mutations.

Familial AD is attractive to study for several reasons. First, it provides homogeneity among affected members of a given family. Second, familial cases are now easier to detect since more relatives are living into the age of risk because of the general increasing survival of the population. Also, restriction fragment DNA polymorphisms, which have recently been applied to localizing the Huntington's disease gene to chromosome 4, have increased the number of genetic markers for linkage studies. This review will discuss the research done previously on familial AD and its implications for future research.

PHENOTYPIC CONSIDERATIONS

The search for the Alzheimer's disease gene begins with the identification of a phenotype that segregates according to mendelian predictions. Our choice of a phenotype came from several sources. First, studies of the distribution of Alzheimer's disease in families and other populations have been aided by the development of diagnostic criteria such as those of Roth and the National Institute for Neurological and Communicative Disorders and Stroke (NINCDS) (12,13). These are comparable with classic descriptions by Alzheimer and Pritchard, and predictive of the pathological features defined by Alzheimer (14-18). Second, Folstein and Breitner (19) conducted a study using the criteria of the *Diagnostic and Statistical Manual*, Ed. 3 (*DSM-III*), along with the exclusion of patients with risk factors for vascular disease. They found a fourfold greater risk for dementia in relatives of patients who were agraphic and had informative pedigrees. The presence of aphasia or agraphia predicts a 55.7% risk of dementia in parents and siblings of those patients (which is consistent with mendelian autosomal dominant inheritance) (20). Thus, we define the phenotype as follows: the diagnosis of Alzheimer's disease will be applied to patients with the insidious onset and gradual progression of amnesia, aphasia, apraxia, and agnosia in the absence of indication of vascular disease or other central nervous system disorders in persons of any age who, on autopsy, are found to have neuronal loss and large numbers of neuritic plaques and tangles in the cerebral cortex.

FAMILY STUDIES

Three types of family studies will be reviewed. All three share the complications that the late onset of AD poses. Since the onset usually occurs in middle age or later, many family members who have the gene may never be affected because of death from other causes. This will tend to increase the number of apparent nonfamilial or sporadic cases. Also, the shorter life span of men biases the sex ratio of manifest cases in families. However, the risk to relatives of affected persons can be estimated using life table statistical procedures, which takes into account the number of individuals at risk during each year of life (21). These will be discussed later.

The first type of family study is the study of twin pairs. The assumption is that the phenotypic expression of the mutant gene in both members will occur more often in a monozygotic twin pair than in a dizygotic twin pair since monozygotic twins share the same genome, whereas dizygotic share, on the average, 50% of the genome. Although studies by Kallman and others suggest high concordance rates in monozygotic twins (22,23), several reports of discordance in monozygotic twin pairs have appeared (24,25). This discordance might be explained by the affected twin having a phenocopy of AD, rather than actually having the AD gene. Another explanation could be that the unaffected twin carried the gene, but died before living to the age of risk. This is supported by the finding that there was more than a 10-year difference in age of onset in one twin pair (5). Nonetheless, no twin studies have been conducted in which strict clinical criteria for Alzheimer's disease have been used, and this would be necessary before any conclusions can be drawn.

The second type of family study pools the data from large numbers of families for analysis of the proportion of cases in close and distant relatives. If the gene were transmitted from one ancestor, the closer relatives will be affected more than distant relatives who share less of the genome and thus are less likely to carry the gene. The assumption in these studies is that the cause and pathological nature of the disorder are the same in different families so that pooling of data is possible. An advantage is that this enables large numbers of cases to be studied despite small family size.

Two types of heterogeneity are possible. The first is the heterogeneity caused by nongenetic disorders that produce a phenotype similar to the genetically transmitted form, that is, phenocopies. For example one phenocopy for AD would be CJD, which in some cases has a several-year course. The second is genetic heterogeneity, in which different loci can cause similar phenotypes. For example, in Friedreich's ataxia there are families with autosomal inheritance and others with X-linked inheritance.

Since 1927 many studies have indicated that in relatives of probands the risk of developing dementia was higher than the risk in the general population. However, few of these used controls from the same cohorts, that is, were concurrently controlled. Some of these studies are discussed below.

Larsson et al. (2) studied probands born in Sweden, registered in a hospital with a diagnosis of senile dementia, and who were subsequently diagnosed as having senile dementia by the criteria of Roth after reexamination. The 217 patients with senile dementia (SD) were compared to patients with arteriosclerotic dementia (ASD) and those with both SD and ASD. The average age of onset was 73. They found 60 secondary cases among 1,412 relatives age 65 and over. However, the number of affected relatives of the 217 patients with SD alone was not specified. Relatives up to the age of 90 were included in the analysis. Several statistical methods were used to calculate the risk of morbidity among relatives. The authors estimated the risk to be 40% by age 90 and they concluded that the disorder aggregated in families in proportions predicted by a mendelian dominant type of transmission (2).

Heston (4) studied the relatives of 125 patients who were diagnosed based on pathological examination as having Alzheimer's disease from a series of 2,204 autopsies conducted in mental hospitals in Minnesota. Pathological criteria were not specified. Average age of onset for female probands was 67 years; of the cases, 40% were familial. The risk to siblings was 20% by age 85, and the risk to parents was 23%. (A recent estimate of the risk to this age group in Baltimore is 8%.) The risk to siblings of patients with an age of onset earlier than age 70 and an affected parent was in the range predicted for an autosomal dominant trait. The risk for relatives of patients with onset later than age 70 was not higher than the rate for the general population. The advantage of this study was the large number of autopsy-verified probands and the examination of the secondary cases. A disadvantage was the reliance on a pathological diagnosis without stated criteria for the number and distribution of plaques and tangles or modern clinical criteria. Since plaques and tangles are nonspecific findings, this method is likely to introduce patients with disorders other than Alzheimer's disease who have plaques and tangles, as well as those persons with normal aging-related changes (4).

Breitner and Folstein (20), and Chase et al. (21) conducted a concurrently controlled family study using new criteria for case definition and new methods for calculating the risk to relatives. They found higher risks than previously reported if risks to relatives by age 90 were estimated. The study tested the hypothesis that relatives of selected patients with Alzheimer's disease would be more often demented than relatives of two control groups. Criteria for affected patients were that they be demented for more than 4 years and unable to write a sentence (as evidence of aphasia and apraxia), and show no evidence of vascular disease, hypertension, diabetes, or other neurological disorder. Controls were defined as individuals in the same nursing homes who were demented but not agraphic or who were not demented. Some 3,500 residents of 15 nursing homes were screened. Multiple interviews were conducted with relatives by interviewers who were unaware of the hypothesis. Relatives of 39 agraphic demented female probands aged 82 ± 7 (89), who had been ill for 7 years, were compared to relatives of 15 nonagraphic demented women aged 84 ± 5 (89), and 33 female nondemented subjects aged 83 ± 6 (89). The risk to siblings and children was 55% by age 90 in the agraphic cases and 7% in the combined controls. The Weinberg morbidity method was used to calculate cumulative risk to probands.[1] A subsequent analysis using the Kaplan-Meier estimator produced similar rates[2] (21). From this study they estimated that 78% of cases of Alzheimer's disease were familial and affected persons probably transmitted the disease as an autosomal dominant trait (20). Subsequent analyses produced a gamma function that closely fits the data (26,27).

A subsequent study by Knesevich et al. (28) reported that the lack of aphasia was associated with a higher prevalence of familial cases. They studied patients with mild dementia and required that relatives have an onset before age 79 (rather than age 90). Thus the studies are not directly comparable. Relatives with AD with onset between 79 and 90 years of age might have been missed. Also, the authors might have included patients with a dementia other than AD since they only required a duration of 6 months or greater (rather than 4 years). The longer duration allows for more diagnostic certainty.

Powell and Folstein (29) studied 21 patients with Alzheimer's disease who had amnesia, apraxia, and aphasia and at least one affected relative. These familial cases represented 75% of patients in the clinic with the informative pedigrees.

---

[1]The Weinberg morbidity table is similar to the life tables used to estimate the cumulative survival probability to a given age, which is calculated by chain multiplication of the interval-specific estimators of survival probability for each interval. For example, in a life table arranged in 5-year intervals, the probability of survival from age 45 to age 60 is estimated by multiplying together the interval-specific estimates for 45-49, 50-54, and 55-59. However, the Weinberg morbidity table differs from the life table in that the principal outcome is not death, but onset of a specific condition that is age-dependent. Deaths, in the framework of the Weinberg method, are analogues to withdrawals (losses to follow-up) in an ordinary life table. Thus, what is estimated is the cumulative probability of escaping the condition and not of survival. Also, the Weinberg method assumes that incident cases are not at risk for the remainder of the interval of onset. Of (a) is the number of persons alive and unaffected at the start of the interval, (b) the number of withdrawals or deaths from competing causes during this interval, (c) the number of incident cases during the interval, and (d) the interval-specific survival probability, the Weinberg formula is $d = [a-(b+c)/2-C]/[a-(b+c)/2]$.

[2]The Kaplan-Meier estimator P(t) of the probability of survival up to time (t) uses only the onset and censoring times (times at which persons are lost because of withdrawal or death from other causes). It does not require that the data be grouped into arbitrary intervals. The estimator is defined as follows: if t1, t2...t are all ⩽t and are the onset times of m affected persons, then with m=n(t),

$$P(t) = \mathop{I}_{j=1}^{N(t)} (N_j-1)/N_j$$

where N_j is the number of cases still under observation at the time of the jth onset, t is earlier than or equal to the time of the last onset, and n(t) is the number of cases with onset up to time +.

The age of onset of familial cases ranged from 25 to 85. There was a significant relationship between the age of onset in patients and their relatives, suggesting genetic heterogeneity with respect to age of onset (29).

The higher prevalence of familial cases and the higher risk to family members found in our studies can be attributed to several methodological variations. The patients were selected by strict clinical criteria that included only those with amnesia and aphasia/agraphia, and eliminated persons with vascular disease. Multiple family members were interviewed. Also, the age of onset for probands and relatives was not restricted. For example, some studies such as that of Heyman et al. (30), restricted their study to relatives with an onset before or at least age 75 and did not use survival analysis. This may account for their relatively low rate of secondary cases (25% of families).

The third type of family study involves the study of many generations and collateral lines of a single family. In these studies large pedigrees or family trees are developed and the segregation/distribution of cases in close and distant relatives is calculated within the same family. The advantage here is the certainty that the same putative gene is being studied. The disadvantage is that only small numbers of families suitable for such an analysis are available. Many biases operate to limit the generalizability of the conclusions; for example, such families are likely to be made up of earlier-onset cases.

More than 50 extended pedigrees have been reported (5). In the pedigrees reported by Lauter and by Feldman, the clinical features of amnesia, apaxia & aphasia were present as well as autopsy evidence of neocortical neuritic plaques and neurofibrillary tangles (6,7). In the pedigree reported by Nee et al. (8) were large numbers of living relatives and affected persons who were available for linkage studies.

These large pedigrees invite the speculation that the disorder is an autosomal dominant trait at least in some families. The presence of similar clinical and pathological features in the majority of clinical cases suggests that the phenotypes are typical of classic Alzheimer's disease of early or late onset. Since so many clinical cases are from families that lack information about relatives, the true prevalence of the familial and genetic forms of the disease will await identification of the gene.

LINKAGE STUDIES

The localization of the gene to a particular chromosome will in all probability require linkage studies. These studies are based on the observation that genes located close together on the chromosome will be more likely to be transmitted together to offspring, since the probability of crossing over of segments of chromosomes increases with the distance between them. Thus, the ratio of the number of cases with a marker trait of known location and the disease gene to the number of cases with a marker trait but without the disease gene is an estimate of the linkage between the two genes. If the linkage is close, the disease gene is near the marker gene. Linkage analysis depends on the capacity to diagnose accurately the presence and absence of the phenotype in the families being studied and a low mutation rate. In a disorder of late and variable onset such as Alzheimer's disease, the identification of escapees (those individuals who have lived through the age at risk without expressing the symptoms of the disease) is difficult. Many linkage studies conducted so far have been inconclusive although several locations on chromosomes 4, 6, and 14 have been suggested (31,32). There has been a recent report that an anonymous Restriction Fragment Length Polymorphism (RELP) DNA probe link to the disease for families of early onset probe has been mapped to chromosome 21 and has also been linked to the probe for the amyloid gene, which is also located on chromosome 21 (33). It remains to be determined whether cases of late onset will also be linked to this particular probe.

CYTOGENETIC STUDIES

Studies of the number or the morphology of chromosomes have not led to the consistent demonstration of abnormalities, except for studies of Alzheimer's disease occurring in individuals with trisomy 21 (34,35). The pathological features of Alzheimer's disease occur in most, if not all, persons with Down's syndrome who have reached the age of 30 (36,37). However, the clinical features of Alzheimer's disease have not been demonstrated in many of these individuals. The failure to confirm the clinical features is in part related to the difficulty in assessing the cognitive state of persons with a low premorbid intelligence.

Schweber proposed the theory that Alzheimer's disease was caused by a duplication of a segment of DNA that would produce a gene dosage effect similar to that found in Down's syndrome but in the presence of a normal carrier type (38). An increased dosage of the amyloid gene has now been reported in three cases of sporadic and late onset disease as well as in one patient with karyotypically normal Down's syndrome (39). This finding has not been confirmed (40).

SUMMARY AND CRITIQUE OF THE GENETIC HYPOTHESIS

We have presented here some of the research supporting the hypothesis that AD is transmitted by a mutant gene. We are applying the term AD only to patients of any age in whom there is an insidious onset and gradual progression of amnesia, aphasia, apraxia, and agnosia in the absence of indications of vascular disease or other CNS disorders. By so defining the term, we describe a population that has been shown to be associated with the pathological findings described by Alzheimer, eliminate many potential phenocopies, and find that a high proportion of the patients have a pedigree consistent with autosomal dominant inheritance of AD with age-dependent expression of the gene.

Nonfamilial AD has an unknown prevalence and may be the result of several factors. First, in some cases the probands might not have any known relatives who lived through the age of risk. Many of the studies that have found a low prevalence of probands with autosomal dominant pedigrees have similarly not taken this into account and/or have failed to use the survival analysis techniques briefly described here. Second, other cases may be phenocopies (i.e., they resemble AD clinically but have another cause). A third possibility would be that there is a substantial new mutation rate. Finally, a fourth possibility would be that the expression of the gene requires one or more other factors that were present more often in some families than in others.

The genetic hypothesis is entirely consistent with and not mutually exclusive of the other hypotheses in the literature. For example, the gene may increase the susceptibility to a virus or increase the potential for aluminum to accumulate in the brain.

By hypothesizing that there is a significant genetic component to the pathogenesis of AD, powerful new methods in molecular biology can be added to neuroscience's methods in the search to understand the pathogenesis of what has become a modern epidemic. However, progress in testing the genetic hypothesis has been impeded by the lack of a gene product that is measurable during life and by the lack of many large families suitable for linkage studies. Even though many pedigrees have been located with several affected members, many of those affected have no longer been alive to donate blood for linkage analysis. Nonetheless, there is hope that the techniques used by Gusella and his colleagues to locate the Huntington's disease gene to chromosome 4 will be useful in finding a marker for the AD gene or genes. Also, although the Down's syndrome model for AD is controversial, it still would be worthwhile to isolate and identify the genes on 21 q 22 required for developing Down's syndrome and the associated pathological change. Thus, the genetic hypothesis opens up several potentially fruitful avenues by which to explore the pathogenesis of AD.

ACKNOWLEDGMENTS

This work was supported in part by the American Philosophical Society, Alzheimer's Disease and Related Disorders, American Federation for Aging Research, NIA AG-05146, John Douglas French Foundation, Meridian Healthcare Systems, NIN CDS-16375, NIH NS-15080, Consolidated Gift Fund for Dementia Research.

We thank Dr. E. A. Murphy for review of the manuscript.

REFERENCES

1. Mortimer, (1981). Epidemiology of dementing illness. In: *The Epidemiology of Dementia*, J.A. Mortimer and L.M. Schuman (Eds.). New York, Oxford University Press, pp. 3-23.
2. Larsson, T., Sjogren, T., and Jacobson, G. (1963). Senile dementia. *Acta Psychiatr. Scand.,* Suppl. 167, 39: 1-259.
3. Heston, L. (1978). Pedigrees of 30 families with Alzheimer disease: Associations with defective organization of microfilaments and microtubules. *Behav. Genet.* 8(4): 315-331.
4. Heston, L., Mastri, A., and Anderson, E. (1981). Dementia of the Alzheimer's type. Clinical genetics, natural history, and associated conditions. *Arch. Gen. Psychiatry* 38: 1085-1090.
5. Cook, R.H., Ward, B.E., and Austin, J.H. (1979). Studies in aging of the brain: IV. Familial Alzheimer disease: Relation to transmissable dementia, aneuplody, and microtubular defects. *Neurology* 29: 1402-1412.
6. Feldman, R.G., Chandler, K.A., Levy, L.L., and Glaser, G.H. (1963). Familial Alzheimer's disease. *Neurology* 13(10): 811-824.
7. Lauter, H. (1961). Genealogische Erhebungen in einer familie mit Alzheimerscher Krankheit. *Arch. Psychiatr. Nervenkr.* 202: 126.
8. Nee, L.E., Polinsky, R.J., Eldridge, R., Weingartner, H., Smallberg, S., and Ebert, M. (1983). A family with histologically confirmed Alzheimer's disease. *Arch. Neurol.* 40: 203-208.
9. Goudsmit, J., White, B.J., Weitkamp, L.R., Keats, B., Morrow, C.H., and Gadjusek, D.C. (1981). Familial Alzheimer disease in two kindreds of the same geographic and ethnic origin. *J. Neurol. Sci.* 49: 78-89.
10. Shore, D., and Wyatt, R. J. (1983). Aluminum and Alzheimer's disease. *J. Nerv. Ment. Dis.* 171(9): 553-558.
11. Glenner, G.G. (1985). On causative theories in Alzheimer's disease. *Hum. Pathol.* 16(5): 433-435.
12. Roth, M. (1955). The natural history of mental disorders arising in the senium. *J. Ment. Sci.* 101: 281-301.
13. McKhann, G., Drachman, D., Folstein, M.F., Katzman, R., Price, D., and Stadlan, E.M. (1984). Clinical diagnosis of Alzheimer's disease: Report of the NINCDS-ADRDA Work Group under the auspices of Department of Health and Human Services Task Force on Alzheimer's Disease. *Neurology* 34: 939-944.
14. Pritchard, J.C. (1837). *A Treatise on Insanity and Other Disorders Affecting the Mind.* Philadelphia, Howell, Barnington and Haswell, pp. 69-80.
15. Alzheimer, A. (1907). Uber eine eigenartige Erkrankung der Hirnrinde. *Allg. Z. Psychiatr. Osychisch-Gericht. Med.* 64: 146-148.
16. Corsellis, J.A.N. (1962). *Mental Illness and the Aging Brain.* London, Oxford University Press.
17. Sjogren, T., et al. (1952). A genetic study of morbus Alzheimer and morbus Pick. *Acta Psychiatr. Scand.* Suppl. 82, 9: 1-152.
18. Constantinidis, J. (1978). Is Alzheimer's disease a major form of senile dementia? Clinical, anatomical and genetic data. In: *Alzheimer's Disease: Senile*

Dementia and Related Disorders (*Aging Vol. 7*), R. Katzman, R.D. Terry, and K.L. Bick (Eds.). New York, Raven Press.
19. Folstein, M.F., and Breitner, J.C.S. (1982). Language disorder predicts familial Alzheimer disease. In: *Alzheimer's Disease: A Report of Progress*, (Aging Vol. 19), S. Corkin, et al. (Eds.). New York, Raven Press.
20. Breitner, J.C.S., and Folstein, M.F. (1984). Familial Alzheimer dementia: A prevalent disorder with specific clinical features. *Psychol. Med.* 14: 63-80.
21. Chase, G.A., Folstein, M.F., Breitner, J., Beatty, T., and Self, S.G. (1983). The use of life tables and survival analysis for testing a genetic hypothesis concerning Alzheimer's disease. *Am. J. Epidemiol.* 117(5): 590-597.
22. Kallman, F., and Sander, G. (1979). Twin studies on senescence. *Am. J. Psychiatry* 106: 29-36.
23. Cook, R.H., Schneck, S.A., and Clark, D.B. (1981). Twins with Alzheimer's disease. *Arch. Neurol.* 38(5): 300-301.
24. Davidson, E.A., and Robertson, E.E. (1955). Alzheimer's disease with acne rosacea in one of identical twins. *J. Neurol. Neurosurg. Psychiatry* 18: 72-77.
25. Hunter, R., and Dayand, W.J. (1972). Alzheimer disease in one monozygotic twin. *J. Neurol. Neurosurg. Psychiatry* 35: 707-710.
26. Breitner, J.C.S., Folstein, M.F., and Murphy, E.A. (1986). Familial aggregation in Alzheimer dementia–I: A model for the age-dependent expression of an autosomal dominant gene. *J. Psychiatr. Res.* 20(1): 31-43.
27. Breitner, J.C.S., Folstein, M.F., and Murphy, E.A. (1986). Familial aggregation in Alzheimer dementia–II: Clinical genetic implications of age-dependent onset. *J. Psychiatr. Res.* 20(1): 45-55.
28. Knesevich, J.W., et al. (1985). Aphasia, family history and the longitudinal course of senile dementia of the Alzheimer type. *Psychiatry Res.* 14: 255-263.
29. Powell, D., and Folstein, M.F. (1984). Pedigree study of familial Alzheimer disease. *J. Neurogenet.* 1: 189-197.
30. Heyman, A., Wilkinson, W.E., Hurwitz, B.J., Schmechel, D., Sigmon, A.H., Weinberg, T., Helms, M.J., and Swift, M. (1983). Alzheimer's disease: Genetic aspects and associated clinical disorders. *Ann. Neurol.* 14: 507-515.
31. Weitcamp, L.R., Nee, L., Keats, B., Polinsky, R., and Guttormsen, S. (1983). Alzheimer disease: Evidence for susceptibility loci on chromosomes 6 and 14. *Am. J. Hum. Genet.* 35: 443-453.
32. Wheelan, L. (1959). Familial Alzheimer's disease. *Ann. Hum. Genet.* 23: 300-310.
33. St. George-Hyslop, P.H., Tanzi, R.E., Polinsky, R.J., Haines, J.L., Nee, L., Watkins, P.C., Myers, R.H., Feldman, R.G., Polen, D., Drachman, D., Growdon, J., Bruni, A., Foncin, J.F., Salmon, D., Frommelt, P., Amaducci, L., Sorbi, S., Placentini, S., Stewart, G.D., Hobbs, W.J., Conneally, P.M., Gusella, J.F. (1987). The genetic defect causing familial Alzheimer's disease maps on chromosome 21. *Science* 235: 885-890.
34. Tanzi, R.E., Gusella, J.F., Watkins, P.C., Bruns, G.A.P., St. George-Hyslop, P., Van Keuren M.L., Patterson, D., Pagan, S., Kurnit, D.M., Neve, R.L.,

et al. (1987). Amyloid B protein gene; cDNA, mRNA distribution, and genetic linkage near the Alzheimer locus. *Science* 235: 880-884.

35. Whalley, L.J. (1982). The dementia of Down's syndrome and its relevance to aetiological studies of Alzheimer's disease. *Ann. N.Y. Acad. Sci.* 306: 39-53.
36. Ropper, A.H., and Williams, R.S. (1980). Relationship between plaques, tangles, and dementia in Down's syndrome. *Neurology* 30: 639-644.
37. Sinex, F.M., and Myers, C.R. (1982). Alzheimer's disease, Down's syndrome, and aging: The genetic approach. *Ann. N.Y. Acad. Sci.* 396: 3-13.
38. Schweber, M. (1985). A possible unitary genetic hypothesis for Alzheimer's disease and Down syndrome. *Ann. N.Y. Acad. Sci.* 450: 223.
39. Delabor, J.M., Goldgaber, D., Lamour, Y., Nicole, A., Huret, J.-L., DeGrouchy, J., Brown, P., Gajdusek, C., and Sinet, P.-M. (1987). "β Amyloid Gene Duplication in Alzheimer's Disease and Karyotypically Normal Down Syndrome." *Science* 235: 1399.
40. Warren, A.C., Robakis, N.K., Ramakrishna, N., Koo, E.H., Ross, C.A., Robb, A.S., Folstein, M.F., Price, D.L., and Antonarakis, S.E. (1987). β-Amyloid gene is not present in three copies in autopsy-validated Alzheimer's disease. *Genomics* 1: 307-312.

2

Neurogenetics and Familial Alzheimer's Disease

THOMAS D. BIRD / *Seattle V.A. Medical Center and University of Washington Medical School, Seattle, Washington*

THOMAS H. LAMPE / *American Lake V.A. Medical Center and University of Washington Medical School, Tacoma, Washington*

In 1907, Alzheimer described a 51-year-old woman with the clinical and pathological characteristics of the disease that now bears his name (1). Alzheimer's disease (AD) was subsequently regarded as a relatively rare cause of presenile dementia. Twenty-five years after Alzheimer's initial report, Schottky published the first detailed account of neuropathologically documented familial AD in more than one generation (2). This family included a 45-year-old woman, her 56-year-old father, her paternal grandmother, and other paternal relatives who all suffered from dementia. The first report of familial AD in the English literature was in 1934, by Lowenberg and Waggoner in Michigan (3). This was soon followed a similar report of familial AD in 1939 by McMenemey et al. in England (4). However, most instances of AD have been regarded as sporadic or nonfamilial, and the influence of genetics has remained unclear. This chapter will review the accumulated evidence that genetic factors play an important role in the pathogenesis of AD.

Five lines of evidence in favor of genetic factors in AD are listed in Table 1. First are the many descriptions since the 1930s of large multiplex and multigeneration families with AD. (Multiplex here simply means several affected persons in the same family.) Fifty such families reported up to 1979 were reviewed by Cook et al. (5). Several additional families have been described subsequently. These large AD families generally meet accepted criteria for autosomal dominant inheritance. That is, the disorder affects every generation, there is male-to-male transmission, there is approximately 50% occurrence of dementia in children of an affected parent, and males and females are equally affected. Most, but not

TABLE 1 Evidence for Genetic Factors in Alzheimer's Disease

Large multiplex families
Suggest autosomal dominant inheritance in some families
Epidemiological studies
Show increased familial incidence
Twin studies
? Increased concordance in identical twins
Down's syndrome
AD neuropathological changes in adults with Down's syndrome
Increased frequency of Down's syndrome in AD families
Sensitivity of AD cells to mutagenic agents
? DNA repair defect

all, such families seem to have the onset of dementia in the "presenile" period, prior to the age of 65 or 70. Such large multiplex families appear to be uncommon, but their actual frequency in the general population is unknown. The existence of such families represents one of the strongest arguments in favor of a genetic factor in at least some cases of AD.

Second, there have been several large epidemiological studies of AD that included investigation of the familial occurrence of the disorder. Of particular note are the studies by Sjogren et al. (6), Larsson et al. (7), Constantinidis et al. (8), Heston et al. (9), Heyman et al. (10), and Amaduoci et al. (11). The diagnostic criteria and study protocols have varied widely. However, a general consensus has emerged that there indeed is an increased familial incidence of dementia in the families of index patients with AD. For example, Heyman and colleagues found that 25% of 68 index patients with presenile AD also had a parent or sibling with dementia (10). Heston has emphasized that early onset of dementia before age 70 in an index patient *and* a similarly affected parent selects for families with a very high frequency of dementia (9). Others have noted that the true frequency of dementia with late onset is probably underestimated in many families because death may occur from other causes prior to the onset of memory loss (12).

Studies of twins with AD represent a third line of evidence supporting the presence of genetic factors in this disease. An early report by Kallman in 1956 showed a high concordance (42%) in monozygotic twins for "senile psychosis" and a much lower concordance in dyzygotic twins (8%) (13). Such figures suggest an important but incomplete genetic factor at work, but the study lacked diagnostic precision and there was no autopsy follow-up. Anecdotal reports of twins with AD have noted both concordance and discordance in monozygotic pairs (14-17). A positive family history for dementia may increase the likelihood for concordance, but this has not been analyzed systematically. It has been demonstrated that a second affected twin may not show signs of dementia until many years after the first twin (16). Additional twin studies of AD are needed and are in progress, including longitudinal studies of aging twins (18).

Fourth, Down's syndrome is the result of a major chromosomal aberration, namely trisomy 21, and persons with Down's syndrome surviving to age 35 or 40 have essentially all demonstrated at autopsy the neuropathological characteristics of AD (19). The severity of these neuropathological changes is often less than that in a typical patient with presenile AD and the adult Down's syndrome patients may or may not show clinical signs of dementia. Nevertheless, the impressive and consistent pathological connection between AD and this major chromosomal disorder is well documented and intriguing. Heston et al. have also reported an increased frequency of Down's syndrome in the relatives of index patients with autopsy-proven AD (20). This finding has been confirmed by some subsequent studies and not others (10,11). The mechanisms underlying the Down's-AD connection remain to be determined.

Fifth, Robbins et al. have reported decreased survival of lymphocytes from AD patients when exposed to X irradiation (21). Similar results using somewhat different techniques have been reported by others (22). The proposed explanation for these findings is that AD cells have a basic defect in DNA repair. Other genetic disorders sometimes affecting the central nervous system have shown even more impressive defects of DNA repair, most notably ataxia telangectasia, Cockayne's syndrome, and xeroderma pigmentosa (23). Studies of DNA repair in AD cells are difficult to replicate because of complex culture techniques, use of differing types of cells, and large numbers of available mutagenic agents. If such studies are consistently confirmed and amplified, they could lead to a better understanding of the genetic pathogenesis of AD and could also demonstrate the usefulness of easily obtained non-nervous-system tissue for further investigation. It should be noted that early reports of gross chromosomal aberrations in AD have not been confirmed (24).

Not all investigators agree that genetic factors play an important role in AD. Table 2 lists some lines of evidence arguing against strong genetic influences in this disease. Although it is not unusual to discover two or three demented relatives in a family, the impressively large multigeneration AD families are uncommon. Also, it is known that environmental or acquired diseases can occur in multiple individuals of a single family. This was well recognized long ago with tuberculosis and rheumatic fever. Kuru occurred in multiple family members of the affected New Guinea tribes and was assumed to be a genetic disorder prior to the demonstration of a "slow virus" as the cause (25). Furthermore, Creutzfeldt-Jakob disease has occurred in multiple relatives over several generations and the explanation for this familial clustering remains undetermined (26). In addition, neuropathological changes of AD (especially neurofibrillary tangles) are not specific for

TABLE 2 Evidence Against Genetic Factors in Alzheimer's Disease

Large multiplex AD families uncommon
Most or many AD cases are "sporadic" or nonfamilial
Acquired diseases can be familial
Neuropathologic changes of AD are nonspecific

TABLE 3 Possible Resolutions of Evidence for and Against Genetic Factors in Alzheimer's Disease

Heterogeneity of causes
Very different causes of AD, some genetic and some non-genetic
Multifactorial inheritance
AD is *combined* result of inherited factor(s) and environmental agent
Polygenic inheritance
AD is net result of the additive effect of several genes

AD and can be found in diseases generally considered nongenetic, such as Parkinson's disease and progressive supranuclear palsy.

How can we reconcile the evidence for and against genetic factors in AD? One possibility is simply that AD is a heterogeneous clinical-pathological syndrome with several distinct and separate causes (see Table 3). One cause could be primarily genetic, even monogenic autosomal dominant, and another cause or causes could be primarily environmental such as toxins or viruses. There might be little or no overlap between the various causes in any individual patient. Another possibility is that some or even most cases of AD are the result of both an inherited predisposition and an environmental agent. The inherited predispoisition and environmental factor or factors are presently unknown, but could be immunological and viral, respectively. This hypothesis fits the so-called "multifactorial" pattern of inheritance. Also, genetic factors in AD could be polygenic, that is, the net result of many genes, none of which has a single major effect. However, polygenic inheritance is not likely to explain the large multigenerational families.

The University of Washington Alzheimer Disease Research Center is ascertaining large multiplex families with AD. The initial criteria for selection of such families are: four or more cases of dementia meeting clinical criteria for AD in two or more generations, one instance of neuropathologically proven AD, at least 10 available potentially informative family members (including affected, unaffected, persons at risk, and spouses of affected individuals). Thus far, we have identified 12 such families. Some of the clinical characteristics of these families are outlined in Table 4. Three of the families have been previously reported (family 6

TABLE 4 Multiplex Families with Alzheimer's Disease

Family	Affected generation	Ethnic background	Pathology confirmed	Age at onset	Male-to-male transmission	Total demented	Living demented
1. L	3	German	Yes	30s-40s	No	11	2
2. V	3	English	Yes	40s	No	7	1
3. P	2	English	Yes	50s-60s	Yes	6	2
4. H	3	German	Yes	50s-60s	No	7	1
5. BK	3	Czech	Yes	40s-50s	Yes	13	6
6. SNW	3	Ashkenazi Jew (Russia)	Yes	40s-50s	Yes	21	4
7. GCSA	5	German/Swiss	Yes	20s-50s	Yes	24	2
8. T	2	Norwegian	Yes	60s	Yes	4 (6?)	1
9. CSF	2	Danish	Yes	60s-70s	No	5	2
10. R	4	German (Russia)	Yes	40s-50s	Yes	19	3
11. KS	3	German (Russia)	Yes	60s	Yes	6	3
12. MG	3	English/Scottish	Yes	40s	Yes	11	1
Total			12/12		8/12	134	28

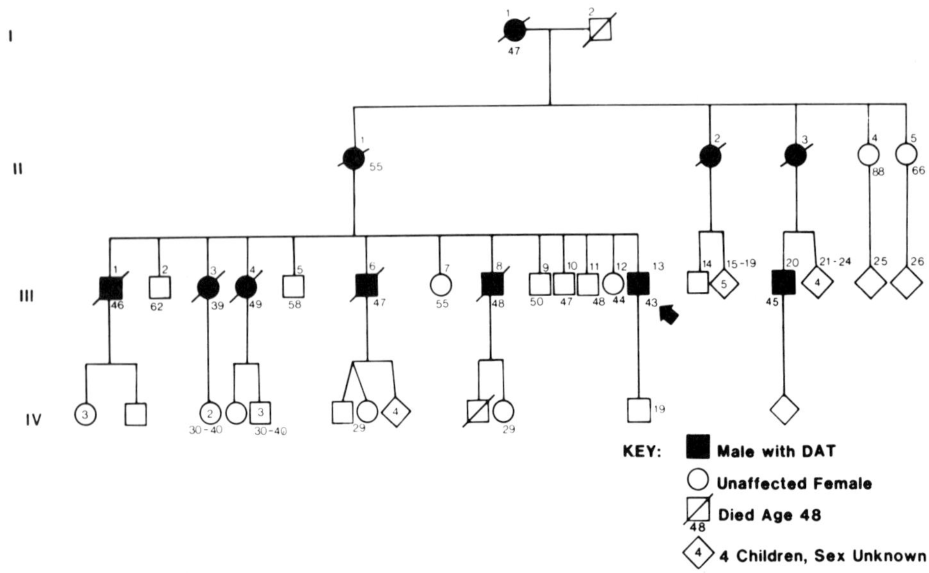

FIGURE 1 Pedigree of family 1 from Table 4, the L family, with dementia of the Alzheimer's type (DAT). Three deceased individuals have had AD documented at autopsy. Note relatively early ages of death ("presenile AD"), both males and females with dementia, and three affected generations.

by Goudsmit et al. [27], family 7 by Heston et al. [28], and family 10 by Cook et al. [5]). Figure 1 shows the pedigree of one of the large new AD families identified by our center. These families generally have early onset, male-to-male transmission, both sexes affected, and high penetrance of the hypothesized AD gene. Such families will prove valuable for clinical, biochemical, and genetic studies of familial AD.

One important aspect of studying large families is that the vast majority of demented individuals are deceased. Living demented persons are relatively few in number. Of the 134 total demented persons in the 12 families identified in Table 3, only 28 are living. This means that pooling of data from several families will undoubtedly be necessary for many scientific studies. Such pooling must be done carefully and thoughtfully because issues of causative and genetic heterogeneity have not been resolved. Past experience shows that a mutation at a single locus may result in different clinical expressions including variable age of onset (for example, the rigid and juvenile forms of Huntington's disease). Also, entirely different mutations at separate loci may have highly similar clinical manifestations (for example, several different inherited lipid storage disorders all produce seizures and mental retardation). Some familial AD families could represent alleles (different mutations at the same genetic locus) and pooling of data from such families for genetic linkage studies would be appropriate. Weitkamp et al. have reported a suggestive linkage between familial AD and the Gm locus on chromosome 14 (29). This study was one on a single large family. Other recent AD linkage studies have pooled data from several different families (30,31). As yet, no chromosomal assignment has been made for a putative AD gene.

Finally, it is of interest that four large AD families all have genetic roots in southwestern Russia, in and around the Ukraine. Two of the families are Ashkenazi Jews originating from the area of Minsk (the SNW family in Table 3 [27] and the MP family in [27]). Two others are of German ancestry and once lived near each other in the vicinity of the Russian city of Saratov (family R in Table 3 and [5] and family KS in Table 3). These families may represent one or two examples of the founder effect (the introduction of AD into the family by a single ancestor many generations ago). The discovery of additional families with origins in this geographic area would be of great interest.

SUMMARY

Several lines of evidence suggest important genetic factors underlying at least some cases of AD. The evidence includes large multiplex AD families, epidemiological studies, reports of concordant twins, associations of trisomy 21 with AD, and a possible defect of DNA repair in AD cells. On the other hand, many instances of AD seem sporadic, environmental diseases can be "familial," and the neuropathologic changes of AD can occur in nongenetic disorders. This conflicting evidence may be resolved by discovering causative heterogeneity in AD or showing that it represents multifactorial or polygenic inheritance. Several AD centers including our own are ascertaining large AD families for further investigation. Data from such families will have to be pooled for some studies because there are so few living affected persons in any one family. Possible genetic heterogeneity will have to be taken into consideration. Some AD families may be the result of a founder effect originating in the southwestern Soviet Union or Germany.

ADDENDUM

Several additional findings of importance to the genetics of AD have occurred since this chapter was written in 1986. St. George-Hyslop et al. have shown that the gene for AD in some families is linked to anonymous DNA markers on chromosome 21 (32). Kang et al. (33) and Tanzi et al. (34) have shown that the gene for amyloid beta protein is also on chromosome 21. However, further investigations have demonstrated recombination between the amyloid gene and the familial AD gene, showing that the mutation in familial AD is not likely to involve the amyloid gene directly (35,36). Numerous factors remain to be determined, including the nature and exact location of the familial AD mutation, the relationship of the AD gene to Down's syndrome and the amyloid gene, the possibility of heterogeneity in familial AD, and the distinction, if any, between familial and "sporadic" AD. Linkage analysis of the families ascertained by our center show evidence for genetic heterogeneity with particular emphasis on pedigrees of Volga German ancestry (37,38). Family #7 (GCSA) in Table 4 has been discovered to have Gerstmann-Straussler Syndrome, not AD.

REFERENCES

1. Alzheimer, A. (1907). Ueber eine eigenartige Erkrankung der Kirnrinde. *Allg. Z. Psychiatr.* 64: 146-148.
2. Schottky, J. (1932). Uber prasenile Verblodungen. *A. Gesamte. Neurol. Psychiat.* 140: 333-397.
3. Lowenberg, K., and Waggoner, R.W. (1934). Familial organic psychosis (Alzheimer's type). *Arch. Neurol. Psychiatry* 31: 737-754.
4. McMenemey, W.H., Worster Drought, C., Flind, J., and Williams, H.D. (1939). Familial presenile dementia: Report of case with clinical and pathological features of Alzheimer's disease. *J. Neurol. Neurosurg. Psychiatry* 2:293-302.
5. Cook, R., Ward, B.E., and Austin, J.H. (1979). Studies in aging of the brain, IV. Familial Alzheimer's disease: Relation to transmissible dementia, aneuploidy and microtubular defects. *Neurology* 29: 1492-1412.
6. Sjogren, J.S., Sjogren, H., and Lindgren, A.G.H. (1952). Morbus Alzheimer and morbus Pick. *Acta Psychiatr. Neurol. Scand.* Suppl. 82: 47-139.
7. Larsson, T., Sjogren, T., and Jacobson, G. (1963). Senile dementia. *Acta Psychiatr. Scand.* 39, Suppl. 167: 1-259.
8. Constantinidis, J., Garrone, G., Tissot, R., and de Ajuriaguerra, J. (1965). The familial incidence of Alzheimer's neurofibrillary change in cortex (in French). *Psychiatr. Neurol.* 150: 235.
9. Heston, L., Mastri, A.R., Anderson, V.E., and White, J. (1981). Dementia of the Alzheimer type. *Arch. Gen. Psychiatry* 38: 1985-1090.
10. Heyman, A., Wilkinson, W.E., Hurwitz, B.J., Schemchel, D., Sigmon, A.H., Weinberg, T., Nelms, M.J., and Swift, M. (1983). Alzheimer's disease: Genetic aspects and associated clinical disorders. *Ann. Neurol.* 14: 507-515.
11. Amaducci, L.A., Fratiglioni, L., Rocia, W.A., Feischi, C., et al. (1986). Risk factors for clinically diagnosed Alzheimer disease: A case-control study of an Italian population. *Neurology* 36: 922-931.
12. Breitner, J.C., and Folstein, M.F. (1984). Familial Alzheimer dementia: A prevalent disorder with specific clinical features. *Psychol. Med.* 14: 63-80.
13. Kallman, F.J. (1956). Genetic aspects of mental disorders in later life. In: *Mental Disorders in Later Life*, O.J. Kaplan (Ed.), Stanford, Stanford Press, pp. 25-45.
14. Hunter, R., Dayan, A.D., and Wilson, J. (1972). Alzheimer's disease in one monozygotic twin. *J. Neurol. Neurosurg. Psychiatry* 35: 707-710.

15. Sharman, J.G., Watt, D.C., Janota, I., and Carrasco, L.H. (1979). Alzheimer's disease in a mother and identical twin sons. *Psychiatr. Med.* 9: 771-774.
16. Cook, R.H., Schneek, S.A., and Clark, D.B. (1981). Twins with Alzheimer's disease. *Arch. Neurol.* 38: 300-301.
17. Kilpatrick, C., Burns, R., and Blumbergs, P. (1983). Identical twins with Alzheimer's disease. *J. Neurol. Neurosurg. Psychiatry* 46: 421-425.
18. Jarvik, L.F. (1978). Genetic factors and chromosomal aberrations in Alzheimer's disease, senile dementia and related disorders. In: *Alzheimer's Disease: Senile Dementia and Related Disorders*, R. Katzman, R.D. Terry, K.L. Bick (Eds.). New York, Raven Press, pp. 273-277.
19. Wisniewski, K.E., Wisniewski, H.M., and Wen, G. (1985). Occurrence of neuropathological changes and dementia of Alzheimer's disease in Down's syndrome. *Ann. Neurol.* 17: 278-282.
20. Heston, L.L. (1977). Alzheimer's disease, trisomy 21, and myeloproliferative disorders: Associations suggesting a genetic diathesis. *Science* 196: 322-323.
21. Robbins, J.H., Otsuka, F., Tarone, R., Polinsky, R., Brumback, R., and Nee, L. Parkinson's disease and Alzheimer's disease: Hypersensitivity to X-rays in cultured cell lines. *J. Neurol. Neurosurg. Psychiatry* 48: 916-923.
22. Robison, S.H., Munzer, J.S., Tandan, R., Bardley, R., and Bradley, W.G. (1985). Repair of alkylated DNA is impaired in Alzheimer's disease cells. *Neurology* 35(suppl.): 217.
23. Robbins, J.H., Brumback, R.A., Polinsky, R., Wirtschaffer, J., et al. (1985). Hypersensitivity to DNA-damaging agents in abiotrophies: A new explanation for degeneration of neurons, photo receptors and muscle in Alzheimer, Parkinson and Huntington diseases, retinitis pigmentosa and Duchenne muscular dystrophy. In: *Molecular Biology of Aging*, A.D. Woodhead, A.D. Blackett, and A. Hollaender (Eds.). New York, Plenum, pp. 315-344.
24. White, B.J., Crandall, C., Goudsmit, J., Morrow, C.H., Alling, D.W., Gajdusek, D.C., and Tijio, J.H. (1981). Cytogenetic studies of familial and sporadic Alzheimer disease. *Am. J. Med. Genet.* 10: 77-89.
25. Gajdusek, D.C. (1979). Observations in the early history of Kuru investigation. In: *Slow Transmissible Disease of the Nervous System*, S. Prusiner and W. Hadlow (Eds.). New York, Academic Press, pp. 7-25.
26. Maaters, C.L., Gajdusek, D.C., and Gibbs, C.J. Jr. (1981). The familial occurrence of Creutzfeldt-Jacob disease and Alzheimer's disease. *Brain* 104: 535-558.
27. Goudsmit, J., White, B.J., Weitkamp, L.R., Keats, B.J.B., Morrow, C.H., and Gajdusek, D.C. (1981). Familial Alzheimer's disease in two kindreds of the same geographic and ethnic origin. *J. Neurol. Sci.* 49: 79-89.
28. Heston, L.L., Lowther, D.L., and Leventhal, C.M. (1966). Alzheimer's disease, a family study. *Arch. Neurol.* 15: 225-233.
29. Weitkamp, L.R., Nee, L., Keats, B., Polinsky, R.J., and Guttormsen, S. (1983). Alzheimer disease: Evidence for susceptibility loci on chromosomes 6 and 14. *Am. J. Hum. Genet.* 35: 443-453.

30. Spence, M.A., Neyman, A., Marazita, M.C., Sparkes, R.S., and Weinberg, T. (1986). Genetic linkage studies in Alzheimer's disease. *Neurology* 36: 581-584.
31. St. George-Hyslop, P., Tanzi, R., Hobbs, W., Gibbons, K., Feldman, R., et al. (1986). Alzheimer's disease: A molecular genetic approach. *Neurology* 36 (Suppl): 227.
32. St. George-Hyslop, P.H., Tanzi, R.E., Polinsky, R.J., Haines, J.L., et al. (1987). The genetic defect causing familial Alzheimer's disease maps on chromosome 21. *Science* 235: 885-890.
33. Kang, J., Lemaire, H.G., Unterbeck, A., Salbaum, J.M., et al. (1987). The precursor of Alzheimer's disease amyloid A4 protein resembles a cell-surface receptor. *Nature* 325: 733-736.
34. Tanzi, R.E., Gusella, J.F., Watkins, P.C., Bruns, G.A.P., et al. (1987). Amyloid β protein gene: cDNA, mRNA distribution, and genetic linkage near the Alzheimer locus. *Science* 235: 880-884.
35. Van Broeckhoven, C., Genethe, A.M., Vandenberghe, A., Horsthemke, B., et al. (1987). Failure of familial Alzheimer's disease to segregate with the A4-amyloid gene in several European families. *Nature* 329: 153-155.
36. Tanzi, R.E., St. George-Hyslop, P.H., Haines, J.L., Polinsky, R.J., et al. (1987). The genetic defect in familial Alzheimer's disease is not tightly linked to the amyloid β-protein gene. *Nature* 329: 156-157.
37. Schellenberg, G.D., Bird, T.D., Wijsman, E.M., Moore, D.K., et al. (1988). Absence of linkage of chromosome 21q21 markers to familial Alzheimer's disease. *Science* 241: 1507-1510.
38. Bird, T.D., Sumi, S.M., Nemens, E.J., Nochlin, D., Schellenberg, G., et al. (In Press). Phenotypic heterogeneity in familial Alzheimer's disease: A study of 24 kindreds. *Annals of Neurology*.

3

Familial and Inherited Forms of Alzheimer's Disease

LINDA E. NEE and RONALD J. POLINSKY / *National Institute of Neurological and Communicative Disorders and Stroke, NIH, Bethesda, Maryland*

It has long been recognized that both sporadic and familial cases of Alzheimer's disease (AD) exist. The familial cases form a minority of the AD population but support the notion that genetics may play a primary role in the causes of this devastating neurological disorder (1). Although the familial form was described approximately 50 years ago (2), there is continued debate about the nature and mode of inheritance. Recent advances in the field of recombinant DNA technology will undoubtedly clarify the genetic contribution to AD, particularly when coupled with a sound clinical approach for ascertaining the inherited form of the disease. This chapter will summarize our efforts towards defining a homogeneous clinical population of AD cases, which serve as an invaluable resource for applying the new methods of molecular biology to elucidate the underlying cause and pathophysiology of AD.

Misdiagnosis is a major obstacle to clinical research in AD: up to 50% of cases turn out to have a different cause for dementia at autopsy (3). The need for uniform application of strict diagnostic criteria culminated in the recommendations of the National Institute of Neurological and Communicative Disorders and Stroke-Alzheimer's Disease and Related Disorders Association (NINCDS-ADRDA) Task Force on Alzheimer's Disease (4). Since the terms *genetic*, *inherited*, and *familial* are often interchanged inappropriately, it is equally important to specify precisely the exact usage. *Genetic* refers to any mechanism or process that involves the genes but does not imply that the result is passed on to future generations, as occurs with *inherited* characteristics. *Familial* means that more than one person in the family has the disease. Not all familial AD cases are inherited. The frequency of AD in the general population reduces the value of studying small familial clusters.

Two approaches we have used for investigating the genetic aspects of AD are the study of twins and of large families with an apparently autosomal dominant form of transmission. There are obvious practical limitations imposed by the relative rarity of such a select patient population. However, the reward of homogenous clinical material is sufficient justification for excluding the bulk of AD patients. Since there are no significant clinical or neuropathological differences between the sporadic and familial forms of AD, it is likely that the findings derived from studying inherited cases will advance our understanding of the disease in general.

TWIN STUDY

Twin studies allow assessment of the contributions from genetic and environmental factors in the expression of disease. A higher concordance rate in monozygotic (MZ) compared to dizygotic (DZ) twins would favor a genetic mechanism. Discordance among MZ twins would implicate other biological, nongenetic, and environmental factors (5). Table 1 summarizes the current literature on twin studies of AD, including our own experience.

Twenty-two of 26 twin pairs ascertained over a 2-year period were considered suitable for our study (6). All medical and family information was reviewed at the

TABLE 1 Literature on Organic Brain Syndrome, Dementia of the Alzheimer's Type in Twin Pairs

Study	Number of pairs	MZ	DZ	Concordant	Discordant
Davidson et al., 1955	1	+	–	No	Yes
Kallmann, 1956	54	?	?	MZ: 42.8% DZ: 8%	MZ: 57.2% DZ: 92%
Hunter et al., 1972	1	+	–	No	Yes
Sharman et al., 1979	1	+	–	Yes	No
Jarvik et al., 1980[a]	12	10	2	MZ: 4-40% DZ: 1-50%	MZ: 6-60% DZ: 1-50%
Cook et al., 1981	1	+	–	Yes	No
Embry et al., 1985	1	+	–	Yes	No
Nee et al. (in press)	22	17	5	MZ: 7-41% DZ: 2-40%	MZ: 10-59% DZ: 3-60%

[a]A follow-up on Kallmann's 1956 study.

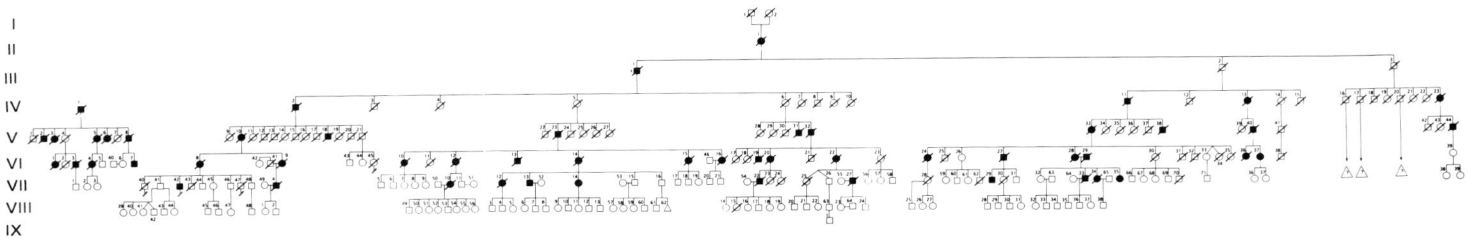

FIGURE 1 Alzheimer's disease family #001. Key: ● = female; ⊘ = male, deceased; △ = unknown sex or both sexes; end of relationship.

National Institutes of Health. Alzheimer's disease was diagnosed if there was a global decline in two or more aspects of cognition for at least 6 months, with an onset between 40 and 90 years of age. Childhood photographs were used to determine zygosity, although this was confirmed by red blood cell phenotyping or HLA in seven twin pairs. The diagnosis of AD was confirmed by autopsy in four patients.

The concordance rates for MZ and DZ twins were not significantly different. Our concordance rate of 41% for MZ twins was similar to that reported by Jarvik (7). An alternative scheme for interpreting the data is also possible, highlighting the uncertainty in mode of inheritance when one is dealing with small pedigrees. In a population of 22 pairs, 8 cases were sporadic, 4 familial, and 10 inherited the trait in an autosomal dominant fashion.

Sporadic cases were so designated if no other family member was known to be affected. Familial, as noted previously, means that more than one person in the family was evidently affected. Involvement of a parent and offspring is consistent with autosomal dominant inheritance. The need to use large families for linkage studies was recognized when studying the twin population; however, among this population no family with extensive affected members was ascertained.

CHARACTERISTICS OF A FAMILY WITH AUTOSOMAL DOMINANT MODE OF INHERITANCE

In 1977, three siblings with AD were referred to NIH for evaluation. Research into the family background revealed that this white Protestant family from England and Scotland emigrated to Canada and now live throughout Canada and the United States.

The family, represented in Figure 1, manifested AD with an autosomal dominant mode of inheritance. The observations supporting this mode of inheritance are no skipped generations as family members became well documented; about 50% of the offspring of affected individuals were affected; close sex ratio of affected individuals; and multiple examples of male-to-male transmission excluding X-linked or cytoplasmic inheritance.

This family first reported in 1983 (8) now has 54 affected family members. The left side of the pedigree could appear to be a separate family; however, family members insist those members are cousins and the names are similar. Autopsies confirming AD have been performed on seven family members. There was no Down's syndrome in this family, although an increased incidence has been observed in other studies (9).

COMMENTS

While sporadic and simple familial cases are widely studied because of their frequency and, hence, availability, those cases would not seem the most fruitful for clinical and genetic research investigations. Twin populations afford the opportunity to examine the contributions of genetic and environmental factors on disease expression. However, among other limitations of AD twin studies, concordance is difficult to establish in an illness with late onset. In addition, histological verification is required to make a definite diagnosis of AD (4).

Single gene disorders continue to be a primary area for genetic research, because they follow the relatively simple and predictable patterns of heredity described by Mendel in 1865 (10). Huntington's disease (HD) is an example of an inherited neurological disorder that causes dementia and is inherited in an autosomal dominant fashion. A genetic marker on chromosome 4 was recently shown to be linked to HD (11).

Using HD as a phenotypic and genetic model, it is interesting to reexamine our twin population. Hayden reported that 13 MZ twin pairs concordant for HD had an intratwin age of onset within 3 years of each other (12). A DZ-concordant HD twin pair was reported in the literature with a 7-year difference in age of onset (13). Thus, apparent single-gene transmission becomes questionable when age of onset among AD twin pairs is taken into consideration. Less than half of the AD twin pairs previously classified as showing single-gene transmission meet the criteria of the HD model. One twin pair had about a 10-year intratwin difference in age of onset. In addition, two twin pairs did not have autopsy confirmation of AD.

A genetic marker has yet to be determined for AD. Initial efforts have focused on chromosome 21 because of the pathological changes similar to AD that are found in older Down's syndrome patients (14). Based on the heterogeneity evident in twin populations, the most fruitful arena for genetic studies is large families with pathological confirmation of AD and a mode of inheritance that is phenotypically autosomal dominant. The importance of the study of large families will potentially become evident with the discovery of an AD biological marker. Hopefulness regarding such a discovery has been fueled by recent molecular biological advances and the finding of an HD genetic marker.

REFERENCES

1. Terry, R.D. (1985). Alzheimer's disease. In: *Textbooks of Neuropathology*, R.L. Davis and D.M. Robertson (Eds.). Baltimore, Williams & Wilkins, pp. 824-842.
2. Cook, R.H., Ward, B.E., and Austin, J.H. (1979). Studies in aging of the brain: IV. Familial Alzheimer's disease: Relation to transmissible dementia, aneuploidy, and microtubular defects. *Neurology* 29: 1402-1412.
3. Garcia, C., Reding, M.J., and Blass, J.P. (1981). Overdiagnosis of dementia. *J. Am. Geriatr. Soc.* 19: 407-410.
4. McKhann, G., Drachman, D., Folstein, M., Katzman, R., Price, D., and Stadlan, E.M. Clinical diagnosis of Alzheimer's disease: Report of the NINCDS-

ADRDA Work Groups under the auspices of Department of Health and Human Services Task Force on Alzheimer's Disease. *Neurology* 34: 939-944.
5. Thompson, S.S., and Thompson, M.W. (1980). *Genetics in Medicine*, 3rd Edition, Philadelphia, W.B. Saunders, pp. 309-310.
6. Nee, L.E., Eldridge, R., Sunderland, T., thomas, C., Katz, D., Thompson, K.E., Weingartner, H., Weiss, H., Julian, C., and Cohen, R. (198?). Dementia of the Alzheimer type: Clinical and family study of 22 twin pairs. *Neurology*.
7. Jarvik, L.F., Ruth, V., and Matsuyama, S.S. (1980). Organic brain syndrome and aging: A six-year follow-up of surviving twins. *Arch. Gen. Psychiatry* 37: 280-286.
8. Nee, L.E., Polinsky, R.J., Eldridge, R., Weingartner, H., Smallberg, S., and Ebert, M. (1983). A family with histologically confirmed Alzheimer's disease. *Arch. Neurol.* 40: 203-208.
9. Heston, L.L., and Mastri, A.R. (1977). Genetics of Alzheimer's disease: Associations with hematologic malignancy and Down's syndrome. *Arch. Gen. Psychiatry* 34: 976-981.
10. McKusick, V.A. (1978). *Mendelian Inheritance in Man: Catalogs of Autosomal Dominant, Autosomal Recessive and X-Linked Phenotypes*, 5th edition. Baltimore, The Johns Hopkins Press.
11. Gusella, J.F., Wexler, N.S., Conneally, P.M., et al. (1983). A polymorphic DNA marker genetically linked to Huntington's disease. *Nature* 306: 234-238.
12. Hayden, M.R. (1981). *Huntington's Chorea.* New York, Springer-Verlag.
13. Rosanoff, A.J., and Handy, L.M. (1935). Huntington's chorea in twins. *Arch. Neurol.* 33: 839-841.
14. St. George-Hyslop, P., Nee, L., Tanzi, R., Hobbs, W., Polinsky, R., and Gusella, J. (198?). DNA Markers in Familial Alzheimer's Disease. Proceedings of the Internation Symposium on New Concepts in Alzheimer's Disease, Pierre Fabre Monograph series, London, MacMillan Press.

4

Neuropsychological Investigation of Dementia of the Alzheimer's Type

LINDA TERI and REBECCA G. LOGSDON / *University of Washington School of Medicine, Seattle, Washington*

INTRODUCTION

The goal of this chapter is to provide an overview of neuropsychological issues in the assessment and early identification of dementia of the Alzheimer's type (DAT). We will introduce readers to fundamental neuropsychological terms, survey the literature on the nature of cognitive dysfunction in DAT, and discuss relevant methods of assessment and early identification, especially as they relate to identifying possible subgroups and/or risk factors for DAT.

DEFINITION OF TERMS

Neuropsychology

Neuropsychology is the study of brain-behavior relationships; it is based on the principle that dysfunction within the brain leads to observable behavioral deficits. The specific expression of these deficits varies considerably as a function of the nature, location, and extent of the brain dysfunction. Individual differences in brain structure, biochemical functioning, medical history, past intellectual functioning, and adaptive ability of the individual also influence the behavioral changes associated with injury or damage to the brain (1). Neuropsychological assessment is used to document the presence of brain dysfunction, draw inferences as to the likely location and type of brain lesion, and make treatment recommendations.

Dementia of the Alzheimer's Type

Dementia of the Alzheimer's type has already been defined earlier in this volume. From a neuropsychological perspective, the cognitive and behavioral functioning of the DAT patient is of particular relevance, and will be reviewed briefly here. Dementia is characterized in the Third Edition of the ***Diagnostic and Statistical Manual*** of the American Psychiatric Association (DSM-III) by memory impairment and intellectual decline of sufficient severity to interfere with social or occupational functioning (2). Other cognitive changes consistent with dementia may include difficulty understanding and using language, problems in planning and executing purposeful motor movements, poor judgement, difficulty with reasoning and problem solving, and altered or exaggerated personality characteristics or behavioral style. In dementia, these changes occur in the absence of psychiatric or metabolic disturbances that might alter or interfere with the individual's ability to accurately perceive his or her environment.

Dementia is a symptom of a number of disorders, one of which is primary degenerative dementia, or dementia of the Alzheimer's type. The cognitive dysfunctions of DAT are characterized by insidious onset with a uniformly progressive deteriorating course. All other specific causes of dementia must be ruled out by history, physical examination, and results of laboratory tests in order to establish a presumptive diagnosis of DAT.

Geriatric Neuropsychology

The field of geriatric neuropsychology is particularly concerned with the differentiation of dementia from normal aging, depression, and other causes of brain dysfunction in older adults (3). Lezak (4) asserts that "degenerative diseases of old age cannot yet be reliably identified by neuroradiologic techniques, so that the most definitive diagnoses are often those arrived at through neuropsychological assessment" (p. 3). Neuropsychological assessment is helpful in establishing the presence and extent of dementia, differentiating treatable from untreatable forms of the disorder, determining the course or progression of the dementia through repeated testing, identifying a patient's relative strengths and weaknesses, and formulating treatment recommendations.

ISSUES IN ASSESSMENT

Deterioration

Before determining that an individual is experiencing cognitive impairment indicative of deterioration, one must know (or infer) something about his or her premorbid functioning. Most geriatric patients have not undergone extensive intellectual assessment prior to the onset of a dementing illness. Therefore, it is necessary to take a number of factors into consideration when estimating the patient's prior intellectual level. The vocabulary subtest of the Wechsler Adult Intelligence Scale-Revised (WAIS-R) is commonly regarded as an index of previous intellectual level. In DAT, however, patients may show dramatic deteriorations on this test

(5). Prior occupational and educational achievement, along with reports from family members as to the patient's level of prior functioning, provide a reasonable guideline for estimating premorbid intellectual ability.

Normal Age-Related Cognitive Changes

It is necessary to preface a discussion of neuropsychological changes that occur in dementing illness with some words of caution. Researchers have documented a variety of physiological and cognitive changes that appear to occur normally as individuals age. Although this chapter's presentation of these changes must necessarily be cursory, readers evaluating older adults are encouraged to read more detailed discussions elsewhere (6-8). In the area of sensory perception, healthy older people do not see or hear as well as younger people. Older adults experience a decline in the ability to discriminate visual details and differentiate colors and brightness. Night vision and the ability to adjust to changes in brightness also decline. Many older people suffer a high-pitch hearing loss, which may lead to difficulty discriminating sounds. Older individuals as a group are more cautious in their responses to problems and/or questions, and less likely to risk failure (9). Response speed and accuracy decline between the ages of 50 and 70 years (10) and older people generally benefit from a slowed rate of presentation and from untimed testing (8). Older persons are, as a group, more susceptible to fatigue, and may demonstrate motivational changes as testing progresses. They may also be unfamiliar with standardized testing procedures, and such procedures may increase their anxiety and affect their test performance adversely (5).

The most widely reported cognitive change with aging is a decreased memory capacity for new material. Although this is also one of the first symptoms of DAT, it is very common for individuals who have no other cognitive deficits to notice and worry about memory problems. In general, short-term memory (less than 30 minutes) appears to decline as a normal consequence of aging, while immediate (less than 1 minute) and long-term (remote) memory appear to remain relatively intact despite increasing age. Interested readers are referred to Poon's excellent review of research in memory changes that occur with normal aging (11).

Defining a "normal" level of performance in a geriatric population is the first step in differentiating the subtle cognitive deficits typical of early stages of dementia from nonpathological age-related cognitive changes. Thus, interpretations of neuropsychological performance must be based upon a clear understanding of normal aging and a confidence in the suitability of the testing environment for a given older adult.

Other Disorders That May Impair Cognition

A number of disorders may present symptoms similar to those of DAT. Multi-infarct dementia is caused by vascular illness in which a number of small infarcts in the brain (occluded blood vessels similar to those that occur in strokes) may cause deterioration in the patient's cognitive functioning. Multi-infarct dementia is suspected in individuals who report a sudden onset and stepwise progression, in patients with known cardiovascular disease or significant hypertension, and in individuals with focal neurological signs. The Hachinski Ischemic Score (12) is often used to assess the presence of symptoms indicative of multi-infarct dementia, but research suggests that its results must be interpreted cautiously (13).

Korsakoff's psychosis is a disorder of memory, learning, and orientation that may appear similar to DAT. Korsakoff's psychosis occurs in some individuals with a long history of sustained heavy alcohol use and is related to a thiamine deficiency during periods of heavy drinking. Clinically, patients with this disorder may retain specific abilities and skills, but demonstrate severe memory deficits, and are unable to learn new material. They typically perform very poorly on memory tests, but their general cognitive functioning may be unimpaired or only mildly impaired (14). Their memory and cognitive deficits are not usually progressive, provided they abstain from further alcohol use.

Depression can also often produce behavioral manifestations that are similar to dementia and can often coexist with DAT (15). Severely depressed individuals often appear apathetic, have difficulty concentrating, have slowed motor responses, and complain of memory loss and confusion. In differentiating depression from dementia, it is important to remember that the primary disturbance in dementia is memory loss; in depression, the primary disturbance is dysphoria or disturbed affect. On standardized testing, depressed adults perform better than demented adults despite subjective reports to the contrary (16) and depressed patients are unlikely to show the neuropsychological deficits evident in demented patients (14).

EVALUATION AT THE GERIATRIC AND FAMILY SERVICES CLINIC OF THE UNIVERSITY OF WASHINGTON

Comprehensive Evaluation

A work group on diagnosis of DAT established by the National Institute of Neurological and Communicative Disorders and Stroke (NINCDS) and the Alzheimer's Disease and Related Disorders Association (ADRDA) proposed that the following areas of functioning be included in the assessment of dementia: attention, orientation, language functioning, memory, purposeful motor movements, visual perception, problem-solving, and social functioning (17). A number of tests are available to evaluate these areas, and the choice of tests depends on the severity of the dementia, the specific characteristics of the patient, the preferences of the examiner, and the evaluation goal. General considerations in choosing tests for the geriatric population are discussed in detail by a number of authors (4,5,18,19).

Major issues include the sensitivity of tests to a variety of dysfunctions, availability of appropriate norms, relevance of tests to aspects of everyday functioning, and the ability of the patient to perform the tasks required by the tests.

The multidisciplinary evaluation process developed at the Geriatric and Family Services Clinic (20) is described here to provide a detailed example of one approach that has proven useful with a variety of geriatric patients. Patients seen in this clinic are typically 60-80 years of age, usually have at least a high school education, and their prior occupational functioning typically ranges from skilled to professional levels. The evaluation begins with a detailed clinical interview with the patient and caregiver(s) to determine the nature, onset, and impact of the problems the patient is experiencing. The interview includes a general assessment of the nature and extent of the patient's cognitive and functional deficits. Brief rating instruments administered at this time include the Kahn-Goldfarb Mental Status Questionnaire to assess orientation and basic information (21) and the Mini Mental State Exam (22), which assesses orientation, memory, reading and oral comprehension, writing, and visual-motor abilities. The Dementia Rating Scale (23) is administered to caregivers to evaluate the patient's ability to perform household tasks, handle small sums of money, find his or her way about indoors or outdoors, recall recent events, and dress, feed, and toilet him or herself.

The initial interview includes an evaluation of any psychiatric symptoms that might complicate diagnostic and therapeutic decisions. As discussed earlier, depression often causes symptoms similar to those seen in dementia and may lead to an inappropriate diagnosis. Depression may also coexist with DAT and exacerbate the patient's cognitive and behavioral deficits (15). Thus, a number of depressive symptoms are carefully evaluated in the clinical interview with both the patient and caregiver. The Hamilton Rating Scale for Depression (24) is an interviewer rating scale included in the initial assessment.

While detailed assessment of medical status is accomplished in a complete physical examination, relevant medical history, including the presence of hypertension, cardiac dysfunction, strokes, and "blacking out" episodes are noted to indicate possible vascular causes of dementia. Other medical issues that are investigated in the initial interview include current and past medications and the relationship of medication status to changes in functioning, history of alcohol or drug abuse, history of head trauma or loss of consciousness, difficulties in ambulation, and visual or hearing problems.

Following the initial assessment, more detailed evaluation of the patient's functioning in a variety of areas is performed. A thorough medical evaluation is provided to rule out any physical cause (including medication complications) that may cause or contribute to the patient's cognitive deficits. An internist specializing in geriatric medicine performs a physical and neurological evaluation, including a review of systems and laboratory tests such as a complete blood count, serum chemistry tests, and thyroid function tests. The internist also reviews the patient's past medical records, including x-rays, computed tomographic (CT) scans, and results of other tests and consultations. He or she obtains additional information from family members, caregivers, and referral physicians. Although not routinely done, electroencephalograms, CT scan, and/or magnetic resonance imaging may be performed if the patient's history or physical exam suggests that these tests would provide additional diagnostic information. For more detailed information about medical evaluation and care of patients with DAT, the reader is referred elsewhere (25).

A social work evaluation is completed in the patient's home to assess environmental factors that may contribute to the patient's difficulty. The social worker evaluates the patient's current living situation, including the availability of support for both patient and caregiver and the need for and availability of community resources (such as adult day centers, housekeeping assistance, or meal preparation services). By conducting the assessment in the patient's home, the social worker is often able to observe first-hand the patient's daily routine and functional abilities, and to note details about the suitability and safety of the current living situation.

Geriatric Neuropsychological Battery

The neuropsychological battery used at the Geriatric and Family Services Clinic was designed to assess the patient's level of functioning in each of the areas discussed by the NINCDS and ADRDA work group. Each of the tests included in the battery will be described briefly and then interpretation of test results will be discussed.

Tests Administered

The Wechsler Adult Intelligence Scale-Revised (WAIS-R) provides a general measure of verbal and nonverbal problem solving ability (Wechsler, 1981). Subscales of the WAIS-R tap a variety of cognitive areas, including concept formation, abstract reasoning, cognitive flexibility, problem solving and judgement, and planning ability. The Dementia Rating Scale (DRS) described by Mattis (1976) is another measure of general level of cognitive functioning specifically designed to evaluate patients with dementia. It includes assessments of attention, initiation and perseveration, construction, conceptualization, and memory. The DRS is useful with patients with moderate or severe cognitive impairments who may be unable to perform many of the tasks required on the WAIS-R.

The Trail Making Test (28) assesses cognitive flexibility, planning, and problem solving. This is a timed test that requires the patient to connect a sequence of numbers in the correct order, and then to alternate between numbers and letters in sequence. Storandt and co-workers (29) reported that Trails A was especially sensitive to cognitive impairment when mildly demented patients were compared with an age-matched normal control group. Age norms are available, allowing comparison of the patient's performance with normal age-appropriate peers (14).

The Wechsler Memory Scale (WMS) evaluates orientation, mental control, immediate recall of logical verbal material, learning of associated word pairs, digit span, and immediate recall of figures (30). Russell's (31) delayed recall procedure is used with the WMS to assess retention of verbal and figural material. The Fuld Object Memory Evaluation (FOME) is a newer test that is particularly useful with the demented older adult (18). It uses simple objects as stimuli to be remembered, employs repeated learning trials with reminders, and assesses the patient's ability to recall and/or recognize items after a delay. The FOME also assesses the ability to name common objects by touch and sight and incorporates a verbal fluency task as an interference procedure.

The Halstead-Wepman Aphasia Screening Test (AST) provides information about language dysfunction, requiring patients to name and spell out common objects, repeat and explain phrases, read, and follow simple instructions (32). In addition to the AST, the Boston Naming Test (BNT) (33) allows evaluation of expressive language. The MMSE and the FOME, as already discussed, provide additional information about language functioning.

The Block Design and Object Assembly subtests of the WAIS-R, the Construction scale of the DRS, and the drawings on the AST provide diverse stimuli to evaluate aspects of constructional and visual-motor skills. Constructional ability involves planning and executing sequences of motor activities, and visual-motor skills involve the coordination of eye and hand movements.

Test Interpretation

The assessment of patients with suspected DAT is a complex procedure, which typically serves several purposes. Testing is often required to assist in differential diagnosis, to indicate the pattern of the patient's relative strengths and weaknesses, to provide treatment recommendations, and to establish a baseline against which to measure changes in cognitive status.

Test scores of patients with DAT are characterized by a generalized reduction in intellectual functioning from a previously higher level. This is often reflected by a discrepancy in prior educational and occupational achievement and current performance on the WAIS-R. The DRS provides additional information as to current level of functioning, and appears to be sensitive to both mild and moderate cognitive impairment (34).

Patients with DAT often perform best on WAIS-R subtests that measure old learning, such as vocabulary and information, and often perform worst on tasks requiring problem solving ability and memory for new material, but individual differences in test performance are very common, and a diagnosis of DAT should not be based on WAIS-R or DRS scores alone. These tests can, however, provide valuable information for treatment planning and for counseling family members of DAT patients. For example, families that question the safety of leaving the patient alone at home may benefit from information as to the patient's judgement and problem-solving skills.

In patients with DAT, memory is globally impaired, and most patients exhibit significant decay of learned verbal *and* graphic material after a 30 min delay. Departures from this expected performance lead to additional testing to rule out other possible causes of their cognitive difficulties. For example, significant memory impairment for verbal material with intact graphic memory or impaired graphic memory with intact verbal memory suggests a possible focal deficit, rather than the more generalized dysfunction typical of DAT. In patients with these patterns of test scores, further medical and neuropsychological testing is conducted to rule out vascular problems, head injury, and tumors, all of which might cause such isolated memory problems. Testing also provides information as to types of assistance that may prove helpful to the patient and family in compensating for memory problems. Some patients, for instance, benefit from repetition of information, while others do not. Some patients may be able to use lists and other memory cues, while others become more confused by such cues. This information can help the family maximize the patient's functioning.

Language testing provides a measure of how much information a patient is able to understand and/or express verbally. Language deficits often accompany strokes, and severe language dysfunction in combination with average or above-average memory and cognitive functioning indicates a need to rule out vascular problems carefully. Families also often find the information obtained in language testing useful as they attempt to facilitate communication with the patient. They may, for example, learn to simplify the words they use or to limit the amount of information they present to maximize the patient's understanding. They may also find that it is helpful to provide multiple choices rather than open-ended questions to a patient with word-finding problems.

Patients with DAT often experience a number of visual-motor deficits that appear to affect their ability to perform many tasks, ranging from very complex activities (such as driving) to relatively basic functions (such as bathing and dressing). Testing provides objective information to families and caregivers as to the kinds of difficulties the patient is experiencing. Test results may be helpful in developing strategies for assisting the patient by changing or simplifying both the environment (e.g., using Velcro rather than buttons) and the task (e.g., using frozen dinners to facilitate meal preparation).

Diagnosis of DAT is conditional upon documented deterioration. If the history is insufficient and test results are inconclusive, testing may be repeated 6 months to 1 year following the initial evaluation to determine whether the cognitive changes are of the global and progressively deteriorating nature that typifies DAT. Retesting also allows evaluation of the effectiveness of any treatments or environmental modifications provided, and provides a basis for further revision of treatment recommendations if appropriate.

Neuropsychological Research and Current Research on Subtypes of DAT

As already discussed, although DAT is characterized by a dementia of insidious onset and progressive course, affected persons may also display a number of different symptoms when they develop DAT, including asphasia (language disorder), agnosia (failure to recognize or identify objects despite intact sensory function), apraxia (difficulty carrying out purposeful motor activity), and personality changes. Recent reports by Mayeux et al. (35), Chui et al. (36), and Hauser et al. (37) suggest that movement disorders such as myoclonus (sudden unsustained muscular contractions) and bradykinesia (abnormally slow movements) are often present in DAT patients regardless of the severity of dementia. Other researchers (38-40) report that motor dysfunction usually does not occur until the latest stages of the disease.

Although many researchers agree that DAT appears to be a heterogeneous group of disorders, no consensus has been reached regarding the identification of clinical subgroups (35,36,41-43). Biological and epidemiological evidence discussed in more detail in Chapter 2 and in recent articles by Amaducci and colleagues (44) and Breitner et al. (45) strongly supports a familial component to some cases of DAT. Researchers, however, are divided as to possible environmental, psychometric, and behavioral distinctions in DAT patients that might help differentiate familial from nonfamilial DAT.

Breitner and Folstein (42) reported on specific clinical features they found associated with familial DAT. In an investigation of 62 DAT patients, these investigators reported that language disorder and apraxia were found in 78% of cases. These symptoms strongly predicted familial aggregation, and relatives of these patients were predicted to be seven times more likely to develop DAT by age 90 than relatives of control subjects. These authors concluded that "language disorder and apraxia specifically identify a distinct clinical entity, Familial Alzheimer Dementia, that is among the commonest [sic] forms of senile dementia" (p. 63).

Another investigation involved 43 DAT patients who were mildly demented (43). Fifty-five percent were found to have probable or definite aphasia, measured by selected subtests of the Boston Diagnostic Aphasia Exam (33). Relationships between aphasia, progression over 2-1/2 years, family history, and mortality were examined. Aphasic subjects had a more rapidly progressive course but a lower prevalence of familial cases than nonaphasic subjects. Contrary to the findings of Breitner and Folstein (42), these authors concluded that the presence of aphasia early in the course of DAT indicated a nonfamilial, rapidly progressive variety of illness.

Mayeux and co-workers (35) investigated possible subtypes of DAT, focusing on movement disorders, rather than language dysfunction, and found evidence for four subtypes of DAT in the group of patients they examined. One group was characterized as "typical," showing steady deterioration over a period of 4 years, with no movement disorder present. Another group, which met DSM-III criteria for DAT at the onset of the investigation, showed no decline over the 4 years of the investigation. A third group was observed to have extrapyramidal movement disorders (most frequently including bradykinesia and rigidity) and greater cognitive impairment than the others. Finally, a fourth group was identified that showed a myoclonic movement disorder. Myoclonus was associated with younger age at onset as well as more severe cognitive impairment. Thirty-seven percent of the patients in this investigation had positive family histories of dementia, but none of the four groups differed significantly as to the presence or absence of family history.

Chui and colleagues (36) evaluated the symptoms of 146 DAT patients. They also found evidence of extrapyramidal and myoclonic movement disorders, which were associated with greater severity and more rapid progression of the disease. Onset prior to age 65 was associated with greater language disturbance and more myoclonus. Forty-five percent had a positive family history of dementia. No significant differences in age at onset, language disorder, duration, severity, or movement disorders were found in the familial compared to the nonfamilial groups.

Cummings et al. (46) excluded patients with movement disorders from a DAT group they investigated. They found that 100% of their DAT patients had some type of language disorder, while none of their normal control group showed evidence of such a disorder. They reported that 20% of the patients they studied had a positive family history of dementia, but they found no significant differences between the familial and nonfamilial groups.

In summary, there exists considerable uncertainty as to the characteristic features of a possible familial subgroup of DAT. Movement disorders do not appear to be a distinguishing characteristic of familial compared to nonfamilial cases of DAT, and the relationship between language dysfunction and family history is a topic currently being investigated and debated by a number of researchers. Some report a positive association (42), some report a negative association (43), and some report no relationship at all (36,46).

DIRECTIONS FOR FUTURE RESEARCH

The next question to be asked is "Why the discrepancy among the research data?" The first factors to be considered are methodological differences in the investigations. Each investigation involved a different group of subjects, and while all subject groups met the requirements for diagnosis of DAT, they differed in other important ways. Age of the subjects and degree of impairment varied considerably among investigations, and would be expected to have a considerable impact on the neuropsychological test performance of the various groups. In some investigations patients with movement disorders were excluded, while in others such patients were included. Each of the different investigations used different neuropsychological measures of language dysfunction, which is also likely to have contributed to their different results. It is clear from these investigations that DAT is not a single static disorder. Symptoms and patterns of dysfunction vary considerably over time and disease progression between individuals and within individuals. Some experience a very slow progression, while for others, progression occurs more rapidly. Some cases of DAT appear to be familial, while others do not. The reasons for these differences are unknown at this time. Because of this variability, it is important that researchers continue to describe carefully their subject groups and methods of evaluation, and exercise caution in generalizing their results to the larger population of DAT patients.

As research into subtypes of DAT continues, more will be learned about patterns of impairment and their relationship to the causes and prognosis of the disorder. Future investigations of neuropsychological risk factors for DAT are likely to benefit from focusing on sensitive tests that are able to detect very subtle early changes in cognitive functioning. A longitudinal prospective approach, studying neuropsychological functioning of persons at risk for developing DAT (i.e., family members) may prove particularly fruitful. Just as a multidisciplinary approach to assessment of DAT has proven effective in clinical practice, a multidisciplinary approach to research into the causes and risk factors of DAT is likely to provide an avenue for a productive, cooperative effort to answer the many remaining questions about the causes and nature of this disorder.

REFERENCES

1. Crockett, D., Clark, C., and Klonoff, H. (1981). An overview of neuropsychology. In: *Handbook of Clinical Neuropsychology*, S.B. filskov and T.J. Boll (Eds.). New York, John Wiley & Sons, pp. 1-38.
2. American Psychiatric Association (1980). *Diagnostic and Statistical Manual of Mental Disorders*, Third Edition. Washington, D.C.: APA.
3. Rosen, W.G. (1983). Clinical and neuropsychological assessment of Alzheimer disease. *Adv. Neurol.* 38: 51-64.
4. Lezak, M.D. (1986). Neuropsychological assessment. In: *Geropsychological Assessment and Treatment*, L. Teri and P.M. Lewinson (Eds.). New York, Springer Publishing Co.
5. Albert, M.S. (1981). Geriatric neuropsychology. *J. Consult. Clin. Psychol.* 49: 835-850.
6. Birren, J.E., and Schaie, K.W. (Eds.). (1985). *Handbook of the Psychology of Aging.* New York, Van Nostrand Reinhold Company.
7. Botwinick, J. (1984). *Aging and Behavior*, Third Edition. New York, Springer Publishing Co.
8. Schaie, K.W. (1981). Psychological changes from midlife to early old age: Implications for the maintenance of mental health. *Am. J. Orthopsychiatry* 51: 199-218.

9. Okun, M.A. (1976). Adult age and cautiousness in decision: A review of the literature. *Hum. Dev.* 19: 220-233.
10. Salthouse, T.A., and Somberg, B.L. (1982). Isolating the age deficit in speeded performance. *J. Gerontol.* 37: 59-63.
11. Poon, L.W. (1985). Differences in human memory with aging: Nature, causes, and clinical implications. In: *Handbook of the Psychology of Aging*, J.E. Birren and K.W. Schaie (Eds.). New York, Van Nostrand Reinhold Co.
12. Hachinski, V., Lassen, N., and Marshall, J. (1974). Multi-infarct dementia: A cause of mental deterioration in the elderly. *Lancet* 2: 207-210.
13. Small, G.W. (1985). Revised ischemic score for diagnosing multi-infarct dementia. *J. Clin. Psychiatry* 46: 514-517.
14. Lezak, M.D. (1983). *Neuropsychological Assessment.* New York, Oxford University Press.
15. Teri, L., and Reifler, B.V. (1986). Depression and dementia. In: *Handbook of Clinical Gerontology*, L. Cartensen and B. Edelstein (Eds.). New York, Pergamon Press.
16. Gallagher, D.E., and Thompson, L.W. (1983). Effectiveness of psychotherapy for both endogenous and nonendogenous depression in older adult outpatients. *J. Gerontol.* 38: 707-712.
17. McKhann, G., Drachman, D., Folstein, M., Katzman, R., Price, D., and Stadlan, E.M. (1984). Clinical diagnosis of Alzheimer's disease. *Neurology* 34: 939-944.
18. Fuld, P.A. (1978). Psychological testing in the differential diagnosis of the dementias. In: *Alzheimer's Disease: Senile Dementia and Related Disorders*, R. Katzman, R.D. Terry, and K.L. Bick (Eds.). New York, Raven Press.
19. Jarvik, L.F. (1980). Diagnosis of dementia in the elderly: A 1980 perspective. *Annu. Rev. Gerontol. Geriatrics* 1: 180-203.
20. Reifler, B.V., Larson, E.B., and Teri, L. (in press). An outpatient geriatric psychiatry assessment and treatment service. *Clin. Geriatrics.*
21. Kahn, R.L., Goldfarb, A.I., Pollack, M., and Peck, R. (1960). Brief objective measures for the determination of mental status in the aged. *Am. J Psychiatry* 117: 326-328.
22. Folstein, M.F., Folstein, S.E., and McHugh, P.R. (1975). Mini-Mental State: A practical method for grading the cognitive state of patients for the clinician. *J. Psychiatr. Res.* 12: 189-198.
23. Blessed, G., Tomlinson, B.E., and Roth, M. (1968). The association between quantitative measures of dementia and of senile change in the cerebral gray matter of elderly subjects. *Br. J. Psychiatry* 114: 797-811.
24. Hamilton, M. (1967). Development of a rating scale for primary depressive illness. *Br. J. Soc. Clin. Psychol.* 6: 278-196.
25. Larson, E.B., Featherstone, H.J., Reifler, B.V., Canfield, C.G., and Chinn, N.M. (1985). Medical aspects of care of elderly patients with cognitive impairment. *Dev. Neuropsychol.* 1: 145-171.
26. Wechsler, D. (1981). *Wechsler Adult Intelligence Scale-Revised.* New York, The Psychological Corporation.

27. Mattis, S. (1976). Mental status examination for organic mental syndrome in the elderly patient. In: *Geriatric Psychiatry: A Handbook for Psychiatrists and Primary Care Physicians*, L. Bellack and T.B. Karasu (Eds.). New York, Grune & Stratton.
28. Reitan, R.M. (1958). Validity of the Trail Making Test as an indicator of brain damage. *Percept. Motor Skills* 8: 271-276.
29. Storandt, M., Botwinick, J., Danziger, W.L., Berg, L., and Hughes, C.P. (1984). Psychometric differentiation of mild senile dementia of the Alzheimer type. *Arch. Neurol.* 41: 497-499.
30. Wechsler, D. (1945). A standardized memory scale for clinical use. *J. Psychol.* 19: 87-95.
31. Russell, E.W. (1975). A multiple scoring method for the assessment of complex memory functions. *J. Consult. Clin. Psychol.* 43: 800-809.
32. Reitan, R.M. (1979). *Manual for Administration of Neuropsychological Test Batteries for Adults and Children.* Tucson, AZ, Reitan Neuropsychology Laboratory.
33. Goodglass, H., and Kaplan, E. (1972). *The Assessment of Aphasia and Related Disorders.* Philadelphia, Lea & Febiger.
34. Vitaliano, P.P., Breen, A.R., Russo, J., Albert, M., Vitiello, M.V., and Prinz, P.N. (1984). The clinical utility of the Dementia Rating Scale for assessing Alzheimer's patients. *J. Gerontol.* 39: 58-64.
35. Mayeux, R., Stern, Y., and Spanton, S. (1985). Heterogeneity in dementia of the Alzheimer type: Evidence of subgroups. *Neurology* 35: 453-461.
36. Chui, H.C., Teng, E.L., Henderson, V.W., and Moy, A.C. (1985). Clinical subtypes of dementia of the Alzheimer type. *Neurology* 35: 1544-1550.
37. Hauser, W.A., Morris, M.L., Heston, L.L., and Anderson, V.E. (1986). Seizures and myoclonus in patients with Alzheimer's disease. *Neurology* 36: 1226-1230.
38. Cummings, J.L., and Benson, D.F. (1983). *Dementia: A Clinical Approach.* Butterworths.
39. Cummings, J.L., and Benson, D.F. (1986). Dementia of the Alzheimer type: An inventory of diagnostic clinical features. *J. Am. Geriatr. Soc.* 34: 12-19.
40. Reisberg, B. (1986). Dementia: A systematic approach to identifying reversible causes. *Geriatrics* 41: 30-46.
41. Heston, L.L., Mastri, A.R., Anderson, E., and White, J. (1981). Dementia of the Alzheimer type: Clinical genetics, natural history, and associated conditions. *Arch. Gen. Psychiatry* 38: 1085-1090.
42. Breitner, J.C., and Folstein, M.F. (1984). Familial Alzheimer dementia: A prevalent disorder with specific clinical features. *Psychol. Bull.* 14: 63-80.
43. Knesevitch, J.W., Toro, F.R., Morris, J.C., and LaBarge, E. (1985). Aphasia, family history and the longitudinal course of DAT. *Psychiatry Res.* 111: 255-263.
44. Amaducci, L.A., Fratiglioni, L., Rocca, W.A., Fieschi, C., Livrea, P., Pedone, D., Bracco, L., Lippi, A., Gandolfo, C., Bino, G., Prencipe, M., Bonatti, M.L., Girotti, F., Carella, F., Tavolato, B., Ferla, S., Lenzi, G.L., Carolei, A., Gambi,

A., Grigoletto, F., and Schoenberg, B.S. (1986). Risk factors for clinically diagnosed Alzheimer disease: A case-control study of an Italian population. *Neurology* 36. 922-931.

45. Brietner, J.C.S., Folstein, M.F., and Murphy, E.A. (1986). Familial aggregation in Alzheimer dementia–II: Clinical genetic implications of age-dependent onset. *J. Psychiatry Res.* 20: 45-55.

46. Cummings, J.L., Benson, F., Hill, M.A., and Read, S. (1985). Aphasia in dementia of the Alzheimer type. *Neurology* 35: 394-397.

5

Notes on the Methods for the Study of Kindreds with Familial Alzheimer's Disease

JEAN-FRANCOIS FONCIN / *Laboratoire de Neurohistologie, Ecole Pratique des Hautes Etudes La Salpêtrière, Paris, France*

DENISE SALMON / *College de France and Centre National de Transfusion Sanguine, Paris, France*

AMALIA C. BRUNI / *Unità Sanitaria Locale 17, Regione Calabria, Italy*

INTRODUCTION

For 15 years we have been studying a large kindred, which we have called family "N" from the historical name of its place of origin. Alzheimer's disease is transmitted in this family in an apparently autosomal dominant manner (1-3); transmission has been established with certitude from the second quarter of the 19th century, and with probability from the mid-18th century. This kindred, one of the largest families with familial Alzheimer's disease (FAD) to have been described, has been the most informative (FAD 4) in the collaborative study that led to the mapping of the FAD gene on chromosome 21 (4). We wish to share our experience with other groups studying or planning to study families with FAD. Following are a succession of short notes on various aspects of the methods involved in the description of AD pedigrees.

THE FIRST CONTACT

The first contact with the family is obviously determinant for the detection and study of FAD. So important is the detection of FAD for progress in AD research in general, and so much depends on the collaborative attitude of the next of kin, that every effort must be made to establish a positive rapport during the first interview with relatives of any patient with possible cognitive impairment. The demonstration of interest on the part of the physician, afforded by thorough family history-taking, is an important step.

On psychological as well as scientific grounds, however, it is important for the interviewer to project a neutral but kind attitude. Direct interrogation about "other cases of the same illness in the family," as often routinely done by junior staff wishing to go straight to the heart of the matter, may be counterproductive both ways: as an effect of (often unconscious) reactive denial, the interviewer is perceived negatively, instances of AD in the family are "forgotten," and the occasion is lost for the detection of FAD. On the other hand, halo effect may lead to spurious "overdiagnosis" by the relatives. From the start, systematic inquiry about matters of public record concerning every relative in memory (even if presumably unaffected) should be pursued, avoiding direct questions concerning mental illness, but registering full names, date and place of birth, maiden name, date and place of marriage, employment, names and addresses of attending physicians and hospitals, date and place of death. Of course, spontaneous indications regarding cases of dementing illness in the family are recorded, but their importance should not be unduly stressed.

Depending on the national law involved and on the relationship formed with the next of kin, it may be desirable at this point to obtain written authorization for communication of medical records of deceased relatives. In France and Italy, such an authorization is not necessary as long as the recipient may be considered the patient's attending physician.

DETERMINING THE AIMS OF THE STUDY

Recording yet another familial cluster of AD is not an aim in itself. After the first contact, a rational decision has to be made regarding the purpose and organization of the study. A number of factors are important in that decision.

The first step is, of necessity, a diagnostic one. Discovery of proven or probable cases of AD in patients with a genetic relationship to the patient is a powerful (and quantifiable) argument in favor of a diagnosis of AD in the patient, especially, one would suspect, if age of onset and clinical appearances are comparable; we do not, however, know whether such correlations have been quantiatively tested. Conversely, the occurrence of at least one proven case of AD in the genetic chain, be it the proband or a relative, is necessary for the validity of any family study from a research point of view.

As indicated above, the importance of FAD for AD research in general would warrant the inclusion of each instance of FAD in a research program. This, however, may be done at various levels. The basic one would be the inclusion of each new instance of FAD in a national or regional registry, the main purpose of which would be to determine the true relative prevalence of FAD and "sporadic" AD. In order to go further, with the aim of providing a pedigree as extensive and as free of bias as possible, and thus suitable as a basis for further applications, more extended inquiries have to be made, which are beyond the ordinary scope of clinical practice. Yet we suspect that the "farming out" of selected AD families to specialized field research teams often does not lead to useful results. The clinical relationship with patient and family is fundamental to the success of the study, and the introduction of "outsiders" may be irremediably deleterious to that relationship. Another reason for maintaining a medical type of relationship is the sensitive nature of the information to be gathered, which ought to be protected by the secrecy rule that is both a tradition and a legal obligation of the medical profession. Outside help, advise, and counsel must be obtained, but the ultimate responsibility, and burden, rests on the clinical team. This may severely limit the aims of any study, and the number of families that can be studied by one team.

SELECTION OF FAMILIES FOR IN-DEPTH STUDIES

Although we had gathered the first elements for a study of several families with related disorders, Gerstmann-Sträussler-Scheinker disease (GSS) (5) or association of signs of AD and of Creutzfeldt-Jakob disease (6), in addition to AD families, we thought it necessary to limit our in-depth investigations to family N. Other groups must be faced with similar choices, and, consequently, criteria have to be determined for the selection of "promising" families.

The first criterion is, of course, the cooperation of family members.

The second group of favorable conditions may be grouped under the heading "accessibility." Records grouped in one place are easier to gather and to compare; field trips to many places are costly and time-consuming: stable families within traditional, rural societies tend to be more favorable to study in those respects. Families with roots in countries where public records were not kept during the 19th century, or where records are inaccessible, such as Soviet Russia, or were destroyed during wars, such as much of central Europe, often lead researchers to frustrating dead ends. Local legal conditions for access to records may also vary.

A prolific family is also an important asset, meaning more significant statistics, and less risk for interruption of transmission in any given branch.

These factors are not specific for FAD research; they were prominent in two recent "success stories" of genetics, namely Huntington's disease in Venezuela and manic-depressive illness among the Amish in the United States. More characteristic of AD is its wide clinical variability. Clear-cut forms of the disease are, of course, easier to trace in old records. This aspects loads the odds for success in AD pedigree tracing heavily in favor of early onset forms, and particularly in favor of those with clear neurological symptoms, such as the first extended AD family to have been recorded, by Van Bogaert in 1940, which featured paraplegia. Whether this bias alone is responsible for the widely notion that early onset AD is much more commonly familial than late-onset forms, is not clear. Actuarial corrections, which have been used by Breitner and Folstein to compute a 0.5

segregation ratio within a collection of small AD clusters, are useless as a tracing tool. The unresolved question of the relevance of results obtained on (early-onset) FAD models to (mainly late-onset) AD in general ought to induce researchers to try tracing late-onset AD pedigrees, in spite of the inherent difficulties.

GATHERING THE DATA

Even if an older cooperating relative with a good memory and interest in family affairs is available, data obtained from interview with members of the nuclear family of the proband are only a small beginning, both from the point of view of reliability and that of extension. Visits to the home of more distant relatives are useful, but still limited in scope. Other methods have to be used, which are outlined here. Many of these methods are not specific to FAD research, and derive from those developed for the tracing of private genealogies, a hobby made popular by books such as *Roots.* Clubs and societies exist from which persons interested in genealogy may receive useful tips and introductions. Members of such groups are usually happy to see their hobby considered as serious scientific business. Membership in a genealogical society is often an asset for workers engaged in tracing medical pedigrees.

The first source is constituted by the municipal registers of birth, marriage, and death (in France, Etat-Civil; in Italy, Stato Civile), which have been organized in most of Europe that was under Napoleonic influence. In southern Italy, these registers date back to 1809, during the reign of Murat. Records dating more than a 100 years may be consulted by all comers and freely copied from the registers; copy of more recent ones may be obtained legally by members of the family (if the existence and date of the document are known). In our case, permission for use of recent registers has been granted by authorities without difficulty, in view of the fact that a public research organization was involved.

When dealing with records of a population in which the relative density of members of the kindred is low, that is, in localities distant from the cradle of the family, it may be cost-efficient to copy only those records in evident relationship with the family under study, that is, to use a "tracing" method. According to this methods, records in which one participant is already known are copied; it privileges the patrilinear link because surnames are more discriminating than given names, and in this way introduces bias. Moreover, when new surnames in matrilinear ascent/descent are identified, further runs of the register are needed. In the use of the registers in the cradle town of the family, we have instead used a "blanket" approach, taking substantial copy of every record in which appears a surname known in the intermarrying population to which the family under study belongs. The creation of a computer database incorporating the whole registers would be the ultimate in blanket covering. It has been done for parts of Quebec (in that case mostly from parish books, Etat Civil being a recent institution in the Province) and is put to use by the IMAGE project (Denis Gauvreau, Montréal). The Church of Jesus-Christ of Latter Day Saints maintains such a database for religious reasons, covering various parts of Europe and America. We have no personal experience, however, in the use of this database, which under French law may require special authorization.

Other registers may be used covering the 19th and 20th centuries. Registers of emigration, kept in Italian minicipal offices, are a link between research at the cradle of the family and on branches that have emigrated. Recent church records may be useful for two reasons: people nowadays tend to be born and to die away from home, whereas baptism and burial take place at their own parish, which is thus a better concentration of documents. Moreover, in countries without an established church, parish books are not covered by the restrictions of access mandated for recent government records. We have found most useful the Status Animarum, which used to be written up by parish priests at fixed intervals: a record of all the households in the parish with a wealth of data on all their members, including the name of the parents and whether they were alive or dead.

Before the 19th century, parish books usually constitute the only available records, regularly covering the 18th century, occasionally the 17th, and rarely the latter part of the 16th. Difficult reading of ancient handwriting, irregular forms of the entries, haphazard variations in spelling make their use awkward for the nonspecialist. We made spot investigations of 18th century parish books in the cradle town of family N. Full use of these records, which would be invaluable for an attempt to pinpoint the mutation at the origin of FAD in family N, would require an analysis by a student of period, and preferably the incorporation of results into a computer database, without which the only practical method would be progressive tracing of ancestry, as usually practiced by amateur genealogists.

A specific source in medical pedigree tracing is, of course, medical records. Copies of records of patients within living memory may be obtained from attending physicians or from hospitals. More specifically, in the case of dementing illness, the records of the State mental hospital system have proven invaluable, in part because they were, by law, kept for 100 years. They may be approached in various ways. From the time of the institution of death certificate transcription, that is, a mention of date and place of death in the margin of the birth certificate (in France from 1926 on), the mention of a locality with a State hospital (often a small community with little other population movement) as the place of death is a presumption of fatal mental disease, and subsequent tracing of the record is easy. We found in this way the record of a long-lost member of a GSS family (5). Records of the State mental hospital serving the cradle town of family N were studied first for patients with surnames known in family N. Later, an attempt was made to study the records of all patients who died within the ages at death of affected members of family N. Unfortunately, an Italian law aiming to abolish mental illness by abolishing the State mental hospital system is now putting in jeopardy the continued accessibility and even existence of these precious records.

The mode of definition of subject status is a recurring question in FAD work. Usual categories of possible, probable, and proven AD are not applicable to FAD. If genetic transmission is demonstrated and one case in the genetic chain is proven, a priori probability for AD may be orders of magnitude higher for at risk subjects, compared with the general population, especially in the case of early onset forms. Bayesian probabilities applied to a priori "possible" cases then result in an a posteriori probability equivalent to quasicertitude. This effect is one of the factors that makes early-onset forms easier to trace. It is one of the reasons that makes FAD precious for AD research in general, allowing us to study patients with early symptoms but nevertheless a firm diagnosis. Errors are still possible: two brothers of the family N proband were hospitalized at the same time in a University neurological clinic for evaluation; both were diagnosed as having AD; the elder subsequently died with dementia, the younger recovered, is now in good health past the maximum age of manifestation of FAD in family N, and is retrospectively believed to have presented pseudodementia as a manifestation of depression in reaction to his brother's illness.

Bayesian probabilities are fundamental in estimating the status of subjects who lived at times when dementia, not to speak of Alzheimer's disease, was not a valid category. Patients with early-onset FAD die within a well-defined age span, and mortality of FAD patients may be compared for each age group with mortality of not-at-risk subjects in the same population (spouses and their families). An a posteriori probability for FAD may be computed for subjects with known age at death and known or estimated a priori genetic risk. In family N, a posteriori probability of AD in subjects at first-degree risk who died between ages 45 and 55 is quite high, approaching 0.9. Compound probabilities applied to sibships may lead to still higher figures. Results of this type are mainly useful when tracing downwards new branches originating from early ancestors, a task now of primary importance with the need for the study of as many as possible living affected and at-risk subjects using Restriction Fragment Length Polymorphisms (RELP).

ORGANIZING THE DATA

Avoiding bias in the construction of pedigrees means that any subject identified through the procedures indicated in the preceding section, and linked to the proband through the transitive set of relationships (consanguinity, marriage), is to be included in the pedigree, being an element of a connected net (generalized genealogical tree) that includes the proband. This method obviously leads to storage of information regarding people without any apparent genetic relationship with the proband. In fact, when applied to approximately closed communities, such as the ones most favorable for pedigree tracing, it leads to the description of a *population* in the population genetics meaning of the term. We have often found that later discovery of new subjects leads to changing the status of relatives by marriage, who would have been lost if not recorded in application of the method, to that of blood relatives, which are of primary interest for Mendelian genetics purposes.

Handling such a rapidly growing mass of data evidently necessitates the use of computer facilities. In fact, we almost stopped working on the N pedigree in the middle 1970s, during the period between the first data gathering by J.F.F. and the introduction of computer treatment by D.S. Our ways of handling the data reflect the changes in computer technology during that period, and certainly would not be the same if the study were designed today. The core of a subject's entry has been modeled on the 80 column IBM punched card standard, which was at that time the usual link between user and (mainframe, of course) computer. A free commentary was later added, using the remaining space on a standard printer line, when it became obvious that paper notes would become useless. Essential in this set-up is an arbitrary but unique subject serial number, usually given by order of entry. To be avoided is the designation of subject by combined generation (vertical) and horizontal number, such as VI-34, which is inevitably ambiguous in large kindreds in which any numbering of generations is bound to be arbitrary. The serial number is the main identification tool for any subject, given the extensive homonymy of surnames and the lack of imagination of 19th century parents for given names. Serial number of parents (0 for "founders," i.e., subjects whose parents are, at the time, not yet recorded) and code numbers for gender and status are the other essential data. The best way to record a marriage without known children is to enter a fictitious child of the couple, with an appropriate code number in lieu of gender.

A more modern approach certainly is to make use of database programs designed for personal computers. In fact, we recently "repatriated" our file via modem in the form of an AppleWorks database file (configuration: Apple IIe with 512K memory extension and hard disk). This rather spartan setup enables one to check permanently with the file in order to incorporate new subjects or to update previous entries, a task which was previously done with the aid of periodically updated (but always behind the times) printout sorted in alphabetical order of subjects, fathers, or mothers. Printouts sorted according to various criteria are now available from the personal computer, primarily for field work. A drawback is that the program we use does not allow for multiple chaining of sorted entries, such as would be necessary for, to take an example, the search for all the ancestors of a given subject. Such work is still done on the mainframe computer with the aid of a series of programs, the ultimate aim of which is the automatic drawing of genealogical trees on paper (7). These trees have been very useful in enabling one to form a mental image of the family, but their future role, except for teaching and publication, is in doubt. The last complete tree was drawn in 1982, when the number of known members of family N was about one-third of the present one; it was already about 10 m long. Since then, only partial trees have been drawn, destined to be used in field work or for communication with colleagues working on other aspects of the genetics of family N. The future probably lies in more powerful and specially adapted database systems, which are already is use by other teams, for instance, in the above-cited Quebec project.

CONCLUSION

The methods described above are means used to achieving a valid and useful model out of a FAD family, to be used for research on AD in general. Description of studies that may be performed on such a privileged material is beyond the scope of this chapter. Let us, however, remind the reader, by way of conclusion, that almost all these studies are dependent on the continued access to living members of the extended family, and in consequence on the clinical relationship established between them and the investigating team.

ACKNOWLEDGMENTS

In addition to the authors of papers cited in reference, we thank Pr. J. Le Beau, who made possible a diagnosis in the index case; Dr. J.E. Gruner, whose encouragements were decisive in the first phase of this work; Mr. C. Molinaro, who guided us in the archives he oversees; and Dr. Fragola, formerly director of the provincial mental hospital.

We acknowledge with thanks grants from Echanges et Recherche Médicale and from Fondation pour la Recherche Médicale.

This work has been supported for various periods by INSERM, CNRS, Ministère de l'Industrie et de la Réchérche and Faculté de Médecine Pitié-Salpèrière. J.F.F. is currently recipient of Réseau INSERM 48 60 11 under contract with Mutuelle Générale de l'Education Nationale. A.C.B. is a Fellow of the John Douglas French Foundation.

REFERENCES

1. Foncin, J.-F., and Supino-Viterbo, V. (1973). Maladie d'Alzheimer familiale: Histopathologie ultrastructurale, étude généalogique. International Congress of Neurology, Barcelona, September 8-15, 1973. *Excerpta Med. Int. Congr. Ser.* 296: 63-64.
2. Foncin, J.-F., Salmon, D., Supino-Viterbo, V., Feldman, R.G., Macchi, G., Mariotti, P., Scoppetta, C., Caruso, G., and Bruni, A.C. (1985). Démence présenile d'Alzheimer transmise dans une famille étendue. *Rev. Neurol. (Paris)* 141: 194-202.

3. Foncin, J.-F., Salmon, D., and Bruni, A.C. (1986). Genetics of Alzheimer's disease: A large kindred with apparent Mendelian transmission; possible implications for a linkage study. In: *New Concepts in Alzheimer's Disease*, M. Briley, A. Kato, and M. Weber (Eds.). London, Macmillan, pp. 242-256.
4. St. George-Hyslop, P.H., Tanzi, R.E., Polinsky, R.J., Haines, J.L., Nee, L., Watkins, P.C., Myers, R., Feldman, R., Pollen, D., Drachman, D., Growdon, J., Bruni, A., Foncin, J.-F., Salmon, D., Frommelt, P., Amaducci, L., Sorbi, S., Piacentini, S., Stewart, G.D., Hobbs, W.J., Conneally, P.M., and Gusella, J.F. (1987). The genetic defect causing familial Alzheimer's disease maps on chromosome 21. *Science* 235: 885-890.
5. Foncin, J.-F., Cardot, J.L., Martinet, Y., and Arnott, G. (1982). Maladie de Gerstmann-Sträussler-Scheinker: Etude anatomo-clinique et généalogique. *Rev. Neurol. (Paris)* 138: 123-135.
6. Gaches, J., Supino-Viterbo, V., and Foncin, J.-F. (1977). Association des maladies d'Alzheimer et de Creutzfeldt-Jakob. *Acta Neurol. Belg.* 77: 202-212.
7. Landre, M.F., Vallat, M.T., and Jutier, P. (1972). Reconnaissance automatique des liens de parenté. Tracé automatique d'arbre génélogique. M.I.S. 10 Villeurbanne, SIMEP.

Part II
Molecular Genetics of Alzheimer's Disease

6

Genetic Heterogeneity in Alzheimer's Disease

V. ELVING ANDERSON / *University of Minnesota, Minneapolis, Minnesota*

INTRODUCTION

Genetic heterogeneity is a potential obstacle that must be considered sooner or later in the study of every medical disorder. The presence of significant genetic heterogeneity may affect diagnosis and treatment. It will also interfere with efforts to establish linkage between a disease and genetic markers, as well as the use of linked markers for genetic counseling.

The evidences for genetic heterogeneity can be assessed at several levels: (a) features of the clinical phenotype, (b) the pattern of inheritance, (c) the primary gene action (a developmental process, an enzyme, or a structural component of cells or membranes), or (d) the genetic code itself. This topic has been recognized for a number of decades and is even more important at present (1-3).

The awareness of possible genetic heterogeneity will affect the way in which data are collected, reported, analyzed, and interpreted. In some instances it may help to resolve difference between studies. Thus it seems preferable to assume heterogeneity and test for it rather than to assume homogeneity at the outset. This strategy, of course, leaves open the option of developing a unifying hypothesis at a more fundamental level.

CAUSES OF GENETIC HETEROGENEITY

One type of heterogeneity is seen when a clinical phenotype may be caused by mutations at two or more genetic loci. This can occur when the mutations involve different steps in an enzymatic pathway, different subunits of a heteromeric protein, a receptor or its corresponding ligand, or regulatory compared to structural genes. Even when only a single locus is involved, significant clinical variations may arise from changes at more than one site within the locus (4).

The deletion or amplification of varying lengths of chromosome segments is an additional source of heterogeneity that is detected more readily through the use of DNA probes (5). The variable clinical features of "microdeletion syndromes" (or continuous gene syndromes) are associated with the nature and extent of the deletions involved (6). Furthermore, there is growing evidence that the various types of leukemia are related to the different types of somatic chromosomal translocations involved (7).

There remains the possibility that nongenetic factors may be responsible for a fraction of the cases of a specific disorder. It must be remembered, of course, that nonfamilial cases may be "chance isolated" instances of a Mendelian trait, while familial cases may reflect the action of a common nongenetic factor. Evidence for genetic heterogeneity is stronger when a direct test for the presence or absence of genetic variation in individuals is available.

GENETIC HETEROGENEITY IN OTHER CONDITIONS

A review of selected examples from other disorders is presented first, as a background for the consideration of Alzheimer's disease itself. Further details and other examples are readily available in McKusick's index of Mendelian traits (8) and in the extensive report on the "molecular biology of *Homo sapiens*" (9).

One of the classic examples is the case of gargoylism, which was the term used earlier to describe a complex set of physical malformations. Careful evaluation of clinical findings showed that the phenotypic features in families with X-linked inheritance were distinguishable from those in families with autosomal recessive inheritance, and these conditions were renamed the Hunter's and Hurler's syndromes, respectively. Some of the related *mucopolysaccharidoses* were shown to be genetically distinct because the mixing of two cell lines in tissue culture corrected the metabolic error (10). Currently, 15 distinguishable conditions are recognized (11).

More recently, molecular studies have helped to explain the heterogeneity found in *Gaucher's disease*, which is caused by a deficiency of lysosomal glucocerebrosidase. Type 1 is characterized by hepatosplenomegaly, anemia, thrombocytopenia, and bone involvement, but the nervous system is not affected. Patients with type 2 have cranial nerve and brain stem abnormalities in addition to hepatosplenomegaly, with onset usually before 6 months of age. Those with type 3 disease have systemic symptoms like those of type 1, but neurologic signs appear during childhood or adolescence. A specific single-base substitution has been identified through the use of DNA probes (12). Four of 5 patients with type 2 disease and all of 11 with type 3 disease had at least 1 allele with the mutation. Only 4 of 20 patients with type 1 had the mutant allele, and they were heterozygotes. Further study is required, of course, to determine if this specific mutation is in some way responsible for expression of the disease in the nervous system.

A different explanation for heterogeneity has been advanced for the *Hartnup* phenotype (13). The Hartnup gene is an autosomal recessive mutation that affects a transport system of intestine and kidney used for a number of amino acids. In a prospective study of 21 subjects identified by newborn screening, all had abnormally elevated amino acid excretion values, but only 2 showed a major disease or developmental problem. Analysis of the data led to the suggestion that the polygenic genetic background modified the effect of the major gene.

Heterogeneity has emerged as a major theme in gene mapping work. The pioneering work on *Huntington's disease* illustrates this point. Through the use of the DNA marker D4S10 detected by probe G8, the mutant gene was determined to be located near the end of the short arm of chromosome 4. This discovery was greatly facilitated by the availability of a very large kindred in Venezuela, since all affected members in that family must have had the same mutant gene. The marker has not yet been used widely in genetic counseling, however, because of the possibility that some families may carry a mutation at another locus and the concern about the possible reaction of family members to the test results (14). No informative family has yet proved to be an exception, but in the absence of effective treatment, the research teams involved have chosen a cautious approach.

Phenylketonuria (PKU) is caused by a deficiency of hepatic phenylalanine hydroxylase (PAH) and is the most common inborn error of amino acid metabolism (15). At the clinical level PKU appears to be a heterogeneous disorder, but thus far all cases appear to arise from mutations of the PAH locus on chromosome 12. In a study of 33 Danish kindreds, as an example of recent work, a total of 12 haplotypes at the PAH locus were identified through the use of restriction enzymes (16). Of 66 mutant chromosomes analyzed, 25 (38%) were associated with haplotype 3, and all of the 25 showed the same single-base substitution at the 5' splice donor site of intron 12. This observation strongly suggested that this specific mutation occurred relatively recently and then spread by founder effect.

Cystic fibrosis (CF) is the most common autosomal recessive disorder in the white population, and the gene responsible has been mapped to chromosome 7 (17). Genetic heterogeneity has been considered as a possible explanation for the high frequency, since the overall frequency might reflect the sum total of several different more rare conditions. As yet, however, there is no evidence for a second CF locus (18).

Studies of *bipolar affective illness* on the other hand, have provided clear evidence that several distinct genetic loci are involved. In a large Amish family (with 19 affected and 62 unaffected in an autosomal dominant pattern of inheritance) the disorder was tightly linked to DNA markers on the short arm of chromosome 11 (19). Close linkage to chromosome 11 markers, however, was excluded in three Icelandic pedigrees (20) and in three non-Amish North American pedigrees (21). Linkage to X-chromosome markers was confirmed in four non-Ashkenazi Jewish families (22) and in nine families from Belgium (23), but not in one Ashkenazi family (22). Thus at least three distinct loci are implicated, one on chromosome 11, one on the X chromosome, and at least one elsewhere.

Duchenne muscular dystrophy (DMD) has shown considerable genetic heterogeneity (24). All cases appear to involve the same locus on the X chromosome, but a number of different mutational changes have been detected. The analysis has been greatly facilitated by the availability of a series of probes known as *pERT*87 (named for the phenol-enhanced reassociation technique) that identify the DXS164 locus close to or within the DMD locus. The DMD locus appears to be extremely large and also subject to a high rate of recombination with adjoining markers (25). About 8% of cases of DMD involve a deletion of part of the DMD locus, and the remainder apparently result from mutations at different points within the same locus or region.

Becker muscular dystrophy (BMD) is a clinically similar but less severe condition. Both DMD and BMD appear to result from two very closed linked loci or from two alleles at the same locus. Identification of the carrier state in DMD and BMD is improved by the combined use of restriction fragment length polymorphisms (RFLPs) together with serum levels of creatine kinase and pyruvate kinase (26).

An X-linked mutation in the mouse, *mdx*, produces a relatively mild form of muscular dystrophy. The close genetic linkage of *mdx* to *G6PD* and *Hprt* on the mouse X chromosome together with the mild features suggested that *mdx* might correspond to Emery-Dreifuss muscular dystrophy (EMD), which is closely linked to *G6PD* on the human X chromosome. It turned out, however, that sequences on the mouse X chromosome that are homologous to a human DMD cDNA clone mapped close to the *mdx* locus but distant from sparse fur, *spf*, the mouse homologue of ornithine transcarbamylase that is closely linked to DMD in the human (27). Another study (28) showed that a region homologous to DMD is close to the phosphorylase b locus in the mouse. This result suggests the possibility that unrecognized deficiencies in phosphorylase kinase may be present in some DMD patients with large deletions. This topic of mouse-human homology is, of course, paralleled in recent studies of Alzheimer's disease and Down's syndrome (29).

The heterogeneity observed in *microdeletion syndromes* has also been detected in studies of DMD. A male patient who showed DMD together with the X-linked phenotypes of chronic granulomatous disease, retinitis pigmentosa, and the McCleod red cell phenotype was shown to have an interstitial deletion (30). Several other patients displayed muscular dystrophy together with congenital adrenal hypoplasia and glycerol kinase deficiency, and analysis with DNA probes showed deletions that include the DMD and neighboring regions (31).

Another example of microdeletion syndromes is seen in studies of loci on chromosome 11 (32,33). The development of Wilms' tumor of the kidney in children has been correlated with deletions of chromosomal band 11p13, but about 2% of the patients also have aniridia. On the other hand, about one-third of children with aniridia also develop Wilms' tumor. Patients with both aniridia and Wilms' tumor often have genitourinary abnormalities and mental retardation as well, a combination termed the *WAGR syndrome.* The majority of these children have a constitutional deletion on one of their chromosomes 11, which always includes band 11p13. Other combinations are correlated with the extent and position of the deletion. Thus the microdeletions can cause complex and variable phenotypes by including varying numbers of contiguous independent genetic loci.

Retinoblastoma (Rb) also involves a chromosomal deletion, but here we find an explanation for the distinction between isolated and familial cases. For some while it has been known that familial cases follow an autosomal dominant pattern of inheritance, are almost always bilateral, and have early onset. Isolated cases are usually unilateral and have later onset. Isolated bilateral cases are always hereditary, while about 85% of isolated unilateral cases are nonhereditary. It is now clear that familial cases inherit one chromosome 13 that has a deletion of band q14. The tumor arises when a mutation affects the function of the allele on the other chromosome 13 (34). This "two-hit" model was proposed by Knudson (35) and also is involved in Wilms' tumor. It is thought that the normal allele on chromosome 13 suppresses tumor formation. Thus retinoblastoma can follow an autosomal dominant pattern of inheritance while functioning as a recessive at the molecular level. Recently the Rb gene has been isolated, and a complementary DNA probe was used to examine 40 retinoblastomas (36). In 16 cases the Rb gene had identifiable structural changes, and in the remainder there was either absence of an Rb transcript or abnormal expression of the Rb transcript.

Nussbaum and Ledbetter (37) have reviewed the complex problems encountered in the *fragile X syndrome*, including types of heterogeneity for which there is no explanation as yet. This syndrome affects nearly 1 in 2,000 males and is responsible for at least 25% of the mental retardation in males. It represents a single-gene, or perhaps more complex, mutation associated with a chromosomal marker. Pedigree analysis, however, suggests that as many as 20% of males who carry the marker X are clinically unaffected, a phenomenon that is most unusual for an X-linked phenomenon. For the mentally normal *mothers* of transmitting males the risk of mental retardation in male offspring is only 9%, whereas, in the male offspring of the mentally normal *daughters* of these transmitting males the risk of retardation is nearly 40%. The linkage between fragile X and the marker F9 is much tighter in families with a transmitting male than in those without, raising the possibility that the fragile X mutation itself increases the recombination frequency in this region. On the basis of these and other considerations, the authors (37) proposed a two-step model. Amplification of the fragile X region, perhaps through unequal meiotic recombination, is hypothesized to be the premutation event. This partially amplified sequence would be a candidate for further amplification and/or deletion, which produces the completed mutation and also enhances the demonstration of fragile-site expression.

Siniscalco (38) also suggested that the fragile X mutations may be the result of relatively common, mistaken crossing-over events. A patient with the fragile X syndrome would be the deficient product of the unequal crossing-over, while the normal transmitting males would be carriers of a tandem duplication. He continued:

> Given the role played by genetic recombination in the generation of these gene clusters, it is natural to wonder whether the deletion-related diseases are the price that the species has to pay for its ability to upgrade its genomic variability through genetic recombination. This is to say that—as J.B.S. Haldane once remarked in one of his writings for the lay public—a significant number of the deleterious mutations known may be genetic holes rather than 'things' and may occur with a frequency considerably higher than those resulting from single-base-pair mutations, such as transversions and transpositions. . . . Moreover, if dreadful diseases may arise from mistaken crossover events in normal individuals, it would make sense to make a special effort to map the hot spots of recombination throughout the entire genome and to study in detail the DNA sequences existing at these sites in hopes of understanding the intimate molecular mechanism of normal and aberrant recombination.

There is good evidence for genetic heterogeneity in the mechanisms leading to *epilepsy* (39). Animal models have clearly demonstrated the role of genetic factors even though the specific causative pathways have not been established. In the human, there are over 140 mendelian traits (including disorders of amino acids, enzymes, hormones, and vasculature) that increase the risk of seizures, although all of these together account for no more than 2% of seizure cases. In the other cases, higher sibling risks are associated with earlier age at onset, generalized epilepsy, and specific electroencephalographic patterns (generalized spike and wave, or photoconvulsive response). Currently DNA markers are being used to study linkage in families with juvenile myoclonic epilepsy and in families with benign familial neonatal convulsions.

Analysis of the variable clinical expression of *Parkinson's disease* (PD) leads to many parallels with Alzheimer's disease. The factors studied in PD include age at onset, rate of progression, isolated or familial nature, cognitive impairment, bradykinesia or tremor, and response to therapy. Martin et al. (40) found that the cumulative risk for siblings approached 30% when there was an affected parent, but was not significantly elevated above control values when no parent was affected. Two major subgroups emerged in a study of 334 patients with PD (41). Tremor as the dominant feature was associated with relative preservation of mental status, earlier age at onset, family history of PD, and a more favorable prognosis. Postural instability, on the other hand, was associated with more pronounced decline in functional and mental status, later age at onset, dysarthria, dysphagia, and more rapid progression.

Cases of osteogenesis imperfecta (OI), or brittle bone disease, can be subdivided on the basis of small differences in clinical and radiographic findings (42). Recent studies of collagen (which is defective in OI) have provided further evidence for heterogeneity among the *collagen disorders* (43,44). There are at least 10 distinct types of collagens, which differ in structure, tissue distribution, physicochemical properties, and function. The biosynthesis involves at least 13 cotranslational and posttranslational modifications requiring more than a dozen enzymes. Gene loci encoding structural proteins and enzymes involved in collagen and other connective tissue metabolism have been mapped to human chromosomes 1, 2, 3, 7, 11, 12, 13, 15, 17, 21, 22, and X. Prockop (45) has emphasized that a defect in a single subunit of collagen can radically alter the structural integrity of a protein containing multiple subunits, a phenomenon he has described as protein suicide.

Finally, it is important to review the genetic syndromes associated with *amyloidosis* (46,47). The majority of the syndromes show an autosomal dominant pattern of inheritance (Table 1), just as in the collagen disorders. There is wide variation in the part of the body affected. Neuropathy, when it is present, may involve the upper limbs, lower limbs, face, or the autonomic system. In other conditions the viscera, skin, eye, heart, gingiva, kidney, or endocrine glands may be the target. This organ and tissue specificity again parallels the collagen disorders. The appearance of a strong ethnic effect results partly from the tradition of naming conditions according to the place of first description, but founder effect may also be involved.

Significant advances in our understanding of the amyloid proteins have resulted from recent studies at the molecular level (48). Familial Mediterranean fever is associated with a specific mutational change in serum amyloid A (49). Amyloidosis VI involves a mutation leading to an amino acid substitution in a serum protein, cystatin C, and is an autosomal dominant form of hereditary cerebral hemorrhage seen in Iceland (50). In a different autosomal dominant form of hereditary cerebral hemorrhage described in Dutch patients the vascular amyloid deposits reacted intensely with an antiserum raised against a synthetic peptide homologous to the AD-related-protein (51). On the basis of this similarity, the authors proposed that this disorder be designated as "familial Alzheimer disease, vascular type."

Amyloidosis I can result from several different point mutations, each of which produces a single amino acid substitution in transthyretin (TTH), formerly called prealbumin because of its electrophoretic mobility in relation to that of albumin. Transthyretin is a major component of the ventricular CSF and is synthesized (apparently exclusively) by the choroid plexus (52). In a study of 6 families, all of the 20 symptomatic members were found to have 1 normal and 1 aberrant gene for TTR (53), an observation consistent with the autosomal dominant mode of inheritance. Moreover, 10 of the 30 asymptomatic individuals were also hetero-

TABLE 1 Genetic Syndromes Associated with Amyloidosis

Autosomal Dominant Phenotypes (N=15)	
10480	Amyloidosis I (Andrade type of familial amyloid neuropathy; Portuguese type of familial amyloid neuropathy; hereditary neuropathic amyloidosis type I; transthyretin abnormality; TTR abnormality; prealbumin defect)
10490	Anyloidosis II (Indiana-type amyloidosis; Rukavina-type amyloidosis; hereditary neuropathic amyloidosis type II)
10500	Amyloidosis III (cardiac-type amyloidosis; Denmark-type amyloidosis)
10510	Amyloidosis IV (Iowa-type amyloidosis; Van-Allen-type amyloidosis)
10512	Amyloidosis V (Finland-type amyloidosis; Meretoja-type amyloidosis)
10515	Amyloidosis VI (cerebral-arterial-type amyloidosis; Iceland-type amyloidosis; cerebral hemorrhage, familial; hereditary cerebral hemorrhage with amyloidosis; defect in metabolism of gamma-trace; cerebral amyloid angiopathy)
10520	Amyloidosis, familial visceral (amyloidosis, type VIII; Ostertag-type amyloidosis; German-type amyloidosis; familial renal amyloidosis)
10521	Amyloidosis VII (oculoleptomeningeal-type amyloidosis; Ohio-type amyloidosis)
10525	Amyloidosis, primary cutaneous (familial lichen amyloidosis; amyloidosis, type IX)
10527	Amyloidosis, Swedish type
12010	Cold hypersensitivity (cold urticaria, familial)
12220	Corneal dystrophy, lattice-type (lattice corneal dystrophy)
13744	Gerstmann-Straussler disease (GSD; encephalopathy, subacute spongiform, Gerstmann-Straussler-type; Gerstmann-Straussler-Scheinker disease; GSSD; cerebellar ataxia, progressive dementia and amyloid deposits in CNS; amyloidosis, cerebral, with spongiform encephalopathy)
17140	Pheochromocytoma and amyloid-producing medullary thyroid carcinoma (PTC syndrome; Sipple syndrome; multiple endocrine neoplasia, type II; MEN2; MEN2A; familial medullary thyroid carcinoma)
19190	Urticaria, deafness, and amyloidosis
Autosomal Recessive Phenotypes (N=4)	
20485	Amyloidosis of gingiva and conjunctiva, with mental retardation
20487	Amyloidosis, corneal
20490	Amyloidosis, cutaneous bullous
24910	Mediterranean fever, familial (FMF)
X-Linked Phenotypes (N=1)	
30122	Amyloidosis, familial cutaneous

From ref. 8.

zygous. The number of asymptomatic individuals with the gene decreased with age, and none was over 40 years. This ability to detect presymptomatic individuals can help in efforts to explain delayed onset of clinical signs. In most (but not all) patients with amyloidosis 1, analysis of the DNA shows an amino acid substitution (methionine for valine) at position 30. The single base change at the DNA level coincidentally creates a new site for the restriction enzyme *NsiI*, thus providing a direct test for the mutation that can be used for preclinical diagnosis of gene carriers, including prenatal diagnosis (54).

Gerstmann-Sträussler syndrome is characterized by spinocerebellar ataxia, progressive dementia, and widespread amyloid plaque deposition in the cerebral and cerebellar cortex. Usually neurofibrillary tangles (NFTs) are absent, but they were numerous in a recently reported atypical patient with features of multiple system atrophy, Alzheimer's disease, spongiform encephalopathy, and cerebrovascular amyloidosis (55). The patient's mother and one brother have a gait disturbance but no signs of mental deterioration. The authors suggest the possibility that this case may represent the association of two nonrelated entities (spinocerebellar ataxia and Alzheimer's disease), but other options might be considered. The association of several distinct phenotypes could result from the simultaneous alteration of continguous gene loci (as described earlier). Alternatively, and in the light of the collagen mutations, a mutation in a different part of an amyloid molecule could alter the distribution of target organs.

The review in this section has covered selective examples of genetic heterogeneity. Perhaps only a few of the mechanisms involved will turn out to be relevant for Alzheimer's disease, but it is important to keep a number of options open for consideration. Recent molecular studies of Alzheimer's disease itself will be discussed later.

GENETIC HETEROGENEITY IN ALZHEIMER'S DISEASE AT THE CLINICAL LEVEL

There have been a number of efforts to define subgroups of AD using various combinations of clinical factors (56,57). In the present context it seems more appropriate to consider whether evidence for genetic heterogeneity as an independent variable is correlated with other variables (58-63).

The limitations on the meaning of a *family history* of AD are well known: relatively late age at onset, difficulty in establishing a firm diagnosis in the absence of a pathological report, and differences in the intensity of family interviewing. Nevertheless some guidelines can assist in the analysis.

1. We can make the simplifying assumption that *familial* cases of AD reflect genetic causes. Even if an infectious agent is sometimes involved, genetic variation in susceptibility is very likely to be important.
2. *Isolated* cases represent an undefined mixture of primarily genetic and primarily nongentic causes (64). It should be noted that in choosing a term to

describe an affected person without affected relatives, *isolated* is a better term than *sporadic*, which infers a low risk, often on a nongentic basis. When this terminology is used, isolated cases are seen to be a mixture of chance isolated and sporadic.

3. In order to permit evaluation of the mode of inheritance, the several categories of first-degree relatives must be recorded separately. It is preferable to sort by parental history (affected or not) and then study siblings of probands.
4. The probands should be classified first by the clinical variable of interest; then the cumulative risk of AD in siblings can be calculated (59,65).

The simple classification of probands by family history (presence or absence of AD in any relative) is less satisfactory, since the size of family is uncontrolled.

The late and variable age at onset of AD continues to raise problems for studies of causes. Essentially all studies report a significant effect of ***age at onset*** of AD in the proband, in the sense that earlier-onset cases tend to be more severe. Some authors (66) have interpreted the data on age at onset as evidence for two distinct subtypes of AD. There is no uniformity in the choice of an age dividing point among various studies, however, thus making comparisons difficult. From a more general point of view, one of the best recent discussions of age at onset as related to causes of disease is by Childs and Scriver (67).

In a study by Heston et al. (59), when the age at onset in the proband was 70 or older, the cumulative risk in siblings by age 90 was 10%, which is the same as in controls. The presence or absence of an affected parent made no difference. In the group of probands with onset before 70, the cumulative risk in siblings by age 90 was 45% when there was an affected parent, compared with 15% when neither parent was affected. Breitner et al. (68) failed to find a difference between early- and late-onset cases in their analysis of the cumulative incidence among first-degree relatives (pooling parents and siblings). Further study is needed to resolve the discrepancy on this important point.

Several reports have studied the relationship of *neurochemical* data to age at onset and clinical characteristics, but with no mention of AD in relatives. The analysis of the brains of 49 AD probands showed that the older patients (at death) had a relatively pure cholinergic deficit confined to temporal lobe and hippocampus, compared with a more severe and widespread deficit in younger patients (69). Seltzer and Sherwin (70) reported that probands with onset before 65 had a higher proportion with language disturbance, left-handedness, and shorter relative survival time. Roth (71) reviewed the data from a number of studies and concluded that the early-onset cases of AD are more severely affected with respect to the nature of the cortical lesions, the range of neurotransmitter deficits, and the neuronal outfall in a number of subcortical nuclei, as well as certain clinical features.

When the family history of AD is noted in a neurochemical study, as in the detailed study of choline acetyltransferase activity by Bird et al. (72), the numbers have been too small for analysis. In view of the tissue specificity of various mutant alleles for amyloidosis and collagen disorders (cited above), it must be strongly recommended that future neuropathological and neurochemical studies report simultaneously the clinical findings in the probands and the history of AD in relatives.

Extrapyramidal signs of Parkinson's disease (PD) have been noted frequently in patients with AD (58,73). Several types of explanation are possible: (a) the presence of these signs may reflect a more severe form of AD (58); (b) such cases might represent the chance occurrence of PD as an independent disease process, but the dementia and PD do not segregate independently among the relatives of these probands (58); (c) these probands may have a genetically variant form of AD. (The possibility of a continguous gene syndrome should be kept in mind.)

In a study of severely affected patients in a nursing home, the presence of *language disorder and apraxia* in the probands was strongly associated with the risk of AD among siblings (74). These results were interpreted as evidence for language disorder and apraxia as specific markers for an autosomal dominant form of AD. Another study (75) found the reverse, namely, that the lack of aphasia was associated with a higher prevalence of familial cases. The issue has not been resolved, but it appears desirable that case reports and larger studies note the presence or absence of these findings.

It is well known that patients with Down's syndrome (DS) often have neuropathological signs of AD and an increased risk of leukemia. Heston and Mastri (76) presented evidence for an increased incidence of DS and immunoproliferative malignancies among relatives of AD probands. An increase in DS among relatives was confirmed by Heyman et al. (62) but not by Whalley et al. (63) or Nee et al. (77). None of the latter three studies found increased numbers of malignancies. A clear test of these hypotheses probably will require molecular data.

Dermatoglyphic studies have produced evidence of a significantly increased frequency of ulnar loops on the fingertips, simian creases on the palms, and other changes that parallel the patterns observed in DS (78). Seltzer and Sherwin (79) found significantly more ulnar loops in AD patients with onset before 65 (compared with controls), but not in patients with later onset. Additional studies to extend these observations would be desirable.

Nee et al. (80) reviewed published *twin* reports and studied 22 additional pairs ascertained through a variety of contacts. The ages at onset were reported and analyzed. Some information has been presented about AD in parents and siblings, but for the concordant pairs there is no indication as to whether one or both were probands. The results to date do not permit an estimate of concordance rates because of problems in ascertaining patients and the small number of DZ pairs. Two additional discordant monozygotic pairs have been reported (81,

82). The latter study incorporated neuropsychological testing, brain imaging, and measures of cerebral glucose metabolism, which are desirable features in case reports about twins.

In addition to the above specific variables, some general points have been made about the evidence for, and the implications of, causative heterogeneity in AD. Jorm (83) concluded that AD research has not yet met the criteria for establishing *qualitatively* different subtypes, but that there appears to be *quantitative* variability in a number of respects. Chui (84). adapted Jorm's theoretical approach, and produced a number of path diagrams illustrating how the clinical heterogeneity observed in AD could be produced. She appropriately emphasized the importance of longitudinal studies to define the meaningfulness of subgroups based on clinical data.

Schweber (85) broadened the scope by including the relationships between AD and DS, and by suggesting that *all* manifestations of AD may be the result of a unitary, single, pathological cause. Alzheimer's disease could result from the tripling of a subsection of the critical segment of chromosome 21 involved in Down's syndrome (a hypothesis that was quite reasonable at that time). In a later section, however, she introduced an essentially different explanation, although still unitary. In this scenario AD could involve the production of a protein product that interacts with the transcription-translation system and hence affects the expression of a number of direct genetic products. The latter hypothesis resembles the proposal by Heston and Morris (86) that transcription of a subset of genes in the 21q22 segment is increased in AD by insertion of a DNA enhancer sequence.

In summary, some interesting hypotheses have been proposed but few firm conclusions can be drawn. There are few studies with sizable samples in which the same variables have been studied and the same methods for analysis used. The data about risk to relatives are not firm enough to be of much help in genetic counseling. A number of studies are underway, however, and further analysis using a common protocol may be possible. Furthermore, these data sets should provide a valuable resource for molecular studies.

GENETIC HETEROGENEITY IN ALZHEIMER'S DISEASE AT THE MOLECULAR LEVEL

Significant developments have taken place recently along two lines: linkage studies using DNA probes, and further delineation of the amyloid deposits in AD. These two lines of research complement and depend upon each other. It is beyond the scope of this chapter to chronicle the sequence of findings as they emerged. Our concern here is with some of the major threads relevant to the continuing search for genetic heterogeneity.

A major event in AD research was the almost simultaneous publication in *Science* (20 February 1987) of four papers reporting recent work, and in *Nature* (19 February 1987) and *Lancet* (14 February 1987) of related papers.

1. Antibodies against amyloid filaments (and their constituent proteins) from AD patients cross-reacted with neuritic plaques and cerebrovascular amyloid deposits from other aged mammals (rhesus and squirrel monkeys, orangutan, polar bear, and dog) (87).

2. With the use of a DNA probe (synthesized to correpond with the first 20 amino acids of the polypeptide that forms the brain amyloid in AD) a complementary DNA clone was isolated from human brain. The corresponding gene was assigned unambiguously to human chromosome 21 (88).

3. A similar cDNA clone (isolated independently) also was assigned to chromosome 21 (89). The correponding RNA was detected in human fetal brain, kidney, heart, and spleen, with lower levels in liver. Within the brain the highest level of expression was in the association cortex. The distribution did not correlate with areas (such as the hippocampus) showing neuritic plaques, but did coincide with the deposition of cerebrovascular amyloid.

4. Ten probes (previously assigned to chromosome 21) were used to analyze DNA from members of four large AD kindreds (of British, German, Russian, and Italian origin, respectively). Affected members had relatively early onset, and the kindreds showed some variation with respect to postmortem pathological appearance, DS in relatives, and myoclonus in the AD probands. Multipoint analysis using two of the markers provided conclusive evidence that a DNA sequence involved in the development of AD does map to chromosome 21, although outside the region essential for Down's syndrome (90).

5. The DNA sequence was established independently for the beta amyloid subunit (A4) and for the larger precursor protein, together with the predicted amino sequence for A4 (42 or 43 amino acids) and its precursor (695 amino acids). The corresponding gene was localized to human chromosome 21. The predicted precursor contains features characteristic of glycosylated cell-surface receptors (91).

6. A clone encoding the amyloid peptide hybridized in situ to chromosome 21 at a position that appeared to be distinct from the region associated with the DS phenotype. Additional, but weaker, hybridization was seen on chromosome 20 in a region containing the gene for another amyloidogenic substance, prion protein (92). A later report (93) showed hybridization also on chromosome 9.

These six papers included reviews of prior work by these authors and others. None provided a complete story, but together they gave an impressive basis for further studies about causative mechanisms.

The major protein subunit (A4) of the amyloid fibril of the tangles, plaques, and blood vessel deposits found in AD and in DS is an insoluble, highly aggregating small polypeptide. This is derived from a larger precursor protein that resembles a cell-surface receptor (91). (It may be of interest that anisotrophy studies (94,95) have led to the suggestion that hippocampal membranes from a subgroup of AD patients are altered in superficial regions near the lipid-aqueous interface, while deeper membrane regions remain unaffected.)

The Alzheimer-like manifestations in DS may result from overexpression of an otherwise normal gene (or genes) on chromosome 21 as a result of increased gene dosage (89,90). The possibility remains, however, of a more complex interaction between other chromosome 21 gene products and the biosynthesis and processing of the A4 precursor in DS (91).

A gene encoding the amino acid sequence of A4 maps to chromosome 21 (88,89,91). This gene is present in several mammalian species (87,88). The expression of this gene (in terms of messenger RNA), however, is not limited to the areas of the brain exhibiting pathological changes in AD (89). This apparent discrepancy has several possible explanations. The precursor protein may be altered in the brain to a component that can form plaque amyloid; other tissues may be able to eliminate amyloidogenic peptides; the brain reads a different part of the gene (89); or the protein produced by the gene may have a function that is not restricted to the brain (89). Subsequent work has shown that a duplication of this gene is found in Down's syndrome but not in sporadic or familial AD (96-100).

A DNA sequence involved in familial AD also maps to chromosome 21 (90). Subsequent work (101,102), however, has shown that this sequence is not identical with, or even closely linked to, the A4 locus.

Familial AD could result from expression of an abnormal protein or from overexpression of a normal protein (from gene duplication or amplification, increased transcription, increased RNA processing, or decreased degradation of the gene product) (90).

A number of other hypotheses have emerged, and it is not yet clear which will turn out to be significant. Furthermore, the diversity of alternative mechanisms may reflect an underlying heterogeneity in causes.

Earlier work had established the critical importance of a detailed understanding of the nature and pathogenesis of the amyloid deposits found in AD (103). The amyloid in plaques and in cerebral blood vessels has similar amino acid composition and shares antigenic determinants (104). There are some superficial resemblances between the plaque core and the scrapie virus, but there are no similarities in amino acid sequences (105). Glenner and Wong (103) proposed the working hypothesis that the cerebrovascular amyloid arises as a variant of a serum protein precursor and then damages capillary walls. The protein procursor seeps out, leading to the formation of the amyloid in neuritic plaques and also blocking strategic receptors of specific cortical neurons (thus leading to the formation of abnormal neurofilaments that cause cell death). An alternative hypothesis is that abnormalities in the synthesis, modification, or aggregation of the tau protein associated with microtubules may interfere with axonal flow and lead to the formation of neurofibrillary tangles (106,107). A ganglioside may also be associated with the neurofibrillary tangles (108).

More recently published reports have amplified the situation but have also added to its complexity. The brains of patients with Guamanian parkinsonism-dementia do not have vascular amyloid deposits or senile plaques, but they do show neurofibrillary tangles containing amyloid with an amino acid sequence identical to that in the amyloid deposits in AD and DS (91,109). In a study using in situ hybridization, the amyloid beta protein messenger RNA was expressed in neurons in the neocortex and hippocampus (similar to amyloid deposits in AD), but the mRNA was also expressed in other brain regions not involved in AD (110). Thus some additional factor may be required to produce the cellular vulnerability seen in AD.

In 10 families with an autosomal dominant pattern of AD, the affected members showed a significant difference in the frequency of a restriction fragment length polymorphism at the apolipoprotein CII locus on chromosome 19 (111). In considering possible hypotheses, the authors pointed out that another amyloid (SAA) is associated with serum high-density lipoportein and that a genetic variant of apolipoprotein AII has been found in liver amyloid deposits in senescence-accelerated mice.

Information about the human proto-oncogenes *ets-1* and *ets-2* may be of interest. An *ets*-1 locus has been mapped to human chromosome 11, mouse chromosome 9, and feline chromosome D1; the *ets*-2 locus is on human chromosome 21 (close to the telomere), mouse chromosome 16, and feline chromosome C2 (112). Constitutive fragile sites have been recognized on human chromosome 11 and 21 at or near the same bands (11q23.3 and 21q22) that map close to the *ets* regions (113). In acute human leukemia, the *ets*-1 locus has been translocated from chromosome 11 to 4, while the *ets*-2 locus has been translocated from chromosome 21 to chromosome 8 (113). Preliminary results show that certain human acute myeloid leukemias with translocated chromosomes 11 or 21 show altered transcriptional expression of *ets*-1 and *ets*-2, respectively (112). Studies in the mouse show that *ets*-2 expression is associated with cell proliferation and follows a pattern similar to other members of the nuclear oncogene family (114). It would be of interest to know how often a translocation involving chromosomes 8 and 21 has been observed in leukemia or other malignancy in DS patients or in relatives of AD patients.

In an important recent development, three laboratories found that the precursor of the amyloid β-protein includes a domain with a high degree of homology to serine protease inhibitors (115-117). The genomic DNA has two axons that are variably transcribed into messenger RNA, presumably by alternative splicing. The lysate from cells transfected with the cDNA including the proteinase-like

TABLE 2 Human Proteinase Inhibitors

Autosomal Dominant	
10395	AL-M (alpha-2-macroglobulin; A2M) chromosome 12
10515	Amyloidosis VI (cerebral-arterial-type amyloidosis; Iceland-type amyloidosis; familial cerebral hemorrhage; hereditary cerebral hemorrhage with amyloidosis; defect in metabolism of gamma-trace; cerebral amyloid angiopathy)
10610	Angioneurotic edema, hereditary (HANE; deficiency of C1 esterase inhibitor) chromosome 11
10728	Antichymotrypsin, alpha-1 (AACT) chromosome 14
10730	Antithrombin III deficiency (AT3; hereditary thrombophilia due to deficiency of AT-III) chromosome 1
10740	Antitrypsin (alpha-1-antitrypsin; protease inhibitor; P1) chromosome 14
17336	Plasminogen activator inhibitor, type 1, chromosome 7
17687	Inter-α-trypsin inhibitor, protein HC, chromosome 9
Autosomal-Recessive	
26285	Plasmin inhibitor deficiency (antiplasmin deficiency; alpha-2-plasmin inhibitor)
X-linked Recessive	
30537	Tissue inhibitor of metalloproteinase (erythroid potentiating activity) chromosome Xp11

From ref. 8.

domain showed an increased inhibition of trypsin activity (117), which provides evidence for the potential functional nature of the insert. In one of the studies (116) the mRNA lacking the sequence was selectively expressed in the association areas of the adult human brain. It is suggested that protease inhibition might be involved in the aberrant processing of the amyloid precursor protein, resulting in the deposit of amyloid β-protein (117). It is of particular interest that amyloidosis VI results from a mutation in the gene for cystatin C, a cysteine protease inhibitor (50). These reports draw attention to the importance of human proteinase and protease inhibitors (118) (Table 2).

A number of efforts are underway to verify and extend these molecular studies. Meanwhile, some tentative conclusions appear justified.

1. Plaque amyloid core and cerebrovascular amyloid are the same protein, but neurofibrillary tangles may be more complex.
2. At least one DNA sequence important for AD is on chromosome 21, but the full development of the condition may involve other gene loci on chro-

mosome 21 or elsewhere. As in other forms of amyloidogenesis, the changes in AD may not be as simple as only one precursor protein playing a major role (119).

3. The association between Down's syndrome and AD is clearly important, but the explanation remains elusive.

IMPLICATIONS FOR FUTURE STUDIES

Genetic heterogeneity should be expected in a phenotype as common as AD, but this does not exclude the possibility of an underlying unitary hypothesis. At the moment the questions are becoming simultaneously simpler and more complex. The future is bright, however, since powerful research methodologies and extremely competent research teams are involved.

Progress will be more rapid if clinical and molecular approaches are carefully integrated. In particular, it would be desirable if patient samples used for molecular studies were identified by the following variables: (a) family history of dementia, parkinsonism, and DS in parents, siblings, children, and more distant relatives of the AD probands; (b) age at onset of AD and nature of first signs; (c) major clinical findings, with special mention of extrapyramidal signs and language disorder. It may not be possible to include all of this information in published reports, but having the data recorded and available would facilitate subsequent analysis or pooling of findings.

In clinical studies, special note should be taken of three familial patterns of AD. In biochemical studies of heterogeneous disorders, it is more efficient to start with *multisib* families: those in which two or more siblings are affected and available for study (120). This strategy enriches the patient sample to ensure a larger proportion with genetic causes and permits the analysis of biochemical results within and between families. After specific hypotheses have been tested and confirmed in these families, the relevant methods can be used to determine if isolated cases involve the same mechanisms.

A second approach involves the identification of all *twin-born* AD patients. The possibility that twin birth increases the risk of AD can be tested by comparing the proportion of twin-born among all AD patients with the expected percentage (about 2%). Some twin pairs will become interesting subjects for case reports, but for certain research questions the pooling of data may become necessary (121).

Finally, an alert should be maintained for those families that have a number of *affected individuals in several generations.* The late onset makes it difficult to find families with affected parents and offspring available for study, but affected cousins or more distant relatives can be informative. Such families deserve careful examination and follow-up (122), and they should be brought to the attention of a research team able to carry out linkage analysis.

SUMMARY

The possibility of genetic heterogeneity is a tool for experimental design rather than a nuisance variable that hinders investigation. It must be considered at a number of points in AD research.

Full-scale evaluation of genetic heterogeneity in AD will require the integration of clinical, cytogenetic, neurochemical, molecular, and other types of data. Helpful insights will come from genetic syndromes associated with amyloidosis, and from other genetic conditions in the human and in the mouse.

REFERENCES

1. Childs, B., and Der Kaloustian, V.M. (1968). Genetic heterogeneity. *N. Engl. J. Med.* 279: 1205-1212.
2. Emery, A.E.H. (1986). *Methodology in Medical Genetics*, 2nd ed. Edinburgh, Churchill Livingstone.
3. Lander, E.S., and Botstein, D. (1986). Mapping complex genetic traits in humans: New methods using a complete RFLP map. *Cold Spring Harbor Symp. Quant. Biol.* 51: 49-62.
4. Myers, R.M., and Maniatis, T. (1986). Recent advances in the development of methods for detecting single-base substitutions associated with human genetic diseases. *Cold Spring Harbor Symp. Quant. Biol.* 51: 275-284.
5. Latt, S.A., Lalande, M., Donlon, T., Wyman, A., Rose, E., Shiloh, Y., Korf, B., Müller, U., Sakai, K., Kanda, N., Kang, J., Stroh, H., Harris, P., Bruns, G., Wharton, R., and Kaplan, L. (1986). DNA-based detection of chromosome deletion and amplification: Diagnostic and mechanistic significance. *Cold Spring Harbor Symp. Quant. Biol.* 51: 299-307.
6. Francke, U. (1987). Microdeletions and mendelian phenotypes. In: *Human Genetics: Proceedings of the 7th International Congress*, F. Vogel and K. Sperling (Eds.), Berlin, Heidelberg, and New York, Springer Verlag, pp. 201-210.
7. Yunis, J. (1983). The chromosomal basis of human neoplasia. *Science* 221: 227-236.
8. McKusick, V.A. (1986). *Mendelian Inheritance in Man*, 7th ed., Baltimore, Johns Hopkins University Press.
9. (1986). Molecular biology of *Homo sapiens. Cold Spring Harbor Symp. Quant. Biol.* 51: 1-1229.
10. Neufeld, E. (1983). Cell mixing and its sequelae. *Am. J. Hum. Genet.* 35: 1081-1085.
11. McKusick, V.A., and Neufeld, E. (1983). The mucopolysaccharide storage diseases. In: *The Metabolic Basis of Inherited Disease*, 5th ed., J.B. Stanbury, J.B. Wyngaarden, D.S. Fredrickson, J.L. Goldstein, and M.S. Brown (Eds.), New York, McGraw-Hill, pp. 751-777.
12. Tsuji, S., Choudary, P.V., Martin, B.M., Stubblefield, B.K., Mayor, J.A., Barranger, J.A., and Ginns, E.I. (1987). A mutation in the human glucocerebrosidase gene in neuronopathic Gaucher's disease. *N. Engl. J. Med.* 316: 570-575.

13. Scriver, C.R., Mahon, B., Levy, H.L., Clow, C.L., Reade, T.M., Kronick, J., Lemieux, B., and Laberge, C. (1987). The Hartnup phenotype: Mendelian transport, disorder, multifactorial disease. *Am. J. Hum. Genet.* 40: 401-412.
14. Meissen, G.J., Myers, R.H., Mastromauro, C.A., Koroshetz, W.J., Klinger, K.W., Farrer, L.A., Watkins, P.A., Gusella, J.F., Bird, E.D., and Martin, J.B. (1988). Predictive testing for Huntington's disease with use of a linked DNA marker. *N. Engl. J. Med.* 318: 535-542.
15. Scriver, C.R., and Clow, C.L. (1980). Phenylketonuria and other phenylalanine hydroxylation mutants in man. *Annu. Rev. Genet.* 14: 179-202.
16. Woo, S.L.C., DiLella, A.D., Marvit, J., and Ledley, F.D. (1986). Molecular basis of phenylketonuria and potential somatic gene therapy. *Cold Spring Harbor Symp. Quant. Biol.* 51: 395-401.
17. Williamson, R., Bell, G., Bell, J., Bates, G., Davies, K.A., Estivill, X., Farrall, M., Kruyer, H., Law, H.Y., Lench, N., Scambler, P., Stainier, P., Wainwright, B., Watson, E., and Worrall, C. (1986). Molecular genetics and the basic defect causing cystic fibrosis. *Cold Spring Harbor Symp. Quant. Biol.* 51: 309-315.
18. Tsui, L.-C., Zengerling, S., Willard, H.F., and Buchwald, M. (1986). Mapping of the cystic fibrosis locus on Chromosome 7. *Cold Spring Harbor Symp. Quant. Biol.* 51: 325-335.
19. Egeland, J.A., Gerhard, D.S., Pauls, D.L., Sussex, J.N., Kidd, K.K., Allen, C.R., Hostetter, A.M., and Housman, D.E. (1987). Bipolar affective disorders linked to DNA markers on chromosome 11. *Nature* 325: 783-787.
20. Hodgkinson, S., Sherrington, R., Gurling, H., Marchbanks, R., Reeders, S., Mallet, J., McInnis, M., Petursson, H., and Brynjolfsson, J. (1987). Molecular genetic evidence for heterogeneity in manic depression. *Nature* 325: 805-806.
21. Detera-Wadleigh, S.D., Berrettini, W.H., Goldin, L.R., Boorman, D., Anderson, S., and Gershon, E.S. (1987). Close linkage of c-Harvey-*ras*-1 and the insulin gene to affective disorder is ruled out in three North American pedigrees. *Nature* 325: 806-808.
22. Baron, A.M., Risch, N., Hamburger, R., Mandel, B., Kushner, S., Newman, M., Drumer, D., and Belmaker, R.H. (1987). Genetic linkage between X-chromosome markers and bipolar affective illness. *Nature* 326: 289-292.
23. Mendlewicz, J., Simon, P., Sevy, S., Charon, F., Brocas, H., Legros, S., and Vassart, G. (1987). Polymorphic DNA marker on X chromosome and manic depression. *Lancet* 1: 1230-1232.
24. Davies, K.E., Ball, S.P., Dorkins, H.R., Forrest, S.M., Kenwrick, S.J., King, A.W., Lavenir, I.J.D., McGlade, S.A., Patterson, M.N., Smith, T.J., Wilson, L., Paulsen, K., Speer, A., and Coutelle, C. (1986). Molecular analysis of human X-linked diseases. *Cold Spring Harbor Symp. Quant. Biol.* 51: 337-343.
25. Pearson, P.L., van Ommen, G.J.B., and Bakker, E. (1986). Carrier detection and gene analysis of Duchenne muscular dystrophy. *Cold Spring Harbor Symp. Quant. Biol.* 51: 353-358.
26. Hyser, C.L., Griggs, R.C., Mendell, J.R., Polakowska, R., Quirk, S., Brooke, M.H., Fenichel, G.M., and Doherty, R.A. (1987). Use of serum creatine

kinase, pyruvate kinase, and genetic linkage for carrier detection in Duchenne and Becker dystrophy. *Neurology* 37: 4-10.

27. Brockdorff, N., Cross, G.S., Cavanna, J.S., Fisher, E.M.C., Lyon, M.F., Davies, K.E., and Brown, S.D.M. (1987). The mapping of a CDNA from the human X-linked Duchenne muscular dystrophy gene to the mouse X chromosome. *Nature* 328: 166-168.
28. Heilig, R., Lemaire, C., Mandel, J.-L., Dandolo, L., Amar, L., and Avner, P. (1987). Localization of the region homologous to the Duchenne muscular dystrophy locus on the mouse X chromosome. *Nature* 328: 168-170.
29. Lovett, M., Goldgaber, D., Ashley, P., Cox, D.R., Gajdusek, D.C., and Epstein, C.J. (1987). The mouse homolog of the human amyloid beta protein (AD-AP) gene is located on the distal end of mouse chromosome 16: Further extension of the homology between human chromosome 21 and mouse chromosome 16. *Biochem. Biophys. Res. Commun.* 144: 1069-1075.
30. Francke, U., Ochs, H.D., de Martinville, B., Giacalone, J., Lindgren, V., Disteche, C., Pagon, R.A., Hofker, M.H., van Ommen, G.-J.B., Pearson, P.L., and Wedgwood, R.J. (1985). Minor Xp21 chromosome deletion in a male associated with expression of Duchenne muscular dystrophy, chromic granulomatous disease, retinitis pigmentosa and McLeod syndrome. *Am. J. Hum. Genet.* 37: 250-267.
31. Francke, U., Harper, J.F., Darras, B.T., Cowan, J.M., McCabe, E.R.B., Kohlschütter, A., Seltzer, W.K., Saito, F., Goto, J., Harpey, J.-P., and Wise, J.E. (1987). Congenital adrenal hypoplasia, myopathy, and glycerol kinase deficiency: Molecular genetic evidence for deletions. *Am. J. Hum. Genet.* 40: 212-227.
32. Housman, D.E., Glaser, T., Gerhard, D.S., Jones, C., Bruns, G.A.P., and Lewis, W.H. (1986). Mapping of human chromosome 11: Organization of genes within the Wilms' tumor region of the chromosome. *Cold Spring Harbor Symp. Quant. Biol.* 51: 837-841.
33. Shows, T.B., Davis, L.M., Qin, S., and Nowak, N.J. (1986). The chromosome 11 gene map: Genes for growth and development, Wilms' tumor deletions, and cancer chromosome breakpoints. *Cold Spring Harbor Symp. Quant. Biol.* 51: 867-877.
34. Cavenee, W.K., and Hansen, M.F. (1986). Molecular genetics of human familial cancer. *Cold Spring Harbor Symp. Quant. Biol.* 51: 829-1835.
35. Knudson, A.G., Hethcote, H.W., and Brown, B.W. (1975). Mutation and childhood cancer: A probabilistic model for the incidence of retinoblastoma. *Proc. Natl. Acad. Sci.* 72: 5116-5120.
36. Fung, Y.-K.T., Murphree, A.L., T'Ang, A., Qian, J., Hinrichs, S.H., and Benedict, W.F. (1987). Structural evidence for the authenticity of the human retinoblastoma gene. *Science* 236: 1657-1661.
37. Nussbaum, R.L., and Ledbetter, D.H. (1986). Fragile X syndrome: A unique mutation in man. *Annu. Rev. Genet.* 20: 109-145.
38. Siniscalco, M. (1986). Genetic recombination and disease. *Cold Spring Harbor Symp. Quant. Biol.* 51: 191-194.

39. Anderson, V.E., Hauser, W.A., and Rich, S.S. (1986). Genetic heterogeneity in the epilepsies. *Adv. Neurol.* 44: 59-75.
40. Martin, W.E., Young, W.I., and Anderson, V.E. (1973). Parkinson's disease—a genetic study. *Brain* 96: 495-506.
41. Zetusky, W.J., Jankovic, J., and Pirozzolo, F.J. (1985). The heterogeneity of Parkinson's disease: Clinical and prognostic implications. *Neurology* 35: 522-526.
42. Sillence, D.O., Barlow, K.K., Garber, A.P., Hall, J.G., and Rimoin, D.L. (1984). Osteogenesis imperfecta type II. Delineation of the phenotype with reference to genetic heterogeneity. *Am. J. Med. Genet.* 17: 407-428.
43. Prockop, D.J. (1986). Genetic defects of collagen. *Hosp. Pract.* Feb. 15: 125-140.
44. Pyeritz, R.E. (1987). Heritable defects in connective tissue. *Hosp. Pract.* Feb 15: 153-168.
45. Prockop, D.J. (1984). Osteogenesis imperfecta: phenotypic heterogeneity, protein suicide, short and long collagen. *Am. J. Hum. Genet.* 36: 499-505.
46. Glenner, G.G., Ignaczak, T.F., and Page, D.L. (1978). The inherited systemic amyloidoses and localized amyloid deposits. In: *Metabolic Basis of Inherited Disorders*, J.G. Stanbury, J.B. Wyngaarden, and D.S. Fredrickson (Eds.), New York, McGraw-Hill, pp. 1308-1339.
47. Araki, S. (1986). Familial amyloidotic polyneuropathies. In: *Amyloidosis*, J. Marrink and M.H. Van Rijswijk (Eds.), Dordrecht, M. Nijhoff, pp. 195-218.
48. Glenner, G.G., Osserman, E.F., Benditt, E.P., Calkins, E., Cohen, A.S., and Zucker-Franklin, D. (Eds.) (1984). *Amyloidosis*, New York, Plenum.
49. Woo, P. (1986). Gene structure of a human serum amyloid A protein and comparison with amyloid A. In: *Amyloidosis*, J. Marrink and M.H. Van Rijswijk (Eds.), Dordrecht, M. Nijhoff, pp. 135-139.
50. Ghiso, J., Vensson, O., and Frangione, B. (1986). Amyloid fibrils in hereditary cerebral hemorrhage with amyloidosis of Icelandic type is a variant of gamma-trace basic protein (cystatin C). *Proc. Natl. Acad. Sci.* 83: 2974-2978.
51. van Duinen, S.G., Castano, E.M., Prelli, F., Bots, G.T.A.B., Luyendijk, W., and Frangione, B. (1987). Hereditary cerebral hemorrhage with amyloidosis in patients of Dutch origin is related to Alzheimer disease. *Proc. Natl. Acad. Sci.* 84: 5991-5994.
52. Herbert, J., Wilcox, J.N., Pham, K.-T.C., Fremeau, R.T., Jr., Zeviani, W., Dwork, A., Soprano, D.R., Makover, A., Goodman, D.S., Zimmerman, E.A., Roberts, J.L., and Schon, E.A. (1986). Transthyretin: A choroid plexus-specific transport protein in human brain. *Neurology* 36: 900-911.
53. Ide, M., Mita, S., Ikegawa, S., Maeda, S., Shimada, K., and Araki, S. (1986). Identification of carriers of mutant prealbumin gene associated with familial amyloidotic polyneuropathy type I by Southern blot procedures: Study of six pedigrees in the Arao district of Japan. *Hum. Genet.* 73: 281-285.

54. Wallace, M.R., Conneally, P.M., Long, G.L., and Benson, M.D. (1986). Molecular detection of carriers of hereditary amyloidosis in a Swedish-American family. *Am. J. Med. Genet.* 25: 335-341.
55. de Courten-Myers, G., and Mandybur, T.I. (1987). Atypical Gerstmann-Straüssler syndrome or familial spinocerebellar ataxia and Alzheimer's disease? *Neurology* 37: 269-275.
56. Chui, H.C., Teng, E.L., Henderson, V.W., and Moy, A.C. (1986). Clinical subtypes of dementia of the Alzheimer type. *Neurology* 35: 1544-1550.
57. Amaducci, L.A., Fratiglioni, L., Rocca, W.A., Feischi, C., Livrea, P., Pedone, D., Braco, L., Lippi, A., Gandolfo, C., Bino, G., Prencipe, M., Bonatti, M.L., Girotti, F., Carella, F., Tavolato, B., Ferla, S., Lenzi, G.L., Carolei, A., Gambia, A., Grigoletto, F., and Schoenberg, B.S. (1986). Risk factors for clinically diagnosed Alzheimer's disease: A case-control study of an Italian population. *Neurology* 36: 922-931.
58. Heston, L.L. (1981). Genetic studies of dementia: With emphasis on Parkinson's disease and Alzheimer's neuropathology. In: *The Epidemiology of Dementia*, J.A. Mortimer and L.M. Schuman (Eds.) New York & Oxford, Oxford University Press, pp. 101-114.
59. Heston, L.L., Mastri, A.R., Anderson, V.E., and White, J. (1981). Dementia of the Alzheimer type. Clinical genetics, natural history, and associated conditions. *Arch. Gen. Psychiatry* 38: 1085-1090.
60. Kay, D.W.K. (1986). The genetics of Alzheimer's disease. *Br. Med. Bull.* 42: 19-23.
61. Kay, D.W.K. (1987). Heterogeneity in Alzheimer's disease: Epidemiological and family studies. *Trends Neurosci.* 10: 194-195.
62. Heyman, A., Wilkinson, W.E., Hurwitz, B.J., Schmechel, D., Sigmon, A.H., Weinberg, T., Helms, M.J., and Swift, M. (1983). Alzheimer's disease: Genetic aspects and associated clinical disorders. *Ann. Neurol.* 14: 507-515.
63. Whalley, L.J., Carothers, A.D., Collyer, S., Demey, R., and Frackiewicz, A. (1982). A study of familial factors in Alzheimer's disease. *Br. J. Psychiatry* 140: 249-256.
64. Breitner, J.C.S., Murphy, E.A., and Folstein, M.F. (1986). Familial aggregation in Alzheimer's disease. II. Clinical genetic implications of age-dependent onset. *J. Psychiatr. Res.* 20: 45-55.
65. Chase, G.A., Folstein, M.F., Breitner, J.C.S., Beary, T.H., and Self, S.G. (1983). The use of life tables and survival analysis in testing genetic hypotheses, with an application to Alzheimer's disease. *Am. J. Epidemiol.* 117: 590-597.
66. Bondareff, W. (1983). Age and Alzheimer disease. *Lancet* 1: 1447.
67. Childs, B., and Scriver, C.R. (1986). Age at onset and causes of disease. *Perspect. Biol. Med.* 29: 437-460.
68. Breitner, J.C.S., Silverman, J.M., Mohs, R.C., and Davis, K.L. (1988). Familial aggregation in Alzheimer's disease: Comparison of risk among relatives of early- and late-onset cases, and among male and female relatives in successive generations. *Neurology* 38: 207-212.

69. Rossor, M.N., Iversen, L.L., Reynolds, G.P., Mountjoy, C.Q., and Roth, M. (1984). Neurochemical characteristics of early and late onset types of Alzheimer's disease. *Br. Med. J.* 288: 961-964.
70. Seltzer, B., and Sherwin, I. (1983). A comparison of clinical features in early- and late-onset primary degenerative dementia. One entity or two? *Arch. Neurol.* 40: 143-146.
71. Roth, M. (1986). The association of clinical neurological findings and its bearing on the classification and aetiology of Alzheimer disease. *Br. Med. Bull.* 42: 42-50.
72. Bird, T.D., Stranahan, S., Sumi, S.M., and Raskind, M. (1983). Alzheimer's disease: choline acetyltransferase activity in brain tissue from clinical and pathological subgroups. *Ann. Neurol.* 14: 284-293.
73. Mayeux, R., Stern, Y., and Spanton, S. (1985). Heterogeneity in dementia of the Alzheimer type: Evidence of subgroups. *Neurology* 35: 453-461.
74. Breitner, J.C.S., and Folstein, M.F. (1984). Familial Alzheimer dementia: A prevalent disorder with specific clinical features. *Psychol. Med.* 14: 63-80.
75. Knesevich, J.W., Toro, F.R., Morris, J.C., and LaBarge, E. (1985). Aphasia, family history, and the longitudinal course of senile dementia of the Alzheimer type. *Psychiatry Res.* 14: 255-263.
76. Heston, L.L., and Mastri, A.R. (1977). The genetics of Alzheimer's disease. Associations with hematologic malignancy and Down's syndrome. *Arch. Gen. Psychiatry* 34: 976-981.
77. Nee, L.E., Polinsky, R.J., Eldridge, R., Weingartner, H., Smallberg, S., and Ebert, M. (1983). A family with histologically confirmed Alzheimer's disease. *Arch. Neurol.* 40: 203-208.
78. Weinreb, H.J. (1986). Dermatoglyphic patterns in Alzheimer's disease. *J. Neurogenet.* 3: 233-246.
79. Seltzer, B., and Sherwin, I. (1986). Fingerprint pattern differences in early- and late-onset primary degenerative dementia. *Arch. Neurol.* 43: 665-668.
80. Nee, L.E., Eldridge, R., Sunderland, T., Thomas, C.B., Katz, D., Thompson, K.E., Weingartner, H., Weiss, H., Julian, C., and Cohen, R. (1987). Dementia of the Alzheimer type: Clinical and family study of 22 twin pairs. *Neurology* 37: 359-363.
81. Renvoize, E.B., Minham, R.H.S., Stewart, M., McDonald, R., and Wallace, D.R.D. (1986). Identical twins discordant for presenile dementia of the Alzheimer type. *Br. J. Psychiatry* 149: 509-512.
82. Luxenberg, J.S., May, C., Haxy, J.V., Grady, C., Moore, A., Berg, G., White, B.J., Robinette, D., and Rapoport, S.I. (1987). Cerebral metabolism, anatomy, and cognition in monozygotic twins discordant for dementia of the Alzheimer type. *J. Neurol.* 50: 333-340.
83. Jorm, A.F. (1985). Subtypes of Alzheimer's dementia: A conceptual analysis and critical review. *Psychol. Med.* 15: 543-553.
84. Chui, H.C. The significance of clinically-defined subgroups of Alzheimer's disease. In: *Proceedings of the Fourth Meeting of the International Study*

Group on the Pharmacology of Memory Disorders Associated with Aging. Zurich, Switzerland, Jan 16-18, 1987, pp. 79-90.
85. Schweber, M. (1985). A possible unitary genetic hypothesis for Alzheimer's disease and Down's syndrome. *Ann. N.Y. Acad. Sci.* 450: 223-238.
86. Heston, L.L., and Morris, M.L. (1986). Family studies of Alzheimer's dementia: Results and prospects. *Can. J. Neurol. Sci.* 13: 432-434.
87. Selkoe, D.J., Bell, D.S., Podlisny, M.B., Price, D.L., and Cork, L.C. (1987). Conservation of brain amyloid proteins in aged mammals and humans with Alzheimer's disease. *Science* 235: 873-877.
88. Goldgaber, D., Lerman, M.I., McBride, O.W., Saffiotti, U., and Gajdusek, D.C. (1987). Characterization and chromosomal localization of a cDNA encoding brain amyloid of Alzheimer's disease. *Science* 235: 877-880.
89. Tanzi, R.E., Gusella, J.F., Watkins, P.C., Bruns, G.A.P., St. George-Hyslop, P., Van Keuren, M.L., Patterson, D., Pagan, S., Kurnit, D.M., and Neve, R.L. (1987). Amyloid beta protein gene: cDNA, mRNA distribution, and genetic linkage near the Alzheimer locus. *Science* 235: 880-884.
90. St. George-Hyslop, P.H., Tanzi, R.E., Polinsky, R.J., Haines, J.L., Nee, L., Watkins, P.C., Myers, R.H., Feldman, R.G., Pollen, D., Drachman, D., Growdon, J., Bruni, A., Foncin, J.-F., Salomin, D., Frommelt, P., Amaducci, L., Sorbi, S., Piacentini, S., Stewart, G.D., Hobbs, W.J., Conneally, P.M., and Gusella, J.F. (1987). The genetic defect causing familial Alzheimer's disease maps on chromosome 21. *Science* 235: 885-890.
91. Kang, J., Lemaire, H.-G., Unterbeck, A., Salbaum, J.M., Masters, C.L., Grzeschik, K.-H., Multhaup, G., Beyreuther, K., and Müller-Hill, B. (1987). The precursor of Alzheimer's disease amyloid A4 protein resembles a cell-surface receptor. *Nature* 325: 733-736.
92. Robakis, N.K., Wisniewski, H.M., Jenkins, E.C., Devine-Gage, E.A., Houck, G.E., Yao, X.-L., Ramakrishna, N., Wolfe, G., Silverman, W.P., and Brown, W.T. (1987). Chromosome 21q21 sublocalisation of gene encoding beta-amyloid peptide in cerebral vessels and neuritic (senile) plaques of people with Alzheimer disease and Down's syndrome. *Lancet* 1: 384-385.
93. Jenkins, E.C., Devine-Gage, E.A., Yao, X.-L., Houck, G.E., Jr., Brown, W.T., Wisniewski, H.M., and Robakis, N.K. (1987). In-situ hybridization of the β-amyloid protein probe to chromosome 9 in patients with familial Alzheimer's disease. *Lancet* 2: 1155-1156.
94. Zubenko, G.S. (1986). Hippocampal membrane alteration in Alzheimer's disease. *Brain Res.* 385: 115-121.
95. Zubenko, G.S., and Ferrell, R.E. (1988). Monozygotic twins concordant for probable Alzheimer's disease and increased platelet membrane fluidity. *Am. J. Med. Genet.* 29: 431-436.
96. St. George-Hyslop, P.H., Tanzi, R.E., Polinsky, R.J., Neve, R.L., Pollen, D., Drachman, D., Growdon, J., Cupples, L.A., Nee, L., Myers, R.H., O'Sullivan, D., Watkins, P.C., Amos, J.A., Ketusch, C.K., Bodfish, J.W., Kinsbourne, M., Feldman, R.G., Bruni, A., Amaducci, L., Foncin, J.-F., and Gusella, J.F. (1987). Absence of duplication of chromosome 21 genes in familial and sporadic Alzheimer's disease. *Science* 238: 664-666.

97. Tanzi, R.E., Bird, E.D., Latt, S.A., and Neve, R.L. (1987). The amyloid protein gene is not duplicated in brains from patients with Alzheimer's disease. *Science* 238: 666-669.
98. Podlisny, M.B., Lee, G., and Selkoe, D.J. (1987). Gene dosage of the amyloid precursor protein in Alzheimer's disease. *Science* 238: 669-671.
99. Murdoch, G.H., Manuelidis, L., Kin, J.H., and Manuelidis, E.E. (1988). β-Amyloid gene dosage in Alzheimer's disease. *Nucleic Acids Res.* 16: 357.
100. Furuya, H., Sasaki, H., Goto, I., Wong, C.W., Glenner, G.G., and Sakasi, Y. (1988). Amyloid β-protein gene duplication is not common in Alzheimer's disease: Analysis by polymorphic restriction fragments. *Biochem. Biophys. Res. Commun.* 150: 75-81.
101. Van Broeckhoven, C., Genthe, A.M., Vanderberghe, A., Horsthemke, B., Backhovens, H., Raeymaekers, R., Van Hul, W., Wehnert, A., Gheuens, J., Cras, P., Bruyland, M., Martin, J.J., Salbaum, M., Multhaup, G., Masters, C.L., Beyreuther, K., Gurling, H.M.D., Mullan, M.J., Holland, A., Barton, A., Irving, N., Williamson, R., Richards, S.J., and Hardy, J.A. (1987). Failure of familial Alzheimer's disease to segregate with the A4-amyloid gene in several European families. *Nature* 329: 153-155.
102. Tanzi, R.E., St. George-Hyslop, P.H., Haines, J.L., Polinsky, R.J., Nee, L., Foncin, J.-F., Neve, R.L., McClatchey, A.I., Conneally, P.M., and Gusella, J.F. (1987). The genetic defect in familial Alzheimer's disease is not tightly linked to the amyloid β-protein gene. *Nature* 329: 156-157.
103. Glenner, G.G., and Wong, C.W. (1987). The nature and pathogenesis of the amyloid deposits in Alzheimer's disease. In: *Amyloidosis*, J. Marrink and M.H. Van Rijswijk (Eds.) Dordrecht, M. Nijhoff, pp. 227-242.
104. Wong, C.W., Quaranta, V., and Glenner, G.G. (1984). Neuritic and cerebrovascular amyloid in Alzheimer disease are antigenically related. *Proc. Natl. Acad. Sci.* 82: 8729-8732.
105. Masters, C.L., Simms, G., Weinman, N.A., Multhaup, G., McDonald, B.L., and Beyreuther, K. (1985). Amyloid plaque core protein in Alzheimer disease and Down's syndrome. *Proc. Natl. Acad. Sci.* 82: 4245-4249.
106. Kosik, K.S., Joachim, C.L., and Selkoe, D.J. (1986). Microtubule-associated protein tau (τ) is a major antigenic component of paired helical filaments in Alzheimer disease. *Proc. Natl. Acad. Sci.* 83: 4044-4048.
107. Wood, J.G., Mirra, S.S., Pollock, N.J., and Binder, L.I. (1986). Neurofibrillary tangles of Alzheimer disease share antigenic determinants with the axonal microtubule-associated protein tau (τ). *Proc. Natl. Acad. Sci.* 83: 4040-4043.
108. Emory, C.R., Ala, T.A., and Frey, W.H. II (1987). Ganglioside monoclonal antibody (A2B5) labels Alzheimer's neurofibrillary tangles. *Neurology* 37: 768-772.
109. Guiroy, D.C., Miyazaki, M., Multhaup, G., Fischer, P., Garruto, R.M., Beyreuther, K., Masters, C.L., Simms, G., Gibbs, C.J. Jr., and Gajdusek, D.C. (1987). Amyloid of neurobrillary tangles of guamanian parkinsonism-dementia and Alzheimer disease share identical amino acid sequence. *Proc. Natl. Acad. Sci.* 84: 2073-2077.

110. Bahmanyar, S., Higgins, G.A., Goldgaber, D., Lewis, D.A., Morrison, J.H., Wilson, M.C., Shankar, S.K., and Gajdusek, D.C. (1987). Localization of amyloid beta protein messenger RNA in brains from patients with Alzheimer's disease. *Science* 237: 77-80.
111. Schellenberg, G.D., Deeb, S.S., Boehnke, M., Bryant, E.M., Martin, G.M., Lampe, T.H., and Bird, T.D. (1987). Association of an apolipoprotein CII allele with familial dementia of the Alzheimer type. *J. Neurogenet.* 4: 97-108.
112. Watson, D.K., McWilliams-Smith, M.J., Kozak, C., Reeves, R., Gearhart, J., Nunn, M.F., Nash, W., Fowle, J.R. III, Duesberg, P., Papas, T.S., and O'Brien, S.J. (1986). Conserved chromosomal positions of dual domains of the *ets* protooncogene in cats, mice, and humans. *Proc. Natl. Acad. Sci.* 83: 1792-1796.
113. Papas, T.S., Watson, D.K., Sacchi, N., O'Brien, S.J., and Ascione, R. (1986). Molecular evolution of *Ets* genes from avians to mammals and their cytogenetic localization to regions involved in leukemia. In: *Gene Amplication and Analysis, vol. 4, Oncogenes,* T.S. Papas and G.F. Vande Woude (Eds.), New York, Elsevier, pp. 207-238.
114. Bhat, N.K., Fisher, R.J., Fujiwara, S., Ascione, R., and Papas, T.S. (1987). Temporal and tissue-specific expression of mouse *ets* genes. *Proc. Natl. Acad. Sci.* 84: 3161-3165.
115. Ponte, P., Gonzalez-DeWhitt, P., Schilling, J., Miller, J., Hus, D., Greenberg, B., Davis, K., Wallace, W., Lieberburg, I., Fuller, F., and Cordell, B. (1988). A new A4 mRNA contains a domain homologous to serine proteinase inhibitors. *Nature* 331: 525-527.
116. Tanzi, R.E., McClatchey, A.I., Lamperti, E.D., Villa-Komaroff, L., Gusella, J.F., and Neve, R.L. (1988). Protease inhibitor domain encoded by an amyloid protein precursor mRNA associated with Alzheimer's disease. *Nature* 331: 528-530.
117. Kitaguchi, N., Takahashi, Y., Tokushima, Y., Shiojiri, S., and Ito, H. (1988). Novel precursor of Alzheimer's disease amyloid protein shows protease inhibitory activity. *Nature* 331: 530-532.
118. Travis, J., and Salvesen, G.S. (1983). Human plasma proteinase inhibitors. *Annu. Rev. Biochem.* 52: 655-709.
119. Schellenberg, G.D., Bird, T.D., Wijsman, E.M., Moore, D.K., Boehnke, M., Bryant, E.M., Lampe, T.H., Nochlin, D., Sumi, S.M., Deeb, S.S., Beyreuther, K., and Martin, G.M. (1988). Absence of linkage of chromosome 21q21 markers to familial Alzheimer's disease. *Science* 41: 1507-1510.
120. Haines, J.L., Panter, S.S., Rich, S.S., Eaton, J.W., Tsai, M.Y., and Anderson, V.E. (1986). Reduced plasma haptoglobin and urinary taurine in familial seizures identified through the multisib strategy. *Am. J. Med. Genet.* 24: 723-734.
121. Anderson, V.E., Wilcox, K., Rich, S.S., Leppik, I.E., and Hauser, W.A. (1988). Twin studies in epilepsy. In: *Genetics of the Epilepsies* G. Beck-Mannagetta, V.E. Anderson, H. Doose, and D. Janz (Eds.), Berlin, Springer.

122. Powell, D., and Folstein, M.F. (1984). Pedigree study of familial Alzheimer disease. *J. Neurogenet.* 1: 189-197.
123. Pericak-Vance, M.A., Yamaoka, L.H., Haynes, C.S., Speer, M.C., Haines, J.L., Gaskell, P.C., Hung, W.-Y., Clark, C.M., Heyman, A.L., Trofatter, J.A., Eisenmenger, J.P., Gilbert, J.R., Lee, J.E., Alberts, M.J., Dawson, D.V., Baertlett, R.J., Earl, N.L., Siddique, T., Vance, J.M., Conneally, P.M., and Roses, A.D. (1988). Genetic linkage studies in Alzheimer's disease families. *Exper. Neurol.* 102: 271-279.

7

Linkage Studies in Alzheimer's Disease Families

M. A. PERICAK-VANCE, L. H. YAMAOKA, C. S. HAYNES, M. C. SPEER, P. C. GASKELL, W. -Y. HUNG, C. M. CLARK, A. L. HEYMAN, J. R. GILBERT, J. E. LEE, M. J. ALBERTS, N. L. EARL, D. V. DAWSON, R. J. BARTLETT, T. SIDDIQUE, J. M. VANCE, A. D. ROSES / *Duke University Medical Center, Durham, North Carolina*

J. A. TROFATTER and P. M. CONNEALLY / *Indiana University School of Medicine, Indianapolis, Indiana*

Alzheimer's disease (AD) is a neurodegenerative disorder that affects millions of people. It is the leading cause of dementia among the elderly. The economic cost in nursing home, medical and ancillary care is greater than 40 billion dollars annually (34). There is no successful treatment or cure for AD. Age of onset is variable and has been reported from the fourth to the ninth decade of life, with the majority of cases occurring in later life. The causes of AD remain unclear. A genetic component has long been implicated in AD due to the familial clustering of AD cases (4,10,14,21). Autosomal dominant inheritance with age-dependent penetrance has been suggested to explain this aggregation. Large multigenerational pedigrees with the rare, early-onset form of AD have been described in which approximately 50% of relatives are affected in several generations (23). Formal segregation analyses have been difficult to perform due to inherent ascertainment biases in the data (35). Despite recent advances in segregation analysis, it is sometimes impossible to make definitive statements regarding inheritance patterns. Linkage analysis is one approach to establishing the existence of a genetic component in the expression of a particular trait. In 1987, linkage of familial Alzheimer's disease (FAD) was reported to two probes on chromosome 21, D21S16 and D21S1/D21S11 (31), thereby locating the gene for FAD to chromosome 21. The families included in the analysis had the early-onset type with mean age of onset (M) of 52.0, 48.7, 49.8, and 39.9 years.

At the Duke Alzheimer's Disease Research Center (ADRDC), we have examined and obtained blood for DNA and paternity studies from 106 members (32 affected) of 13 FAD families each with multiple affected family members (Figure 1) to test

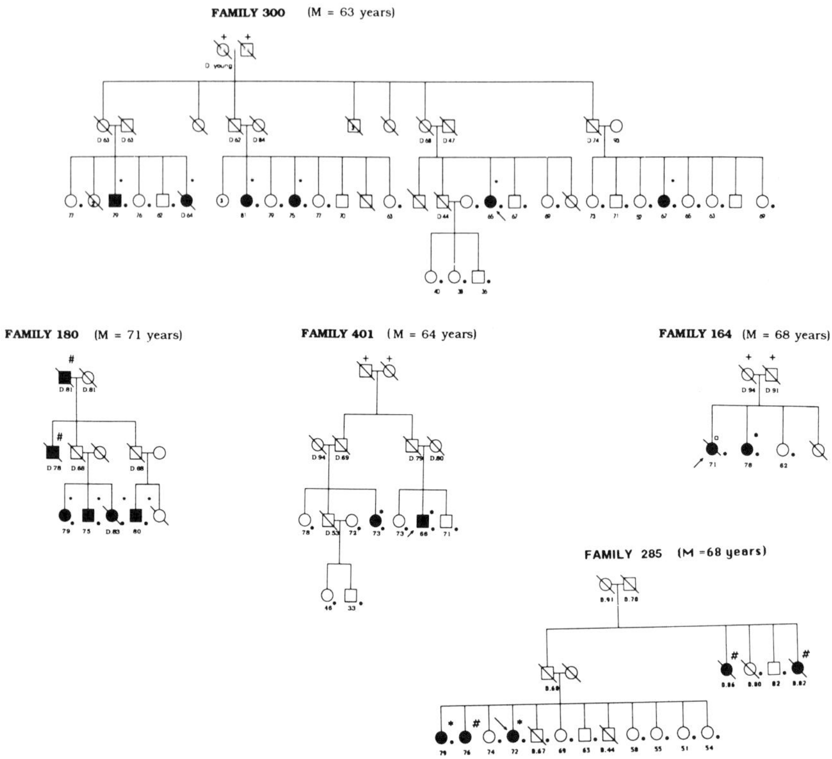

(a)

Figure 1 The 13 Alzheimer's disease families used in the linkage analysis. The pedigrees of these families have not been published previously.

the previously reported linkage findings (31). Paternity was tested by standard methods using a series of blood group and serum proteins (29) to identify parental exclusions where possible, and by examining the results of several multiallelic marker systems (i.e., ABO, MNS, D21S1/D21S11) to identify allelic exclusions among the sibs. The total number of affected persons, living and deceased, in these families is 49. Five of the families have autopsy-confirmed AD. Nine of the 13 families have 3 or more family members affected with AD and 4 families have 2 AD affected family members. The majority of the affected individuals were first-degree relatives. Sampled individuals from the 13 families were evaluated by a neurologist and associated diagnostic personnel of the ADRDC and the clinical diagnosis of probable AD made as described previously (20). Unpublished data from the Duke ADRC show confirmation of the clinical diagnosis of AD by

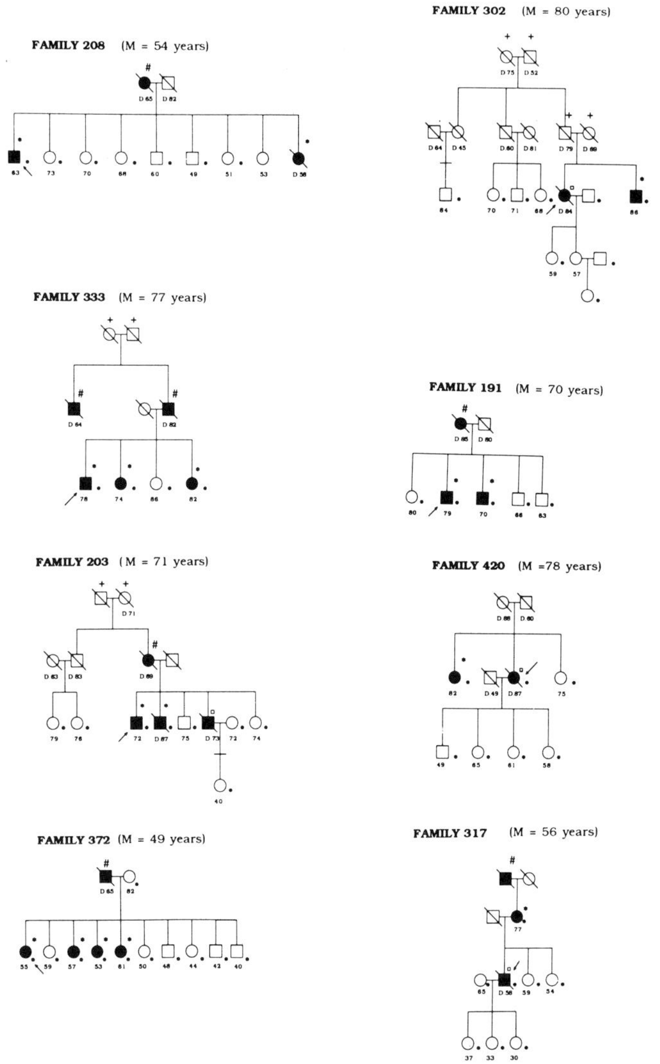
FAMILY 208 (M = 54 years)
FAMILY 302 (M = 80 years)
FAMILY 333 (M = 77 years)
FAMILY 191 (M = 70 years)
FAMILY 203 (M = 71 years)
FAMILY 420 (M =78 years)
FAMILY 372 (M = 49 years)
FAMILY 317 (M = 56 years)

(b)

pathological findings at autopsy in 10 of 10 independent individuals from families with multiple affected members.

Of the 49 affected family members included in the present study only 12 were not examined by ADRC personnel. Most of these are deceased family members (i.e., parents of living affected patients). Of those individuals not available for examination, medical records were obtained and reviewed by a neurologist before clinical status was assigned. In making the diagnosis of AD, care was taken to exclude confounding causes of dementia such as depression and multiple infarct disease.

The mode of inheritance in these families is consistent with autosomal dominance with age-dependent penetrance. Age of onset was determined based on the history of the onset of documented memory disorder. In 10 families, M ranged from 60 to 80+ years. Two families (317 and 208) have M = 56 and M = 54 years, respectively, and one family (372) has exceptionally early age of onset (M = 49), similar to the FAD families reported in the linkage study (31). Because the majority of the families in our study have late-onset AD, we were interested in testing the previously reported chromosome 21 linked probes (31) for linkage in our data set. Linkage of late onset FAD to the above proves is of critical significance in determining the overall causes of AD since late-onset AD represents the most common clinical form of the disease. Exclusion of linkage to this region of chromosome 21 would necessitate the further screening of other chromosome regions for linkage to identify the gene(s) involved in late-onset FAD.

The markers included in the linkage analysis were the chromosome 21 probes, D21S1/D21S11 and D21S16. High-molecular-weight genomic DNA was prepared from lymphocytes as previously described (1,29). The restriction endonuclease digestion, agarose gel electrophoresis, Southern blotting, DNA probe labeling, and hybridization are as outlined previously (29,31). Genetypes were assigned accordingly. Specifically. DNA from each member within the pedigree was isolated from blood or from Epstein-Barr virus (EBV)-transformed lymphoblast cell lines. This genomic DNA was digested with the appropriate restriction enzyme and the resultant fragments were size-separated by submarine, agarose gel electrophoresis in TAE buffer (40 mM tris-acetate, 2 mM EDTA). The DNA fragments were transferred from the gel to a nylon filter support (Gene Screen Plus, New England Nuclear) by capillary action using the alkaline transfer procedure (7). DNA probes were labeled with α-[^{32}P] deoxycytidine triphosphate (New England Nuclear) by random oligonucleotide priming (Amersham). Labeling probes were hybridized to the filters for 18-24 hr at 42°C in 50% formamide, 10% dextran sulfate, 1% SDS, 1 M NaC1; 20 mM sodium phosphate buffer, pH 7.0, 5X Denhardts; and 100 μg/ml salmon sperm DNA. The filters were washed twice in 2 X SSC at room temperature and then twice in 2 X SSC-1% SDS at 65°C. The filters were exposed to X-ray film (Kodak XAR-5) with a Dupont Cronex intensifying screen at -80°C for 24-72 hr.

The data were analyzed for linkage using both the LIPED (15,24) and LINKAGE (17-19) computer programs. An autosomal dominant mode of inheritance with age-dependent penetrance was assumed for FAD. The age curve used in the analysis was calculated from the overall pedigree data (13,28). A normal distribution was constructed using the sample mean (M) and variance (S^2) for age of onset as calculated from the pedigree data. Age-on-onset data were available on 45 family members, resulting in M = 66.1 ± 8.6. The age curve generated by this approach is similar to the data obtained through epidemiological studies (5).

In addition to the age risk curve calculated from the sample data, a low penetrance curve was examined on the two-point analyses. Use of the low penetrance curve has the effect of reducing the information contributed by unaffected individuals who may actually carry the gene but may not have yet manifested symptoms; even older unaffected individuals are given a substantial probability of developing AD. For example, for individuals ≥ 80 years of age, the probability of being unaffected given genotypes Aa (A = FAD allele and a = normal allele) was set as 0.40. Individuals < 80 years of age were assigned an even higher probability of being unaffected, given their age. This is an important consideration in late-onset FAD, since these individuals would provide evidence against linkage. Finally, the data were analyzed for both the two-point and multipoint analyses using only affected family members in the analysis (i.e., at-risk family members were coded as unknown with respect to disease status for FAD), thereby eliminating any information contributed by at-risk individuals whose genotype with respect to the FAD locus is not known with certainty.

For three of the families (372, 300, and 285) in whom age-of-onset data were available on several family members, family specific age curves were examined for their effects on the two-point logarithm of the odds of linkage (lod) score results. Using previously described methodology (13,27), the mean and variance of age of onset for the individual pedigrees was estimated by maximum likelihood. A normal distribution was then constructed for each family using the estimated M and S^2.

For comparison with the previous study, a gene frequency of 0.0001 was initially incorporated for the AD locus (31). D21S16 was analyzed in the individual families using the LIPED program (15,24) while LINKAGE (17-19) was used to analyze the complex D21S1/D21S11 marker. This marker detects four polymorphisms (BamH1, Msp1, EcoR1, Taq1) that can be combined into a haplotype for the linkage analysis. Haplotypes can be constructed by hand in some cases, but this frequently results in loss of data, since not all individuals can be uniquely haplotyped (28). This is particularly true in late-onset FAD pedigrees, where many family members are missing and/or deceased. To circumvent these problems, the MLINK subprogram of the LINKAGE package (17-19) was used in the D21S1/D21S11 analysis, with the recombination fraction between the BamH1, Msp1, EcoR1, and Taq1 sites fixed at 0.0 (18). Because the sites are in disequilibrium (31), individual frequencies were calculated for each of the possible haplotypes.

Two-point lod scores for the markers were calculated for each pedigree at each of the recombination fractions (θ males = θ females) 0.001, 0.05, 0.10, 0.20, 0.30, and 0.40. The results were tabulated and then summed over the various pedigrees. A lod score $\geqslant$ +3 is significant evidence for linkage, while a lod score $\leqslant$ -2 is significant evidence for exclusion of linkage (22).

In addition, multipoint analysis using the LINKMAP subprogram of the LINKAGE package (17-19) was used to maximize the available information. The multipoint approach (interval mapping) increases the power of the analysis and decreases the amount of data needed to find a significant linkage result. The location of AD was varied with respect to a fixed map for the D21S16-D21S1/D21S11 loci. The D21S16 locus was chosen as the arbitrary origin set at 0.0. The D21S1/D21S11 locus was then set at a map distance of 0.087 based on previously reported recombination between the two loci (31). Haldane's formula was used to determine the genetic distances (location) of the loci (19). The distance for the AD locus is given relative to the origin. The EcoR1-Taq1 sites of the D21S1/D21S11 marker are in complete disequilibrium (31). Thus, for ease in computation, only the BamH1, Msp1, and EcoR1 sites were used in constructing the D21S1/D21S11 haplotype for the multipoint analysis.

The resulting two-point lod scores between FAD and D21S1/D21S11 and D21S16 are given in Table 1. Families are listed in order of their decreasing mean age of onset (M). Linkage is excluded between FAD and D21S1/D21S11 up to approximately 20± centimorgans (cM) ($\theta \leqslant 0.20$, $z < -2.0$). This exclusion region includes the amyloid gene (33). The highest individual lod score ($z = 0.90$ at θ = 0.0) is found in family 372, with M = 49. The results of the linkage analysis between FAD and D21S16 are inconclusive. D21S16 is considerably less informative than the haplotype D21S1/D21S11 marker (36). While the overall maximum lod score for D21S16 is positive ($\theta = 0.0$, $z = 0.77$), the largest single contribution ($z = 0.65$) came from family 372. The other two early-onset FAD families were not informative for D21S16. No obligate recombinants were seen with D21S16, a probable result of its low PIC (polymorphism information content) value.

The analyses were repeated with the disease gene frequency (p) and the age-of-onset curve being varied, including mutation (α) in the model and using only affected individuals in the linkage study. Varying the gene frequency should allow for the possibility that the AD gene entered the pedigree through married-in individuals, and the use of mutation would aid in circumventing the confounding occurrence of sporadic AD. The range of the estimates used in the analyses were p = 0.0001-0.06 (16) and μ = 0.0-0.00013. The value 0.00013 was chosen for μ because it represents one of the highest estimated mutation rates in humans (6). Table 2 gives the lod scores from these various tests at the selected recombination value of 0.10, summed over all families and summed over just the late-onset FAD families (M > 60 years). As expected, elimination of the early-onset FAD families

Table 1 Two-point lod scores for linkage of familial Alzheimer's disease with the DNA markers D21S1/D21S11 and D21S16

Family	M[a]	0.001	0.05	0.10	0.20	0.30	0.40
Recombination Fraction (θ) Alzheimer's disease vs. D21S1/D21S11							
302	80	−0.06	−0.05	−0.04	−0.03	−0.02	−0.02
420	78	−2.39	−0.72	−0.44	−0.19	−0.08	−0.02
333	77	−0.22	−0.13	−0.08	−0.02	−0.00	0.00
180	71	−3.00	−1.24	−0.77	−0.34	−0.13	−0.03
203	71	−0.49	−0.40	−0.31	−0.17	−0.07	−0.02
191	70	−0.28	−0.23	−0.18	−0.10	−0.04	−0.01
154	68	−0.41	−0.30	−0.22	−0.11	−0.05	−0.01
285	68	−2.40	−0.76	−0.49	−0.22	−0.09	−0.02
401	64	−0.52	−0.48	−0.40	−0.22	−0.09	−0.02
300	63	−4.00	−1.40	−0.86	−0.38	−0.16	−0.04
317	56	0.00	0.00	0.00	0.00	0.00	0.00
208	54	−0.14	−0.11	−0.09	−0.05	−0.02	−0.01
372	49	+0.90	+0.81	+0.72	+0.52	+0.30	+0.09
Total all families		−12.88	−4.90	−3.06	−1.97	−0.42	−0.09
Alzheimer's disease vs. D21S16							
302	80	+0.03	+0.03	+0.02	+0.01	+0.01	+0.00
420	78	−0.03	−0.03	−0.03	−0.01	−0.01	+0.00
333	77	+0.06	+0.05	+0.04	+0.02	+0.01	+0.00
180	71	+0.16	+0.13	+0.10	+0.05	+0.02	+0.01
203	71	−0.22	−0.15	−0.10	−0.04	−0.01	+0.00
191	70	+0.00	+0.00	+0.00	+0.00	+0.00	+0.00
164	68	−0.02	−0.03	−0.02	−0.01	−0.01	+0.00
285	68	+0.00	+0.00	+0.00	+0.00	+0.00	+0.00
401	64	+0.26	+0.23	+0.19	+0.11	+0.05	+0.01
300	63	−0.09	−0.09	−0.09	−0.08	−0.05	−0.01
317	56	+0.00	+0.00	+0.00	+0.00	+0.00	+0.00
208	54	+0.00	+0.00	+0.00	+0.00	+0.00	+0.00
372	49	+0.65	+0.58	+0.50	+0.35	+0.19	+0.06
Total all families		+0.77	+0.70	+0.61	+0.41	+0.21	+0.06

[a]M = Mean Age of Onset.

Table 2 Lod scores for familial Alzheimer's disease and the DNA markers D21S1/D21S11 and D21S16 when the age of onset curve and gene frequency (p) used are varied, including mutation (μ) in the model

			D21S1/D21S11: $\theta = 0.10$		D21S16: $\theta = 0.10$	
Age curve	q	μ	All Families	Late-onset Families	All Families	Late-onset Families
Pedigree data[a]	0.0001	0	−2.16	−2.79	0.605	0.105
	0.0001	0.00013	−2.12	−2.75	0.605	0.105
Low penetrance[b]	0.06	0	−2.21	−2.71	0.474	0.044
	0.06	0.00013	−1.79	−2.28	0.474	0.044
	0.0001	0	−1.37	−2.13	0.584	0.126
Affecteds only[c]	0.06	0	−0.81	−1.33	0.410	0.070
	0.0001	0	−1.64	−2.35	0.610	0.150

[a]Age risk curve generated from overall pedigree data (normal distribution, 66.1 ± 8.6 years).
[b]Age risk curve shifted to allow for low penetrance (e.g., for individuals ⩾80 years of age the probability of being normal given genotype Aa = 0.40 when A equals the Alzheimer's disease allele and a equals normal allele).
[c]Only affected individuals were included in analysis. At-risk individuals were coded as unknown with respect to status for Alzheimer's disease.

from the summer score increased the exclusion region for D21S1/D21S11 and decreased the overall score for D21S16 similarly, due to family 372's linkage result. The results remained consistently negative for FAD and D21S1/D21S11 across the various analyses. The results for D21S16 remained inconclusive. Throughout all analyses, linkage could not be established between AD and the markers used.

The multipoint results are shown in Figure 2. Two graphs are depicted. The solid line represents the use of an age curve (M = 66.1 ± 8.6) for at-risk individuals. The dashed line represents the analysis when only affected individuals were included for study. The multipoint results support the two-point findings. The area of exclusion (solid line) includes 15 cM to the left of D21S16 as well as the area between the two markers, and up to 27 cM distal from D21S1/D21S11. Family 372 gave the highest lod score: $\hat{z} = 0.98$. The results when only affected individuals were included (dashed line) peaked with a lod score of 0.08. Again, family 372 produced the highest score: $\hat{z} = 0.90$.

The results of the linkage studies showed these data fail to support linkage of autosomal dominant late onset AD to the D21S1/D21S11-D21S16 region of chromosome 21 as reported for the early-onset AD families (31). Although a peak lod

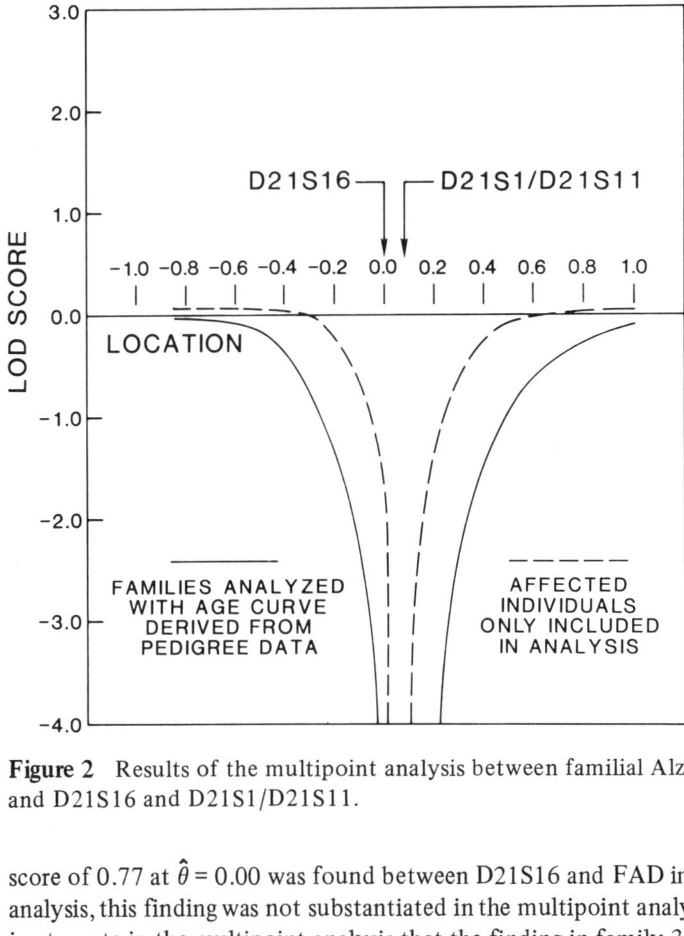

Figure 2 Results of the multipoint analysis between familial Alzheimer's disease and D21S16 and D21S1/D21S11.

score of 0.77 at $\hat{\theta} = 0.00$ was found between D21S16 and FAD in the two-point analysis, this finding was not substantiated in the multipoint analysis. It is interesting to note in the multipoint analysis that the finding in family 372 of $\hat{z} = 0.98$ supports the previously reported linkage data (31) from the early-onset families. Testing for heterogeneity (25) in these data using the multipoint results was not significant. In addition, genetic heterogeneity was also examined by combining our linkage results for D21S1/D21S11 with the published results (31). Testing the null hypothesis of homogeneity was not significant (25).

Genetic heterogeneity is known to exist in a number of neurological disorders including Charcot-Marie-Tooth (CMT) disease (2), limb girdle muscular dystrophy (11), and the hereditary ataxias (8). The original CMT1 families analyzed for linkage were found to show linkage to the Duffy locus on chromosome 1 (3,12,32). Subsequent analyses identified non-Duffy-linked families. The above FAD linkage results may be representative of genetic heterogeneity at the FAD locus. Although testing of this hypothesis was not significant, it is often difficult to detect heterogeneity and large numbers of families can be required for analysis (26).

Several different approaches to age of onset were examined in the analyses using a variety of age curves including information obtained from only affected individuals. Varying the age of onset curves did not significantly alter the lod score results. These findings confirm earlier studies on Huntington's disease linkage data (28), which showed that variation of the age-of-onset distribution used in the analysis resulted in small changes in the lod score values while the estimate of the recombination fraction remained intact.

The usefulness of the multipoint approach has been indicated in recent studies (16) that have shown that the ability to detect linkage is optimized even in small families when interval mapping is used. The amount of data needed for the analysis can be reduced anywhere from 5 to 50 times. Since the majority of the FAD families have the late-onset type and thus have limited data available, the use of the multipoint approach makes a linkage study feasible even in families structured as in late-onset FAD.

The failure to detect linkage of autosomal dominant late onset FAD to the region of chromosome 21 where the early onset FAD gene was localized, together with the exclusion of linkage to a large portion of that same region, suggests the possibility that more than one cause for FAD may exist. These differences between early-onset FAD and late-onset FAD are consistent with observations of both clinical and neurochemical differences between the two types (9,30). These findings indicate the need for the screening of both additional families and chromosome 21 markers as well as the examination of chromosomal areas for linkage. The eventual localization of late-onset FAD will provide the basis for studies aimed at determining the basic defect in this common form of familial AD.

ACKNOWLEDGMENTS

The authors thank Drs. J. F. Gusella and G. D. Stewart for providing the DNA probes D21S1/D21S11 and D21S16; Drs. Michael Boehnke, Jonathan Haines, and R. C. Elston for their helpful comments; Wendy Smith, Fiona Francis, James Koh, Edward Hanson, Kenneth M. Wilkinson, and Sharon Musick for expert assistance with the polymorphism and DNA analysis; Peggy Pate and Helen Harbett for technical assistance with the family data analysis; Laurita Melton for manuscript preparation. This work was supported by the Joseph and Kathleen Bryan Alzheimer's Disease Research Center (AGO5128), by NS19999 and NS23008 from the NINCDS, by a grant from the Denver Foundation for Health and Research, and by Clinical Research Unit MO1-RR-30 from the NIGMS. R. J. Bartlett is a recipient of an ADRDA/Allied Signal Faculty Scholar Award.

REFERENCES

1. Bartlett, R. J., M. A. Pericak-Vance, L. H. Yamaoka, J. R. Gilbert, M. H. Herbstreith, W-Y. Hung, J. E. Lee, T. K. Mohandas, G. Bruns, C. Laberge, M-C. Thibault, D. A. Ross, and Roses, A. D. (1987). A new probe for the diagnosis of myotonic muscular dystrophy. *Science* 235: 1648-1650.

2. Bird, T. D., J. Ott, and E. R. Giblett (1982). Evidence for linkage of CMT neuropathy to the Duffy locus on chromosome 1. *Am. J. Hum. Genet.* 34: 388-394.
3. Bird, T. D., J. Ott, E. R. Giblett, P. F. Chance, S. M. Lumi, and Kraft, G. H. (1983). Genetic linkage evidence for heterogeneity in CMT neuropathy (HMSN Type I). *Ann. Neurol.* 14: 679-684.
4. Breitner, J. C. S., and Folstein, M. J. (1984). Familial Alzheimer's dementia: A prevalent disorder with specific clinical features. *Psychol. Med.* 14: 63-80.
5. Breitner, J. C. S., J. M. Silverman, R. C. Mohs, and Davis, K. L. (1988). Familial aggregation in Alzheimer's disease: Comparison of risk among relatives of early-and-late-onset cases, and among male and female relatives in successive generations. *Neurology* 38: 207-212.
6. Cavalli-Sforza, S., and Bodmer, W. F. (1971). *The Genetics of Human Populations*. San Francisco, W. H. Freeman.
7. Chomczynski, P., and Qasba, P. K. (1985). Alkaline transfer of DNA to Gene Screen Plus Membrane. New England Nuclear Publication.
8. Farris, B. K., J. L. Smith, and Ayyar, D. R. (1986). Neuro-ophthalmologic findings in vestibulocerebellar ataxia. *Arch. Neurol.* 43: 1050-1053.
9. Filley, C. M., J. Kelley, and Heaton, R. K. (1986). Neuropsychologic features of early and late onset Alzheimer's disease. *Arch. Neurol.* 43: 574-576.
10. Folstein, M. F., and Powell D. (1984). Is Alzheimer's disease inherited: A methodologic review. *Integr. Psychiatry* 2: 163-175.
11. Gilchrist, J. M., M. A. Pericak-Vance, J. Stajich, L. Silverman, and Roses, A. D. (1988). Clinical and genetic investigation in autosomal dominant limb-girdle muscular dystrophy. *Neurology* 38: 5-8.
12. Guiloff, R. J., P. K. Thomas, J. Contreras, S. Armitage, G. Schwarz, and Sedgwick, E. M. (1982). Linkage of autosomal dominant type I hereditary motor and sensory neuropathy to the Duffy locus on chromosome 1. *J. Neurol. Neurosurg. Psychiatry* 45: 669-674.
13. Haynes, C. S., M. A. Pericak-Vance, and Dawson, D. V. (1986). Analysis of Huntington disease linkage and age-of-onset distributions. *Genet. Epidemiol. Suppl.* 1: 236-239.
14. Heyman, A., W. E. Wilkinson, J. A. Stafford, M. J. Helms, A. H. Sigmon, and Weinberg, T. (1984). Alzheimer's disease: A study of epidemiologic aspects. *Ann. Neurol.* 15: 335-341.
15. Hodge, S. E., L. A. Morton, S. Tideman, K. K. Kidd, and Spence, M. A. (1979). Age-of-onset correction available for linkage analysis (LIPED). *Am. J. Hum. Genet.* 31: 761-762.
16. Larsson, T., T. Sjogren, and Jacobson, G. (1963). Senile dementia: A clinical, sociomedical and genetic study. *Acta Psychiatr. Scand.* 39: (Suppl 167).
17. Lathrop, G. M., and Lalouel, J. M. (1984). Easy calculations of lod scores and genetic risks on small computers. *Am. J. Hum. Genet.* 36: 460-465.
18. Lathrop, G. M., J. M. Lalouel, C. Julier, and Ott, J. (1984). Strategies for multilocus linkage analysis in humans. *Proc. Natl. Acad. Sci. (USA)* 81: 3443-3446.
19. Lathrop, G. M., J. M. Lalouel, C. Julier, and Ott, J. (1985). Multi-locus linkage analysis in humans: detection of linkage and estimation of recombination. *Am. J. Hum. Genet.* 37: 482-498.

20. McKhann, G. D. Drachman, M. Folstein, R. Katzman, D. Price, and Stadlan, E. (1984). Clinical diagnosis of Alzheimer's disease: report of the NINCD-ADRDA Work Group under the auspices of the Department of Health and Human Services Task Force on Alzheimer's disease. *Neurology* 34: 939-944.
21. Mohs, R. C., J. C. S. Breitner, J. M. Silverman, and Davis, K. (1987). Alzheimer's disease: Morbid risk among first degree relatives approximates 50% by age 90. *Arch. Gen. Phychiatry* 44: 405-408.
22. Morton, N. E. (1956). Detection and estimation of linkage between genes for elliptocytosis and RH blood type. *Am. J. Genet.* 7: 277.
23. Nee, L. E., R. J. Polinsky, R. Eldridge, H. Weingartner, S. Smallberg, and Ebert, M. (1983). A family with histologically confirmed Alzheimer's disease. *Arch. Neurol.* 40: 203-208.
24. Ott, J. 1984. Estimation of the recombination fraction in human pedigree: Efficient computation of the likelihood for human linkage studies. *Am. J. Hum. Genet.* 27: 588-597.
25. Ott, J. (1985). *Analysis of Human Genetic Linkage*. Baltimore/London, The Johns Hopkins University Press.
26. Ott, J. (1986). The number of families required to detect or exclude linkage heterogeneity. *Am. J. Hum. Genet.* 39: 159-165.
27. Pericak-Vance, M. A., R. C. Elston, P. M. Conneally, and Dawson, D. V. (1983). Age of onset heterogeneity in Huntington's disease. *Am. J. Med. Genet.* 14(1): 49-60.
28. Pericak-Vance, M. A., and Meyers, D. A. (1986). Genetic analysis workshop IV: Huntington disease linkage analysis summary. *Genet. Epidemiol. Suppl.* 1: 197-209.
29. Pericak-Vance, M. A., L. H. Yamaoka, R. I. F. Assinder, W-Y. Hung, R. J. Bartlett, J. M. Stajich, P. C. Gaskell, D. A. Ross, S. Sherman, G. H. Fey, S. Humphries, R. Williamson, and Roses, A. D. (1986). Tight linkage of apolipoprotein C2 to myotonic dystrophy on chromosome 19. *Neurology* 36: 1418-1423.
30. Seltzer, R., and Sherwin, I. (1983). A comparison of clinical features in early and late-onset primary degenerative dementia. One entity or two? *Arch. Neurol.* 40: 143-146.
31. St. George-Hyslop, P. H., R. E. Tanzi, R. J. Polinsky, J. L. Haines, L. Nee, P. C. Watkins, R. H. Meyers, R. G. Feldman, D. Pollen, D. Drachman, J. Growdonn, A. Bruni, J. F. Foncin, G. Salmon, P. Fromheld, L. Amaducci, S. Sorgi, S. Placentini, G. D. Stewart, W. Hobbs, P. M. Conneally, and Gusella, J. F. (1987). The genetic defect causing familial Alzheimer's disease maps on chromosome 21. *Science* 235: 885-890.
32. Stebbins, N. B., and Conneally, P. M. (1982). Linkage of dominantly inherited CMT neuropathy to the Duffy locus in an Indiana family. *Am. J. Hum. Genet.* 34: 195A.
33. Tanzi, R. E. (1985). A genetic linkage map of human chromosome 21. Eighth International Workshop on Human Gene Mapping. *Cytogenet. Cell Genet.* 40: 760.
34. U. S. Congress, Office of Technology Assessment (1987). *Losing a Million Minds: Confronting the Tragedy of Alzheimer's Disease and other Dementias*. OTA-BA-323. Washington, D.C., U.S. Government Printing Office.

35. Weitkamp, L. R., L. Nee, B. Keats, R. J. Polinsky, and Guttormsen, S. (1983). Alzheimer's disease: Evidence for susceptibility loci on chromosomes 6 and 14. *Am. J. Hum. Genet.* 35: 443-453.
36. Willard, H., M. Skolnick, P. Pearson, and Mandel, J. L. (1985). Human gene mapping by recombinant DNA techniques: Report on polymorphic DNA segments. Eighth International Workshop on Human Gene Mapping. Cytogenet. *Cell Genet.* 40: 360-390.

8

Familial and Sporadic Alzheimer's Disease: Molecular Genetic Approaches

P. H. ST. GEORGE-HYSLOP, R. J. POLINSKY, R. E. TANZI, J. L. HAINES, L. NEE, J. GROWDON, D. POLLEN, D. DRACHMAN, R. H. MYERS, R. G. FELDMAN, D. O'SULLIVAN, J.–F. FONCIN, S. A. BRUNI, D. SALMON, L. AMMADUCCI, S. SORBI, S. PIACENTINI, P. FROMMELT, P. M. CONNEALLY, J. F. GUSELLA / *Massachusetts General Hospital, Boston, Massachusetts*

Until recently, the causes of Alzheimer's Disease (AD) has largely been studied using conventional clinical, epidemiological, or biochemical methods (1-6). While these methods have produced several important observations, they have been unsuccessful in identifying the primary cause of AD. However, among the significant results produced by the clinical and epidemiological studies has been the discovery that relatives of AD patients show a higher than expected incidence of this disorder (7-14). It is significant that the risk of AD in these relatives approximates that of an illness inherited as an autosomal dominant trait with incomplete penetrance due to late age of onset (7-14). Although this familial aggregation of cases does not necessarily prove the presence of a genetic basis for AD, several pedigrees have now been described in which the disorder appears to result unequivocally from a dominantly inherited defect in an autosomal gene (15-26).

With certain caveats to be discussed later, the chromosomal location of the genetic defect causing at least the clearly inherited FAD could be determined using molecular genetic linkage strategies. These techniques have recently lead to localization of the gene defects causing other inherited neurological disorders such as Huntington's chorea, and Duchenne muscular dystrophy (3). Definition of the chromosomal region carrying the FAD gene would support subsequent attempts to clone and characterize functionally the normal and disease alleles of the FAD gene. An understanding of the biochemical function of the normal homologue, and of the effects of the FAD mutation upon this function, should provide useful insights into the pathophysiology of at least FAD, and possibly also of sporadic

AD. Such knowledge could then be applied to the development of rational therapeutic and diagnostic tools to combat this disorder.

MOLECULAR GENETIC STRATEGIES

Current molecular genetic techniques used to locate the gene defect causing autosomal dominant disorders such as FAD are based on a modification of classic genetic linkage studies and Mendelian laws of inheritance. Simply stated, one attempts to show that the disease gene is coinherited with a polymorphic genetic marker. The observation that the disease gene and the genetic marker cosegregate in a given family implies that they are situated very close together on the same chromosome, and are only very infrequently separated by recombination during gametogenesis. Consequently, if one already knows the chromosomal location of the genetic marker, one can infer the chromosomal location of the disease gene.

Classic genetic linkage studies have used expressed genes coding for polymorphic proteins such as the ABO blood group antigens. Unfortunately, the restricted number and informativeness of the classic protein markers make them of only limited usefulness. However, it has recently been observed that the nucleotide sequence of DNA itself contains naturally occurring variations that can be used as polymorphic genetic markers (27). These nucleotide variations, which can be as small as a single nucleotide substitution, can be recognized by the fact that they may alter the recognition sequence for restriction endonuclease enzymes that cleave DNA at specific nucleotide sequences. The consequent destruction or creation of recognition sequences leads respectively to the production of longer or shorter fragments when genomic DNA is cleaved with that restriction enzyme, thereby generating restriction fragment length polymorphisms (RFLPs). Since these naturally occurring nucleotide sequence variations occur very frequently throughout the genome (approximately 1 every 500 base pairs), and since they are inheritable, they can be used as genetic markers.

Genetic linkage is usually assessed statistically by computing a logarithm of the odds score (lod score), which is the logarithm of the ratio of the likelihood that the observed pattern of inheritance of the marker and the disease occurred due to linkage, compared to the likelihood that the pattern of inheritance occurred by chance alone (5). By convention, lod scores of greater than +3.0, which imply more than a thousandfold odds in favor of linkage, are taken to prove linkage. Lod scores of less than −2.0 are taken to refute the presence of linkage since they imply 100-fold odds in favor of random chance association. Lod scores between these two extremes are usually considered indeterminate, although they do have some statistical value. For instance, empirical and theoretical observations suggest that with the subsequent acquisition of more data, initial lod scores of between +2 and +3 are later found to be correct about 90% of the time (28).

LIMITATIONS OF GENETIC LINKAGE STUDIES IN FAD

The clinical course of FAD produces a number of difficulties not usually encountered in most other dominantly inherited neurogenetic disorders. Because of the patients' late onset of symptoms and the short subsequent life span, most FAD pedigrees have few living affected members available for study at any given time. Furthermore, it is unlikely that an unaffected parent and an affected child will be alive at the same time. As a consequence, FAD pedigrees typically give considerably less genetic information than do comparably sized pedigrees of patients with other neurogenetic disorders.

Several strategies must be used to maximize the amount of genetic information yielded by FAD pedigrees. The simplest strategy is to sum the lod scores generated by several independent pedigrees to generate a significant cumulative lod score. This strategy, which simply allows one to assess a larger number of meiotic events for the presence or absence of cosegregation of the marker and the disease, is statistically valid (28). This strategy requires the assumption that all of the pedigrees included in the analysis have genetic defects at the same chromosomal locus. If one or more of the pedigrees has genetic defects at different loci, linkage will be more difficult to identify. This difficulty arises because positive scores in the pedigrees with genetic defects at the test locus will be offset by negative scores from pedigrees with defects at other loci.

Another useful strategy is to used DNA probes that reveal RFLPs with many alleles, each allele having a low frequency in the general population. The significance of concordance between affected members for one allele of a marker depends heavily upon the population frequency of that allele. If the allele is very infrequent in the general population, it would be likely that the concordance occurred because the marker and the disease gene were inherited together from a common affected ancestor (i.e., due to linkage). However, if the concordant allele is very common in the general population, it is also possible that the allele may have been acquired instead from several different married-in members of the pedigree (i.e., nonlinkage). This uncertainty, which must be accounted for in the analysis, will result in lower lod scores. Consequently, linkage is easier to detect if highly polymorphic probes with multiple low-frequency alleles are used as genetic markers.

The final strategy that can be used to facilitate the detection of linkage is multipoint linkage analysis (29). It is not unusual for a probe to yield genetic information from only some branches of a pedigree, and to be uniformative in other branches due to homozygous matings. Frequently, other nearby probes will be informative in different portions of the same pedigree. Consequently, if the genetic information from several nearby probes could be summed, the maximum amount of information could be gleaned from each pedigree. To perform such multipoint linkage analysis, however, it is necessary that the genetic relationships between the marker loci be known (i.e., that a genetic map of the chromosomal region be constructed). Such genetic maps have been constructed for a small number of chromosomes, and are being actively pursued for several other chromosomes. Thus multipoint linkage analysis strategies can now be applied to improve further the potential to discover the chromosomal locus of the FAD mutation.

CURRENT RESULTS IN FAD

The FAD gene could have been located on any of the 22 autosomal chromosomes. However, two chromosomal sites appeared to merit particular attention. Chromosome 14 had previously been suggested as a potential locus for the FAD gene, based on minimally positive lod scores with the classic protein marker *Gm* in one large pedigree (30). We reexamined the same pedigree, using both *Gm* and a more highly polymorphic DNA marker *D14S1* (probe pAW101), which is located about 3 cM from *Gm* (31-33). Using both of these markers, as well as additional members of the pedigree collected subsequent to the previous analysis, we obtained lod scores sufficiently negative to refute linkage to this region of the genome (manuscript in preparation).

The high incidence of Alzheimer-like neuropathological findings in elderly patients with Down's syndrome (DS) suggested that chromosome 21 was another potential site for the FAD gene (34-44). Consequently, we tested a series of chromosome 21 DNA markers for linkage to FAD. These markers had previously been mapped to various regions of chromosome 21 by both physical and genetic means, thereby allowing the construction of a genetic linkage map of chromosome 21 (45-47).

Contrary to initial expectations, all the probes from the distal half of chromosome 21 (21q22-21qter) gave negative lod scores, thereby allowing us to exclude the "obligate" DS region of chromosome 21 as the site of the FAD gene (48). However, when markers mapped to the proximal portion of chromosome 21 (21cen-21q21) were studied, two markers *D21S1/D21S11* (probes pPW228C and pPW236B) and *D21S16* (probe pGSE9) gave lod scores between +2.0 and +3.0 (48). Since these scores do not reach the critical level of +3.0, they can only be considered as strongly suggestive of linkage rather than actual proof. Nevertheless, as noted earlier, previous studies have suggested that lod scores between +2.0 and +3.0 are correct about 0-% of the time (28). Since *D21S1/D21S11* and *D21S16* are located close to each other on chromosome 21, the likelihood that both markers would give positive yet erroneous scores is quite small (<1%). To test further the possibility that the FAD gene may be located near these markers, we used multipoint linkage analysis to calculate lod scores for various possible locations between and to either side of these two markers. This analysis calculated a peak lod score of +4.25 for a location between the markers, with a secondary peak of +4.06 for a location to one side of both markers (Fig. 1). These calculations therefore confirm with a reasonable certainty ($1:10^4$) that the FAD mutation in the four pedigrees examined is located in the proximal region of chromosome 21. Because the lod scores generated for locations between and to one side of the markers are not significantly different, it is not yet possible to establish precisely the location of the gene defect with respect to these markers.

The discovery of the approximate chromosomal location of at least one gene defect capable of causing FAD is important for several reasons. Most significantly, this knowledge will serve as basis for cloning the defective and normal alleles of the FAD gene without the need for any prior knowledge of the likely function of FAD gene. Second, as will be discussed later, it may now be possible to address directly the hypothesis of a genetic basis for "sporadic" AD. An answer to this question will likely determine the extent to which environmental agents must be sought to explain the high incidence of AD. Third, the discovery of polymorphic genetic markers linked to FAD raises the possibility of presymptomatic or prenatal diagnosis. However, before such testing can be carried out meaningfully, unequivocal answers must be reached both for the precise location of the FAD gene relative to a battery of flanking DNA markers and for the possibility of genetic heterogeneity between different families with FAD.

AMYLOID: A CANDIDATE FAD GENE?

The gene coding for the B-amyloid precursor peptide (BAP) that accumulates in brain tissue of normal elderly individuals, and of patients with AD and DS, has recently been cloned and mapped to the 21q21 region of chromosome 21 (49-52). This observation has led to speculation that the BAP gene may be the site of the FAD mutation. In support of this notion, preliminary investigations in a small number of sporadic AD cases appeared to show the presence of an extra copy of the BAP gene, similar to that observed in DS (53). This result would imply not only that the mutation causing FAD may reside in the BAP gene, but also that "sporadic" AD really has a genetic basis (gene duplication). The thesis that AD may result from cryptic duplication of portions of chromosome 21 received additional support with the independent description of triplication of the *SOD 1* gene (54). To confirm these preliminary observations, we have assessed gene dosage in cerebral cortex and peripheral tissues from 63 cases of sporadic AD and 4 independent FAD pedigrees, as well as in similar tissues from normal, DS, and non-AD neurological controls. Using a variety of techniques we were unable to document the presence of gene duplication in either brain or peripheral tissues at the BAP or *SOD 1* loci. Furthermore, no evidence of chromosomal duplication was observed in the vicinity of the DNA markers linked to FAD, or at the *D21S17* locus within the DS region of chromosome 21 (55). This would suggest that chromosomal duplication at the sites tested is an infrequent event in AD, and is unlikely to be related causally to the occurrence of either FAD or sporadic AD.

Further evidence that the BAP gene is not the site of the FAD mutation comes from four other sources. First and most definitive is the observation that several recombination events have been observed between the FAD gene and the BAP gene by two independent groups (56,57). Second, with certain provisos, if the BAP gene were the site of a mutation causing "sporadic" AD, one might expect that particular RFLP alleles of the BAP gene would be more common in AD than in the normal population. No such allelic association was observed (55). Furthermore, elderly DS patients with evidence of cognitive decline did not differ from age-matched DS patients without cognitive decline in terms of which alleles of the BAP gene were duplicated or triplicated (55). Finally, the appearance of amyloid deposits in normal elderly brain tissue, and the reports of isolation of the A4 peptide from tissues with Parkinsonian dementia of Guam (56) add further circumstantial evidence against a causal role for the BAP gene in AD.

HETEROGENEITY IN FAD AND THE CAUSES OF SPORADIC AD

Several investigators have reported clinical, pathological, and neurochemical observations that suggest that AD might be a heterogeneous group of illnesses (58-60). Obviously, before AD can be considered a single uniform illness, it will be necessary to show not only that sporadic AD is due to an incompletely penetrant gene defect at the FAD locus, but also that no cases of FAD result from mutations at other chromosomal loci.

The question of heterogeneity within FAD should be fairly readily addressed by examination of many additional FAD pedigrees for linkage to chromosome 21. The inclusion of small nuclear families with several AD cases, but without clar inheritance through several generations, should initially be treated with caution in the analysis of heterogeneity in FAD. Single recombinant events in these very small families do not by themselves necessarily constitute good evidence for heterogeneity, particularly when the currently available genetic markers are located at some distance from the FAD gene (~8 cM). Furthermore, in these small families the precise mode of inheritance is often difficult to ascertain. Such pedigrees could represent chance occurrence of several cases of a common, truly nongenetic illness within the same family. Indeed this latter possibility is a major concern in the analysis of the genetic causes of sporadic AD.

The discovery of DNA markers linked to young-onset FAD may allow more direct examination of the inheritability of late-onset "sporadic" AD. However, several features of the late-onset type of AD will make a definitive answer difficult. Late-onset patients with AD typically do not have large extended pedigrees, with the result that in any particular family it may be difficult to decide if and how the disorder is inherited. Multiple cases of late-onset AD within the same family could result from an incompletely penetrant autosomal dominant gene; a high-frequency recessive disorder masquerading as a dominant disorder (pseudo-dominant inheritance); or simply chance occurrence of multiple nongenetic cases. Clearly, correct analysis of the data will require identification of the true mode of inheritance.

If one assumes that multiple cases of AD in the same family are in fact due to an inherited defect (dominant or recessive), the chromosomal location of the genetic defect could be discovered by allelic association studies in addition to classic genetic linkage studies. These allelic association studies attempt to show that a particular allele of an RFLP occurs more commonly in patients with AD than in the general population. This is achieved either by examining multiple sets of affected siblings for concordance (sib pair method), or by examining a cohort of affected individuals in comparison to the general population of the same ethnic/genetic origin. Although these strategies have the advantage that they do not require extended pedigrees, they do require that the marker allele be situated very close to the disease mutation. As noted earlier, we have used this strategy to determine whether late-onset "sporadic" AD was associated with particular alleles of the BAP gene or of the DNA markers linked to FAD (55). The absence of a demonstrable association between "sporadic" AD and any of these loci obviously fails to provide support for the hypothesis that these loci are the *exact* site of the "sporadic" AD-causing mutation. However, since we already know that none of these loci are precisely at the site of even the FAD mutation, this result is not surprising, and certainly does *not* negate the hypothesis that "sporadic" AD may be inherited, or even that the "sporadic" AD gene defect may reside on chromosome 21. Clearly, at the current time, the issue of a genetic cause for the more common sporadic cases of AD has not been definitively studied at the molecular level.

SUMMARY

Genetic linkage analysis has provided reasonable evidence that a gene causing the familial form of Alzheimer's disease in four large pedigrees is located on the proximal portion of chromosome 21. The major significance of this result is that knowledge of the chromosomal location of the FAD gene will serve as a basis for attempts to clone and characterize the defective and normal alleles of this gene. An understanding of the biochemical functions of the normal and disease alleles may permit the construction of better diagnostic and therapeutic tools to combat the disorder. Additionally, even before the actual FAD gene is cloned, it may be possible in the future to consider presymptomatic testing in appropriate families, providing that the question of genetic heterogeneity can be resolved, and that additional informative DNA markers flanking the FAD gene can be generated. Finally, knowledge of the chromosomal location of at least one type of FAD should allow direct examination of the hypothesis concerning a genetic basis for even late-onset "sporadic" AD. Currently available evidence incicates that neither FAD nor sporadic AD result from inherited defects in the β-amyloid precursor gene.

ACKNOWLEDGMENTS

This work was supported by NIH grants ADRC P50 AGO5134-02, and NS20012, by the McKnight Foundation, by the Julieanne Dorn Fund for Neurological Research, and by a generous donation from Mr. J. Freudenberger. P. St. G. H. was a Medical Research Council of Canada Fellow, and is presently a John Douglas French Foundation Fellow. J. A. A. is supported in part by a grant from the Charles H. Hood Foundation. J. F. G. is a Searle Scholar of the Chicago Community Trust.

The authors thank W. W. Tourtellotte, R. Thompson, I. Rosario, and T. Hedley-White for AD and control brain tissue; G. D. Stewart and R. Hallewell for supplying chromosome 21 probes; M. E. MacDonald and V. Ramesh for technical advice; S. Healey for technical assistance; and C. Altshuler and B. Williamson for assisting in the collection of the FAD pedigrees.

REFERENCES

1. Wurtman, R.J. (1985). Alzheimer's disease. *Sci. Am.* 252: 62-75.
2. Katzman, R. (1986). Alzheimer's disease. *N. Engl. J. Med.* 314: 964-973.
3. Whitehouse, P.J., Price, K.L., Clark, A.W., Coyle, J.T., and DeLong, M.R. (1981). Alzheimer's disease: Evidence of loss of cholonergic neurons in the nucleus basalis. *Ann. Neurol.* 10: 122-126.
4. Lewis, P.N., Lukiw, W.J., DeBoni, U., Crapper McLachlan, D.R. et al. (1984). Changes in chromatin structure associated with Alzheimer's disease. *J. Neurochem.* 37: 1193-1202.
5. Sajdel-Sulkowska, E.M., and Mrrotta, C.A. (1984). Alzheimer's disease brain: Alterations in RNA levels and in a ribonuclease inhibitor complex. *Science* 225: 947-949.
6. Morrison, J.H., Rogers, J., Scherr, S., Benoit, R., and Bloom, F.E. (1985). Somatostatin immunoreactivity in neuritic plaques of Alzheimer's patients. *Nature* 314: 90-92.
7. Heston, L.L., Mastri, A.R., Anderson, V.E., and White, J. (1981). *Arch. Gen. Psychiatry* 38: 1985.
8. Heyman, A., Wilkinson, W.E., Hurwitz, B.J., Schmechel, D., Sigmon, A.H., Weinberg, T., Helms, M.J., and Swift, M. (1983). Alzheimer's disease: Genetic aspects and associated clinical disorders. *Ann. Neurol.* 14: 507-515.
9. Oliver, C., and Holland, A.J. (1986). *Psychol. Med.* 16: 307.
10. Mortimer, J.A., and Schuman, L.M. (Eds.). (1981). *The Epidemiology of Dementia.* New York, Oxford University Press.

11. Rocca, W.A., Amaducci, L.A., and Schoenberg, B.S. (1986). Epidemiology of clinically diagnosed Alzheimer disease. *Ann. Neurol.* 19: 415-424.
12. Chase, G.A., Folstein, M.F., Breitner, J.C.S., Beary, T.H., and Self, S.G. (1983). The use of life tables and survival analysis in testing genetic hypothesis with an application to Alzheimer's disease. *Am. J. Epidemiol.* 117: 590-597.
13. Breitner, J.C.S., and Folstein, M.F. (1984). Familial Alzheimer dementia: A prevalent disorder with specific clinical features. *Psychol. Med.* 14: 63-80.
14. Mohs, R.C., Breitner, J.C., Silverman, J.M., and Davis, K.L. (1987). *Arch Gen. Psychiatry* 44: 405.
15. Lowenberg, K., and Waggoner, R.W. (1934). Familial organic psychosis (Alzheimer's type). *Arch. Neurol. Psychiatry* 31: 737-754.
16. McMenemy, W.H., Worster-Drought, C., Flind, J., and Williams, H.G. (1939). Familial presenile dementia; report of case with clinical and pathological features of Alzheimer's disease. *J. Neurol. Psychiatry* 2: 293.
17. Delay, J., Deselaux, P., Perrin, J., and de Burat, J.F. (1945). Demence atrophique familiale. Aspects encephalographiques analogues de deux collateraux. *Rev Neurol* 77: 85.
18. Nee, L., Polinsky, R.J., Eldridge, R., Weingartner, H., Smallberg, S., and Ebert, M. (1983). A family with histologically confirmed Alzheimer disease. *Arch. Neurol.* 40:203-208.
19. Worster-Draught, C., Greenfield, J.G., and McMenemy, W.H. (1944). A form of familial presenile dementia with spastic paralysis. *Brain* 67: 38-43.
20. Feldman, R.G., Chandler, K.A., Levy, L.L., and Glaser, G.H. (1963). Familial Alzheimer's disease. *Neurology* 13: 811-823.
21. Heston, L.L., Lowther, D.L., and Leventhal, C.M. (1966). Alzheimer's disease: A family study. *Arch. Neurol.* 15: 225-233.
22. Foncin, J.F., Salmon, D., Supino-Viterbo, V., et al. (1985). Démence présenile D'Alzheimer transmise dans une famille étendue. *Rev. Neurol. (Paris)* 141: 194-202.
23. Lauter, H. (1961). Genealogische Erhebungen in einer Familie mit Alzheimerschen Krankheit. *Arch. Psychiatr. Z. Ges. Neurol.* 202: 126-139.
24. Goudsmit, J., White, B.J., Weitkamp, L.R., Keats, J.B., Morrow, C.H., and Gajdusek, D.C. (1981). Familial Alzheimer's disease in two kindreds of the same geographic and ethnic origin. *J. Neurol. Sci.* 49: 79-89.
25. Cook, R.H., Ward, B.E., and Austin, J.H. (1979). Studies in aging of the brain: V. Familial Alzheimer disease: Relation to transmissible dementia, aneuploidy, and microtubular defects. *Neurology* 29: 1402-1412.
26. McKusick, V.A. (1983). *Mendelian Inheritance in Man*, 6th edition, Baltimore, Johns Hopkins University Press, pp. 30-31.
27. Botstein, D., White, R.L., Skolnick, M., Davis, R. (1980). Construction of a genetic linkage map in man using restriction fragment length polymorphisms. *Am. J. Hum. Gen.* 32: 314-331.
28. Ott, J. (1985). *Analysis of Human Genetic Linkage.* Baltimore and London, Johns Hopkins University Press.

29. Lathrop, G.M., Lalouel, J.M., Julier, C., and Ott, J. (1985). Multilocus linkage analysis in humans; Detection of linkage and estimation of recombination. *Am. J. Hum. Genet.* 37: 482-498.
30. Weitkamp, L.R., Nee, L., Keats, B., Polinsky, R.J., and Guttormsen, S. (1983). Alzheimer's disease: Evidence for susceptibility loci on chromosome 6 and 14. *Am. J. Hum. Genet.* 35: 443-453.
31. Wyman, A.R., and White, R. (1980). A highly polymorphic locus in human DNA. *Proc. Natl. Acad. Sci. U.S.A.* 77: 6754-6758.
32. Linsley, P., Bech-Hansen, N.T., Siminovitch, L., and Cox, D.W. (1983). Analysis of a break in chromosome 14 mapping to the region of the immunoglobulin heavy chain locus. *Proc. Natl. Acad. Sci. U.S.A.* 80: 1997-2001.
33. Balazs, I., Purrello, M., Rubinstein, P., Alhadeff, B., and Siniscalco, M. (1982). Highly polymorphic DNA site D14S1 maps to the region of Burkitt lymphoma translocation and is closely linked to the heavy chain immunoglobulin locus. *Proc. Natl. Acad. Sci. U.S.A.* 79: 7395-7399.
34. Jervis, G.A. (1948). Early senile changes in mongoloid idiocy. *Am. J. Psychiatry* 105: 102-106.
35. Crapper, D.R., D'Alton, A.J., Skpotiz, M., Scott, J.W., and Hachinski, V.L. (1975). Alzheimer degeneration in Down's syndrome. *Arch. Neurol.* 32: 618-623.
36. Heston, L.L. (1982). Alzheimer's disease and Down's syndrome: Evidence suggesting an association. *Ann. N.Y. Acad. Sci.* 396: 3-13.
37. Wisniewski, K.E., Dalton, A.J., Crapper McLachlan, D.R., Wen, G.Y., and Wisniewski, H.M. (1985). Alzheimer's disease in Down's syndrome: Clinicopathologic studies. *Neurology* 35: 957-961.
40. Sinex, F.M., and Myers, R.H. (Eds.). Alzheimer's disease, Down's syndrome and aging: The genetic approach. *Ann. N.Y. Acad. Sci.* 396: 3-13, 1982.
41. Burger, P.C., and Vogel, F.S. (1973). The development of the pathologic changes of Alzheimer's disease and senile dementia in patients with Down's syndrome. *Am. J. Pathol.* 73: 457-476.
42. Yates, C.M., Simpson, J., Maloney, A.F.J., et al. (1980). Alzheimer-like cholingergic deficiency in Down's syndrome. *Lancet* 2: 979.
43. Heston, L.L., and Mastri, A.R. (1977). The genetics of Alzheimer's disease: Associations with hematologic malignancy and Down syndrome. *Arch. Gen. Psychiatry* 34: 976-981.
44. Eisner, D. (1983). *Psychol. Rep.* 52: 119.
45. Stewart, G.D., Harris, P., Galt, J., and Ferguson-Smith, M.A. (1985). *Nucleic Acids Res.* 13: 4125.
46. Watkins, P.C. et al. (1985). *Nucleic Acids Res.* 13: 6075.
47. Tanzi, R.E., et al. (1985). Cytogenet. Cell Genet. 40: 760.
48. St. George-Hyslop, P.H., Tanzi, R., Polinsky, R., et al. (1987). The genetic defect causing familial Alzheimer's disease maps on chromosome 21. *Science* 235: 885-890.
49. Kang, J., Lemaire, H.G., Unterbeck, A., et al. (1987). The precursor of the Alzheimer's disease amyloid A4 protein resembles a cell-surface receptor. *Nature* 325: 733-736.

50. Golgaber, D., Lerman, M.I., McBride, O.W., Saffiotti, U., and Gadjusek, D.C. (1987). Characterization and chromosomal localization of a cDNA encoding brain amyloid of Alzheimer's disease. *Science* 235: 877-880.
51. Tanzi, R.E., Gusella, J.F., Watkins, P.C., Bruns, G.A.P., St. George-Hyslop, P.H., et al. (1987). Amyloid B protein gene: cDNA, mRNA distribution, and genetic linkage near the Alzheimer locus. *Science* 235: 880-884.
52. Robakis, N.K., Wisniewski, H.M., Jenkins, E.C., et al. (1987). Chromosome 21q21 sublocalization of gene encoding B-amyloid peptide in cerebral vessels and neuritic (senile) plaques of people with Alzheimer disease and Down syndrome. *Lancet* 1: 384-385.
53. Delabar, J.M., Goldgaber, D., Lamour, Y., et al. (1987). B-Amyloid gene duplication in Alzheimer's disease and karyotypically normal Down syndrome. *Science* 235: 1390-1392.
54. Schweber, M., Tuson, C., Shiloh, R., Ben-Neriah, Z. (1987). Triplication of chromosome 21 material in Alzheimer's disease. *Neurology* 37: 222.
55. St. George-Hyslop, P.H., Tanzi, R.E., Polinsky, R.J., et al. (1987). Absence of duplication of genes on chromosome 21 in familial and sporadic Alzheimer disease. *Science.* in press.
56. Van Broeckhoven, C., Genthe, A.M., Vandenbeghe, A., et al. (1987). Failure of familial Alzheimer's disease to segregate with the A4-amyloid gene in several European families. *Nature* 329: 153-155.
57. Tanzi, R.E., St. George-Hyslop, P.H., Haines, J.L., et al. (1987). The genetic defect in familial Alzheimer's disease is not tightly linked to the amyloid B-protein gene. *Nature* 329: 156-157.
58. Guiroy, D.C., Miyazaki, M., Multhaup, G., et al. (1987). Amyloid of neurofibrillary tangles od Guamanian parkinson-dementia and Alzheimer disease share identical amino acid sequence. *Proc. Natl. Acad. Sci. U.S.A.* 84: 2073-2077.
59. Personal communication.
60. Bondareff, W., Mountjoy, C.Q., Roth, M., Rossor, M., Ivefsen, L.L., and Reynolds, G.P. (1987). *Arch. Gen. Psychiatry* 44: 412.
61. Nee, L.E., Eldridge, R., Sunderland, T., et al. (1987). Dementia of the Alzheimer type: Clinical and family study of 22 twin pairs. *Neurology* 37: 359-363.

9

Down's Syndrome and the Measurement of Chromosome 21 DNA Amounts in Alzheimer's Disease

MIRIAM SCHWEBER / *Boston University School of Medicine, Boston, Massachusetts*

INTRODUCTION

Recombinant DNA (RDNA) techniques have been available for almost 20 years and have provided enormously powerful new ways to investigate biological problems at the molecular level. The effect must be analogous to the invention of the compound microscope; suddenly, the possibility of exploring entire new worlds is presented. Utilization of RDNA methods has provided tremendous increases in molecular knowledge and concepts at a rate described as "a frenetic pace of new discoveries" (1). However, there have been relatively few direct uses of the methods for genetic diagnostic purposes, despite early optimistic predictions of their applicability (2). There was a time lag between the invention of compound microscopes and improvements sufficient to permit widescale use; in similar fashion, the application of RDNA methods to genetic analysis and diagnosis of the hundreds of known genetic conditions has been relatively slow, despite intense efforts.

In some conditions with well-established genetic bases, RDNA analysis has provided a detailed understanding of the molecular changes involved, as in the thalessemias (3). However, so far, sickle cell anemia is the only genetic disorder involving a single base substitution that can be routinely diagnosed by RDNA techniques; this is possible because the change provides an altered, restriction enzyme site (4,5). Explorations of alternative approaches are continuing (6). For conditions with strong family patterns but unknown genetic location, the main strategy has been to establish alterations in restriction enzyme sites linked to the genetic locus, that is, by restriction fragment length polymorphism (RFLP) analysis (7). This approach has permitted relative localization for a number of genetic diseases (8) and has provided diagnostic capability for some, including Huntington's disease (9). Predictions of future applicability of RDNA methods in medical genetics has centered on such methods (10). These approaches assume a mutational model of genetic control. However, an appreciable number of genetic conditions involve only a change in the relative abundance of otherwise apparently normal DNA sequences. The most well known of these is Down's syndrome (DS), in which there are three instead of two copies of a specific segment on chromosome 21 (11,12).

It seems almost patently obvious that if the disorder being looked for involves only a change in the amount of certain DNAs present in the genome, the simplest way to test for that disorder is to measure the amount of those DNAs present in an individual. Despite numerous attempts, this has not been possible with RDNA methods until now because of methodological problems. This chapter is an account of the problems involved in the accurate quantification of individual samples by RDNA methods, the system developed to overcome them, and the use of such methods in the analysis of the causes of Alzheimer's disease (AD). The hypothesis that such measurements could be relevant to the causes of AD evolved from an examination of the evidence for a relationship between AD and the effects of aging in Down's syndrome (DS).

ALZHEIMER'S DISEASE AND THE EFFECTS OF AGING IN DOWN'S SYNDROME

In 1876, an article by Fraser with an appendix by Mitchel reported the occurrence of dementia among adults with DS; Mitchel also noted the effects of birth order on the frequency of DS in families (13). In 1929, Struwe suggested that the dementia seen in DS adults was of the AD type (14). Data were accumulated demonstrating that most DS adults over age 40 exhibited brain neuropathological changes similar to those found for AD (see 15-18). Thus, in 1966, Woodard stated that, for AD, "a genetic abnormality, such as trisomy 21, may be an important contributing factor" (p. 1164, 19). During the early 1980s, similarities of biochemical alterations in the brain in AD patients and older persons with DS were reported for a variety of neurotransmitters, metabolites, precursors and others (reviews in 18,20). At the epidemiological level, an interconnection between AD and DS was claimed because of an increased incidence of DS in families of familial AD probands when second- and third-degree relatives were included (21-24). Thus, a diverse body of evidence had been accumulated implying some kind of relationship between AD and the effects of aging in DS by 1982 when the first symposium on the topic was presented (25).

Reviews through the early 1980s stressed the limitations of various studies and generally concluded that exploring a relationship between AD and DS would not be informative. Thus, in that first symposium in 1982, Whalley argued that "the similarities, however, are relatively superficial" for AD and DS. The reasons advanced were the exceptional occurrence of older persons with DS who did not have the AD-type brain neuropathological changes, the absence of birth order effects in AD, and the lack of consistent chromosomal abnormalities in AD (26). His argument was supported by data showing no increase in DS in AD families in England, but the sample size was small and only included first-degree relatives (27); nonetheless, he maintained this position in 1984 (28). C. Epstein in 1983 considered that "pursuit of these relations has not been fruitful" (p. 173, 29) and concluded that "there is at present no evidence to support the notion that the genetic abnormalities in DS . . . directly cause[s] the AD changes" (p. 173, 29). Ingrahm agreed in 1984, mainly because of the discrepancy in reported rates of AD-type brain neuropathological changes in older persons with DS and the rates of clinically diagnosed dementia (30).

This lack of correspondence between laboratory findings of neuropathology (near to or at 100%) and those of overt dementia (estimated at 25-35%) (16,31-33) has been puzzling. Some neuropathologists simply stated that all DS adults develop AD on anatomical grounds (34); they include the author of a recent text (35). Others have argued that the neuropathological appearance in DS could not be caused by AD because of the behavioral findings, suggesting, instead, that the anatomical changes were due to a mimicking condition (31,32). Another proposed explanation for both the neuropathological and behavioral changes in adults with DS was that premature aging occurs in DS (32,36-40). Various editorials, articles, and reviews have favored this concept to explain the AD-type brain manifestations that occur with aging in persons with DS (15,20,41-44). A number of physical indicators have been adduced as evidence of premature aging in DS (reviewed in 15,20) but each has also been challenged (see 20,29). To explain the early development of AD in all DS adults by premature aging implies that AD should also be a normal part of the aging process and not a disease; such a concept has been regarded as incorrect for some time. If dementia is no longer regarded as an inevitable concomitant of normative aging (45), the development of dementia in adults with DS cannot be explained by an acceleration of normal aging processes. Even if there are physical changes in DS consistent with premature aging, the behavioral changes involved in dementia should not also be ascribed to them. Progeria, the classic condition of premature aging, involves no mental deterioration (46). The most sensitive indicator of aging in the central nervous system is the accumulation of lipofuscin granules (47); no undue increase was found in the brains of adults with DS (48). Thus, there is no evidence for premature aging in the brain of older persons with DS, nor does that concept explain the overt dementia that does develop in some adults with DS.

Subtle declines in cognition and reaction times have been reported as a function of aging in adults with DS (17,33,38,49-55), but interpretations have varied as to their extent and significance. The difficulties in determining the early signs of dementia in retarded persons have been stressed (16,51,54) and attention has recently focused on defining appropriate stages (55,56).

In comparing the effects of AD and aging in DS, it is important to differentiate irrelevant from meaningful evidence. A survey of autopsy data concluded that all persons with DS over age 36 exhibited full neuropathological signs of AD and that claimed exceptions were indefensible (16). Given the expected rate of DS in the general population of 1/1000 live births (57-59), reports of no increase in the DS frequency in AD families, based on small populations (60,61) and/or not including second- and third-degree relatives (27) are not material. In particular, arguments purporting to support (or negate) a relationship between DS and AD because of the presence (or absence) of parental age effects (particularly maternal ones) and/or birth order are totally irrelevant (26,61-66). These effects influence the rate of nondisjunction (67,68) that produces trisomy 21* (~96% of all DS; 58,59,67); they are *not* intrinsic to the basic cause of DS itself. Translocation DS* (~3% of all DS) is not due to nondisjunction and its incidence decreases with advancing maternal age (58,69,70). Whether there are parental age or birth order effects in AD may be of interest, but such data have no relevance to any relationship between AD and DS. Reports that equate DS with trisomy 21 (71, 72) do not clarify the relation to AD. Similarly, theories that purport to explain the relationship of AD and DS by postulating some type of effect on cell division as a cause of AD (72,73) confuse the effects of nondisjunction with those of the basic cause of DS.

Using the evidence from a variety of disciplines, it was possible to conclude that what all persons with DS develop with age was AD itself (74). The discrepancy in the rates of clinical diagnosis of dementia and neuropathological changes for adults with DS could be discounted by arguing that most of the early stages of AD involve losses in abilities that persons with DS never had (75). This argument implied that there should be a unitary genetic bases for both AD and DS. Given that DS is due only to a triplication of a limited segment of chromosome 21, if all persons with DS developed AD but not the reverse, the simplest explanation was that AD was caused by a triplication of a small subsection of DNA on chromosome 21 near to or within that DS DNA (74). The problem was to measure that amount.

QUANTITATIVE MEASUREMENTS OF DNA ON SOUTHERN BLOTS

The most frequent RDNA method involves Southern blot analysis. In standardized procedures, isolated genomic DNA is digested, electrophoresed, transferred to a filter, and probed with radioactively labeled sequences of interest with registration

*Trisomy 21 produces Down's syndrome due to the presence of three complete copies of chromosome 21 per nucleus. In translocation Down's syndrome, only a limited section of the long arm of chromosome 21 is present three times. Translocation Down's syndrome can be phenotypically identical to trisomy 21.

of the resultant hybrids' signal on x-ray film. Almost all of the immense amounts of molecular information garnered with this method have involved qualitative analyses, expressed as changes in position of the bands produced on the film. Quantitative results have been previously done to distinguish DS samples, but only with pooled measurements and extensive statistical treatment. Because measurements on individual samples were not possible, these could be used for neither diagnostic nor prospective purposes.

The problem of accurate quantification of single samples on Southern blots is complex because two sets of factors must be controlled: those arising from optical problems due to the film registration of the signal on film and those due to the biochemical procedures needed to generate the signal (76). The response of any film to an impinging signal is described by the Hurter-Driffield (H-D) equation of classic optics. As shown in Figure 1, this describes an S-shaped curve with well-defined, separate regions of response. To obtain reliable quantification, it is necessary to control the exposure of the signal so that it lies within the linear range of response of the film used (77). A measuring system is needed to calibrate the appropriate exposure, as a light meter does for a camera. Control of signals deposited on a film was studied in the 1950s in early bubble chamber experiments, since measurement of the width of the tracks produced on film can be used to determine the energy level of the particle making the track (78,79). In the studies described here, exposure control for Southern blots was achieved by incorporating the image of a silvered step-wedge gradient on each piece of film before the radioactive signal was deposited. Densitometric tracings of the step-wedge image permitted determination of the linear range of the response of the film used. The exposure of the filter could then be adjusted to regulate the intensity of the image produced by the radioactivity. The requirement for quantitative measurements is that the peak height of the densitometric tracing of each image from the filter be confined to the film's linear range of response, which is deter-

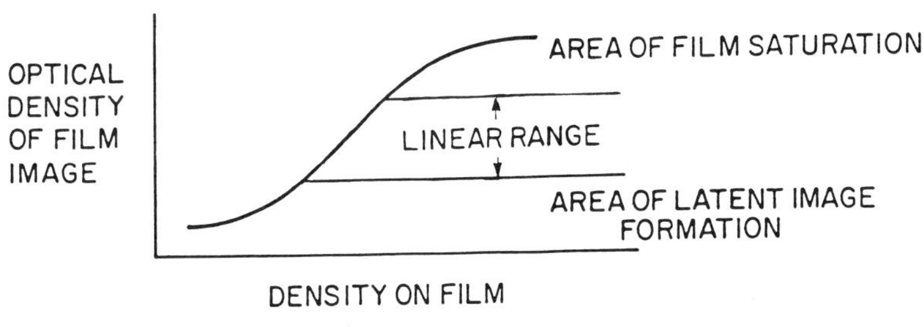

FIGURE 1 Idealized form of the Hurter-Driffield (H-D) curve showing the limited linear region of film response.

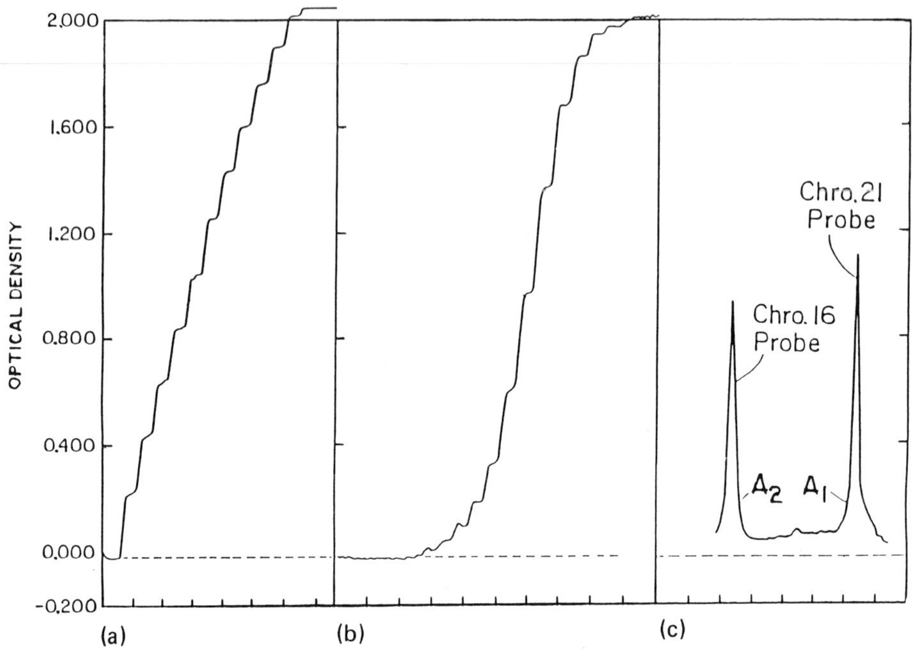

FIGURE 2 Computerized densitometric tracing directly of the step-wedge (a) and of its image (b) as registered on film (Kodak X Omat AR). The image produces the H-D curve. Only images whose heights lie within the linear range can provide accurate quantification (from the areas subsumed). Part (c) shows a Southern blot tracing of an expsure controlled for quantification (Eco RI digest probed with the SOD–1 subclone and ϵ-globin fragment).

mined by the tracing of the step-wedge image on that same piece of film. The limitation of the linear range of the standard Kodak x-ray film used for Southern blot analyses (i.e., its H-D curve) is shown in Figure 2.

The effects of the biochemical procedures were extensively tested. To determine the criticality of control, measurements were done on karyotyped fibroblast cell lines containing differing chromosomal 21 constitutions, specifically monosomy 21, disomy 21 (normals), and trisomy 21 (DS) cells. The number of chromosome 21s present relative to the number of other autosomes in each of these lines is 1/2, 2/2, and 3/2. However, these numerical relations of numbers of chromosomes are not to be expected when one measures amounts of DNA at the molecular level. (For example, if one used a probe for chromosome 21 that was size S and one from a reference chromosome present in normal amounts that was size 2S, the expected ratio for DS would be 0.75 [3S/⟦2 X 2S⟧], not 3/2.) When the criterion of discrimination between karyotyped fibroblast cell lines was used, blood and brain tissues were taken from normal, DS, and non-DS mentally retarded adults. Each was examined with a variety of enzymes, including those whose cutting patterns reversed the position for control and reference probe attachment; this ensured that differential transfer effects due to differences in molecular size of the genomic fragments on the gel did not affect the results.

The intensity of the signal produced on the film by a labeled DNA fragment on a Southern blot can be measured by the area subsumed under the peak it produces on a densitometric tracing. For each gel, there are a variety of effecting biochemical factors, some of which cannot be known. By using both a test and a reference chromosome, many of these can be cancelled so that:

$$A_1/A_2 = f[D_1/D_2]$$

where 1 refers to a test probe from chromosome 21 and 2 indicates a reference chromosome sequence, A is the area under the peaks generated by tracings of the bands produced on the film, and D is the amount of DNA measured by each probe. One would like to determine the ratio of D_1/D_2 directly, but the only parameter that can be measured is A_1/A_2. It is clear that there must be a relationship between the number of chromosomes present and the comparative amounts of D_1/D_2 and, as shown, there is a relationship between A_1/A_2 and D_1/D_2. Thus, determinations of A_1/A_2 can be informative for comparative purposes, but not for absolute values. Because some biochemical factors are exponential in nature (especially the radioactive decay curve of beta particles), the slope of the determinations of area ratios for different chromosome 21 constitutions potentially can differ in each gel run. Thus, the direct, numerical area ratios can only be compared within a single gel.

The reference chromosome probe used was an ϵ-globin insert of 1.2 Kb (80). For chromosome 21, a unique sequence fragment covering the Vth exon near the end of the 3' coding strand of superoxide dismutase-1 (SOD-1) was subcloned for us by Dr. Yoram Groner, Weizmann Institute, Israel, from the SOD-1 sequence (81,82). When exposures and biochemical conditions are controlled, differences are evident even before the areas are determined on both blots (Fig. 3) and tracings (Fig. 4) of cell types of different chromosomal composition. Repeat determinations of the ratios of different chromosome 21 cell lines are shown in Figure 5. Results from each individual gel produce a different curve of values; hence comparisons of the numerical values between gels are meaningless. However, within each gel there is distinct and reproducible differentiation of the individual samples from the different chromosome 21 cell lines. The numerical values of the area ratios generated by the two probes can be used directly to characterize an unknown sample if it is run on the same gel with at least two standards of known chromosomal constitution under controlled optical and biochemical conditions. Identification is made directly from the single tracing of a

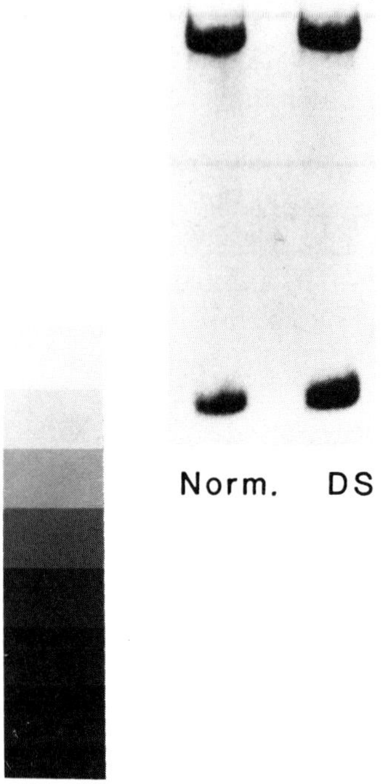

FIGURE 3 Film image of a controlled Southern blot from white blood cells of a normal and an adult with Down's syndrome (DS). The step-wedge image extends through the top of Fig. 3, but only the central steps can be registered on the film.

single gel lane containing the DNA from a single individual. There are no problems with differential gel loading in different lanes, relative intensity of labeling of the two fragments, differential transfer of fragments with differing molecular weight, or other factors. Coded, blind samples of DS and normal bloods were successfully differentiated using this approach. Such determinations provided the assurance that examination of AD samples could be meaningful.

FIGURE 5 A_1/A_2 ratios of areas subsumed under controlled conditions as described with repeated testing of karyotypes fibroblast cell lines. The results discriminate between chromosomal types consistently within a gel, but the absolute values vary between gels.

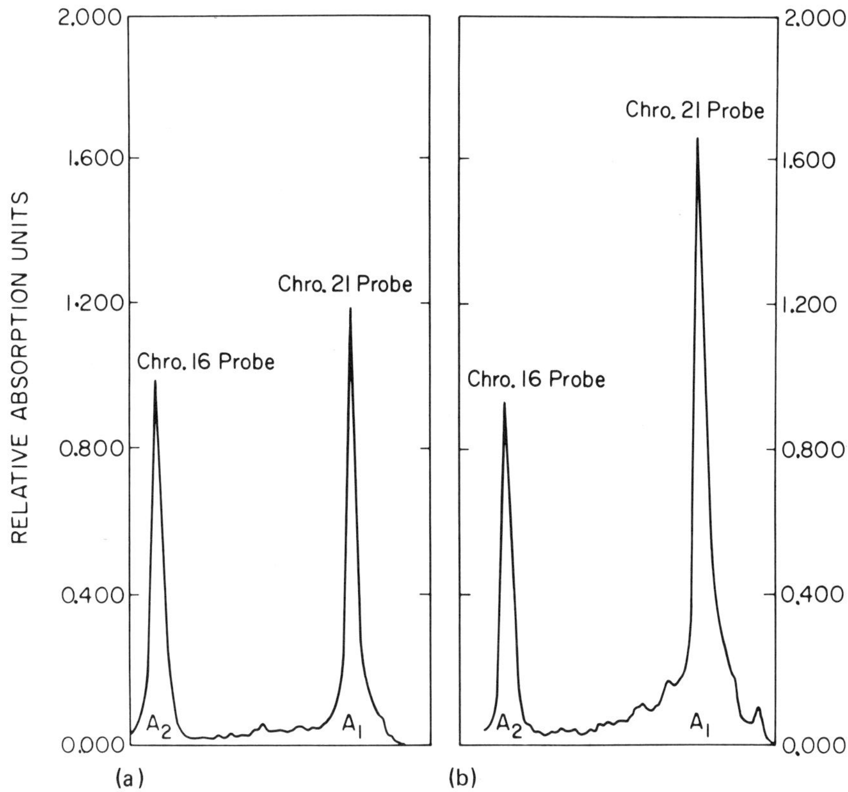

FIGURE 4 Computerized densitometric tracing (Shimadzu Dual-Wave length TLC scanner CS-930CS) of the Southern blot in Fig. 3. Chromosome 16 DNA amounts (detected by the ϵ-globin probe) are similar in both samples; the difference in chromosome 21 amounts (from the SOD-1 subclone) is evident. Ratios are obtained directly from area print-outs. Normal (a) and Down's syndrome (b).

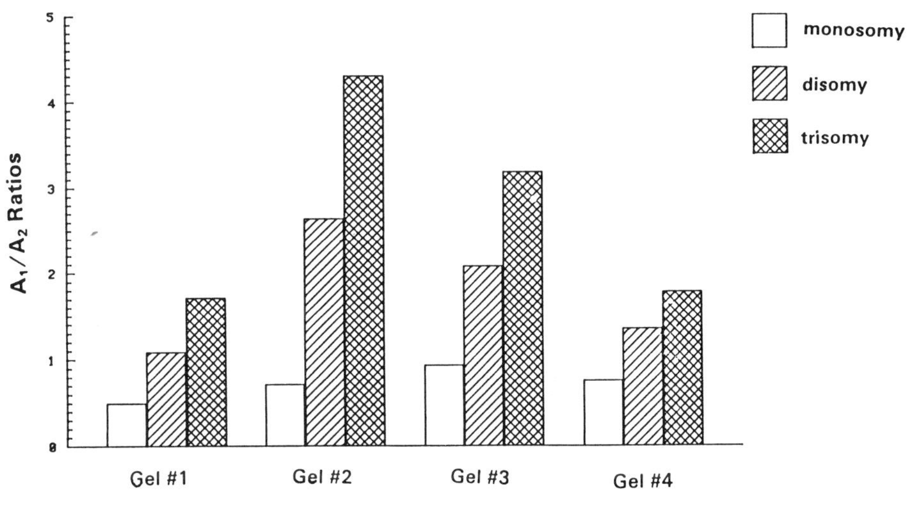

TABLE 1 Tissue Samples Examined

Chromosomal Type	Characteristics	Tissue	N	Age	Sex	Source
Monosomy 21	Karyotyped	Fibroblasts	1	6 mo	M	a
Disomy 21 (normals)	Fully functional	White cells	10	53 yr	F+M	b
	Autopsied	Brain	2	64/61 yr	F/M	c
	Autopsied	Brain	2	73/73 yr	M/M	d
	Karyotyped	Fibroblasts	2	1 mo/8 mo	M/M	e
(non-DS)	Retarded	White cells	4	36-40 yr	F+M	f
Trisomy 21-DS	Karyotyped	Fibroblasts	2	3 mo/12 hr	M/M	e
	Clinical DS	White cells	6	26-40 yr	F+M	f
Alzheimer's disease	Autopsy; fam.	Fibroblasts	2	53/47 yr	F/F	g[1,2]
	Autopsy, 3 sporadic, 1?	Brain	4	56-96 yr	M+F	c,d,h[1,2]

	Clinical AD, fam.	White cells	4	47-76 yr	All M	i,j[1,2,3]
	Clinical AD, sporadic	White cells	4	62-72 yr	All M	j[4,5,6,7]
	Autopsy, family	Immortalized lymphoblasts	1	81 yr	F	k

There was full autopsy verification of brain samples of both normals and persons with Alzheimer's disease (AD) and also for the AD cell lines of fibroblasts (two sisters) and the lymphoblast line immortalized with Epstein-Barr virus. The eight AD white blood cell samples were from clinically diagnosed patients; the four of these classified as sporadic had fingerprint patterns similar to those of Down's syndrome and long-lived parents and siblings with no indication of dementia. The four classified as familial had close family relatives diagnosed as having AD, many with autopsy verification. For the total of 15 persons with Alzheimer's disease, 7 had familial disease (from 6 unrelated families), 7 had sporadic-type, and 1 was unknown; in classification by age of onset, 10 were early-onset ($<$age 65) and 5 late-onset ($>$65).

Sources: [a]Cell line GM 0137A from Human Cell Repository, Camden, NJ. [b]Blood Bank, University Hospital, Boston University Medical Center, Boston, MA. [c]Dr. Edward Bird, Brain Bank, Belmont, MA. [d]Dr. Judith Marquis, Department of Pharmacology, Boston University School of Medicine, Boston, MA. [e]Repository for Mutant Human Cell Strains, Montreal Children's Hospital, Montreal, QUE. [f]Dr. Florence Lai, Eunice K. Shriver Center, Waltham, MA. [g]Lines #AG4401B and AG4402 (sisters) from the Cell Repository, Camden, NJ, via Dr. Frank Zemlan, Department of Genetics, University of Cincinnati, OH. [h]Dr. Brent Vogt, Department of Anatomy, Boston University School of Medicine, Boston, MA. [i]Dr. Robert Feldman, Department of Neurology, Boston University School of Medicine, Boston, MA. [j]Dr. Benjamin Selzer, GRECC Unit, Veterans Administration Hospital, Bedford, MA. [k]Dr. Gerard Schellenberg, Division of Neurology, University of Washington, and Dr. Thomas Bird, Division of Neurology, Veterans Administration Medical Center, Seattle, WA.

[1-4]Specific patients with Alzheimer's disease identified in Table 2.

TABLE 2 Examples of A_1/A_2 Ratios of Chromosome 21/16 Probe Signals

Samples		Gel 1	Gel 2	Gel 3	Gel 4	Gel 5	Gel 6	Gel 7	Gel 8	Gel 9
Disomy 21	White cells	1.10		1.07	0.47		1.53	1.76	1.45	1.38
	Fibroblasts		1.80							
	Brains			1.04		1.73				
non-DS	White cells		1.80							
Trisomy 21	White cells	2.73	2.86	1.61	1.24	2.89	2.29	3.70	2.07	2.56
	White cells			1.63						
	Fibroblasts		2.80		1.22					
Alzheimer's brains		2.69[d]	2.70[d]	1.67[d]	1.19[d]	2.68[h1]				
Brains		2.45[c]		1.69[c]		2.65[c]				
Fibroblasts				1.70[g1]						
Immortalized lymphoblasts										2.6[k]
White cells		2.64[i]					2.32[j2]	3.71[j2]	2.06[j1]	
White cells							2.24[j4]	3.60[j6]	2.04[j3]	
White cells							2.28[j7]		2.10[j5]	
Enzyme used		Eco	Eco	dIII	PST	Eco	Eco	Eco	Eco	Eco

Each ratio shown was directly obtained from a single tracing of a single lane containing genomic DNA of a single individual. Within a gel, the ratios of Alzheimer's disease samples were similar to those of the patients with Down's syndrome, both differing from the normals. For comparisons between gels (i.e., horizontally), normalization of this direct data is required.

Non-DS, mentally retarded persons without Down's syndrome; white cells, mostly leukocytes with some lymphocytes from fresh blood samples; Eco, Eco RI; dIII, Hin dIII; PST, PST *T*. Superscripts designate specific Alzheimer's disease samples listed in Table 1.

ALZHEIMER'S DISEASE

Measurements were made on carefully selected samples from a variety of sources (Table 1). All AD tissues produced area ratios of amounts of DNA similar to that of trisomy 21 tissues, not that of disomy 21 when all three were run on the same gel (76,83). Sample results are shown in Figures 6 and 7 and Table 2. The 15 AD samples included 4 different tissue types and all classifications of AD (7 sporadic cases, 7 familial ones from 6 unrelated families, and one unknown: 10 early and 5 late onset). Seven samples had AD diagnosis confirmed at autopsy. Eight blood samples were taken from living patients. Of these, four had strong family patterns; the other four appeared to be sporadic and were chosen because their fingerprint patterns displayed a high frequency of ulnar loops as found in DS (84-86). All samples were tested with various enzymes. All AD tissues examined produced results

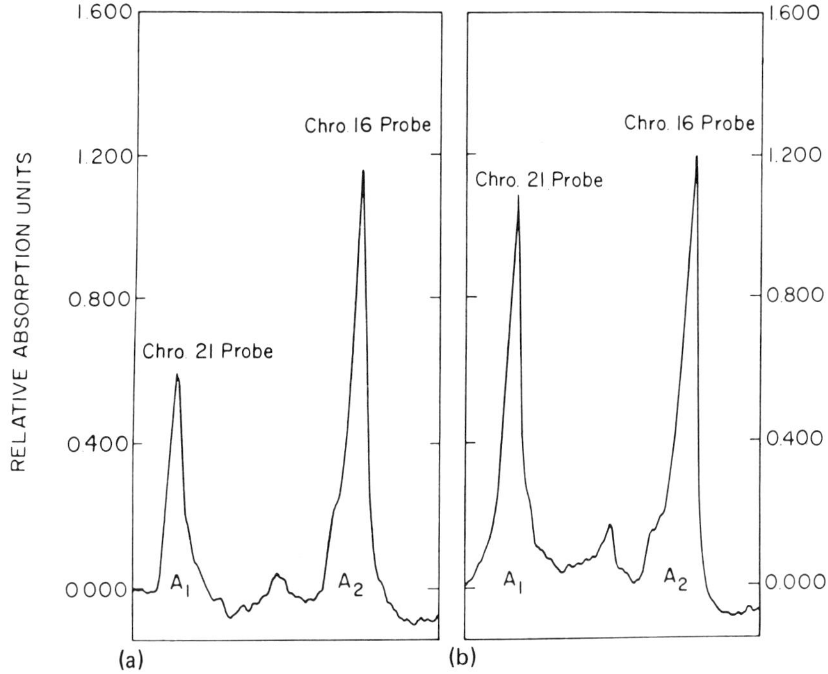

FIGURE 6 Tracings of controlled Southern blot films of brain DNA of a normal individual (a) and an Alzheimer's disease (AD) victim (b), both with full neuropathological verification. Chromosome 16 amounts are comparable; increased amount of chromosome 21 probe attachment in the AD sample is evident. (PST *T* digests).

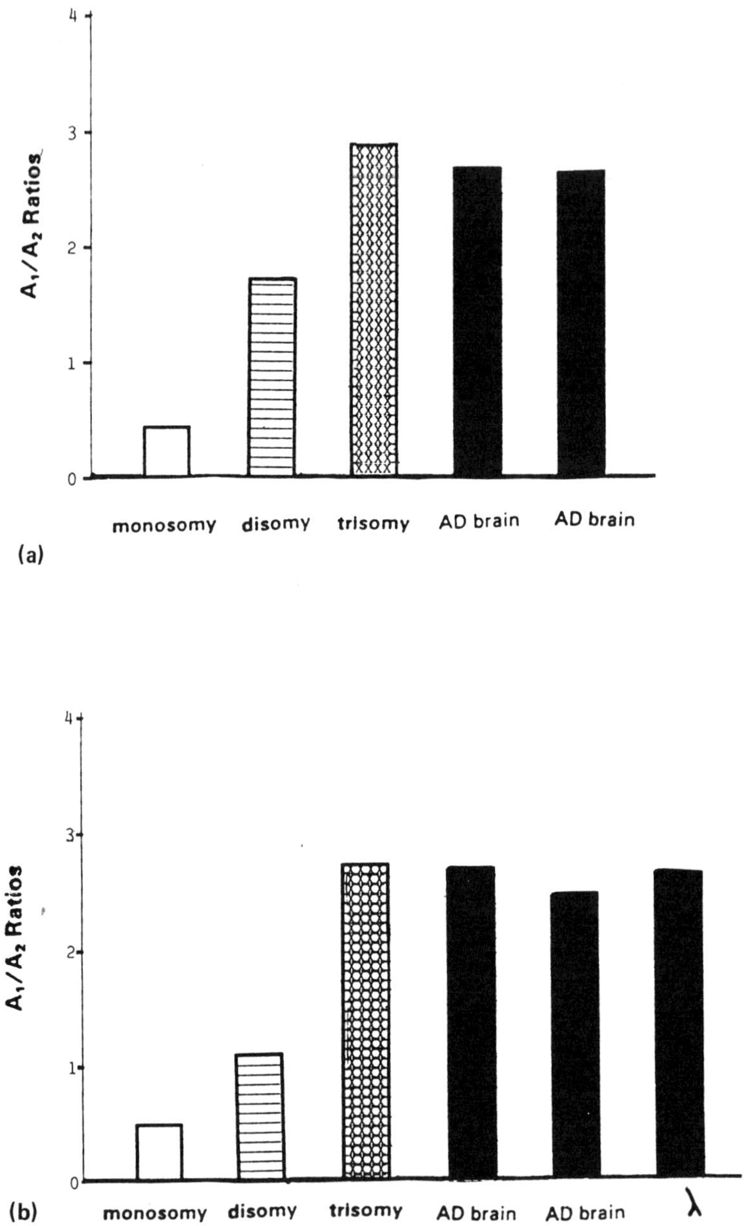

FIGURE 7 A1/A2 ratios obtained on individual gels. Values obtained for AD are similar to those of the trisomy 21 cells. Area ratios of gel 5 on Table 2 plus monosomy value of 0.44 (7a); of gel 1 plus monosomy value of 0.5 (7b).

similar to those found for DS. There were minimal differences between repeated tracings of the same lane or between different lanes on the same gel containing samples with the same chromosomal classification (see Table 2).

With the establishment of consistency of determinations within a gel, normalization of the data between gels could be justified. Because extrapolations of data obtained upon repeated examinations of the known chromosome 21 lines do not pass through the origin (Fig. 5), a log relation could not be used. A simple equation was formulated to normalize the numerical results obtained on different gels

TABLE 3 Statistical Treatment

A_1/A_2 Data Normalized

Category	Number	Expected $\bar{R}$	Observed $\bar{R}$	Standard deviation
Monosomy 21	15	>1	1.91	0.27
Disomy 21	18	1.0	1.007	0.068
Trisomy 21 (Down's syndrome)	30	0.0	-0.004	0.09
Alzheimer's disease	62	?	0.009	0.11

Probability that Differences in Observed $\bar{R}$ are Due to Chance

Categories Compared	Probability
Monosomy 21 vs. disomy 21	<0.0001
Monosomy 21 vs. trisomy 21	<0.0001
Monosomy 21 vs. Alzheimer's disease	<0.0001
Disomy 21 vs. trisomy 21	<0.0001
Disomy 21 vs. Alzheimer's disease	<0.0001
Trisomy 21 vs. Alzheimer's disease	0.56

To compare the area ratios from different experiments, the observed data were normalized by calculating a factor, R, using the formula:

$$R = \frac{(A_1/A_2)_{DS} - (A_1/A_2)_X}{(A_1/A_2)_{DS} - (A_1/A_2)_n}$$

where DS, Down's syndrome; X, the unknown; n, the normal. It is clear that if the A_1/A_2 value of X is the same as that of the DS, R = 0, whereas if the value of X is the same as that of the normal, R = 1. There is no significance in the differences in sign observed between A_1/A_2 values obtained.

Comparisons of the mean R values obtained were done using t tests with provision for unequal variance. It was highly unlikely that the observed difference between the mean Rs for any of the categories could be due to chance effects except for that between trisomy 21 and Alzheimer's disease.

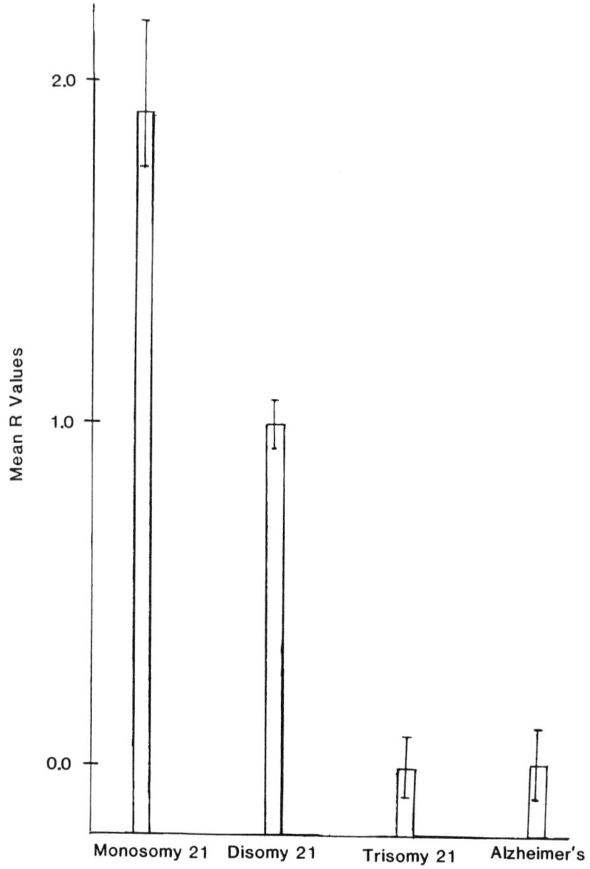

FIGURE 8 Graphic representation of mean R values shown in Table 3. Bars denote standard deviations.

(Table 3). Probabilities were obtained using t-test comparisons of the means of the compilations. These indicated that differences observed between all categories were highly unlikely to be due to chance except in the case of DS compared with AD (Table 3; Fig. 8). The likelihood that the difference observed between the compiled means for AD and DS was only a chance effect argues that the DNA is present in similar amounts in these two categories on chromosome 21 near the 3' end of SOD-1.

The results obtained suggest that a possible basis of all types of AD may be an increase in amount of a small subsection of DNA on chromosome 21 to the level of DNA present in DS; the simplest hypothesis is that triplication of that DNA occurs in both conditions. Since the gene for SOD-1 has been localized to chromosome band 21q22 (87-89), the same site as DS DNA (11,12), the data further argue that the DNA region increased in AD is located near the DS DNA. The development of dementia and autopsy confirmation of AD-type neuropathological changes in two translocation DS individuals (76) further support this localization.

No increase in DNA at the SOD-1 locus was reported from the blood of three AD cases by Delabar et al. (90), who used a dot blot series as an exposure standard and pooled five repeats for each measurement. The cloned DNA used was pS61-10 (D. Goldgaber, personal communication, 1987), isolated by Y. Groner (81,82). In similar fashion, no increase in SOD-1 DNA in AD was found by RFLP analysis using a full-sequence clone (91). We had not found DNA increases in AD cases using pS61-10 several years ago. There were several possible reasons for this, including the inclusion on pS61-10 of sequences homologous to four pseudogenes located on four other chromosomes (92,93). Moreover, the reported lack of increased SOD-1 in the brains of AD victims (94) made it unlikely that increased DNA levels in AD would extend through the complete SOD sequence. Thus, we proceeded to use the subclone at the end of the SOD-1 locus discussed here. It should be noted, however, that the two AD fibroblast cell lines tested here have been found to have high SOD-1 levels, comparable to those of DS individuals (F. Zemlan, personal communication, 1987). Thus, it may be that DNA triplication extends through the SOD-1 locus in some AD cases.

With the recent finding that the amyloid β-protein deposited in AD is coded by a gene on chromosome 21 (71,95-98), the possibility has been examined that amplification at that locus in AD results in overexpression (90,91,99,100; and Chapters 6, 11, 12, and 13). My theoretical presentation in 1985 of a unitary genetic hypothesis for AD and DS reasoned that an increased DNA level in AD should involve *only* a very minute sequence located near to or within the DS DNA location (74). From comparisons with DS, specific regulatory effects were suggested without overexpression of complete structural genes due to increased dosage. With no appreciable increase in SOD in the brain in AD and the localization of the amyloid locus millions of bases away from the DS chromosomal site, amplification of either locus in AD would be unexpected on the basis of the original hypothesis. Other implications of chromosome 21 in AD include the existence and location of a FAD gene defined by RFLP analysis (91, 101, 102, and Chapters 6, 8, and Invited Editorial Comments for Part II). This seems to be located even farther from the DS site than the amyloid locus and, thus, would be even less likely to be implicated by the results reported here. Another chromosome 21 debate concerns the ETS-2 location that Delabar et al. reported was increased in AD (90). The results reported here raise other questions including whether the increase in DNA for AD occurs only at the 3' end of the coding strand of SOD-1; whether there are variable breakage points and triplication extents along chromosome 21 in AD; whether such genetic variability can be related to the heterogeneity of the clinical manifestations of AD; and determination of the relation of the DS and AD DNA locations.

DISCUSSION

The results reported here suggest that familial AD is initiated by a germ line event that produces triplication of a subsection of chromosome 21. A variety of genetic mechanisms could be responsible. Although not required, the simplest model would be the doubling within chromosome 21 of a DNA subsegment. Persons who inherit this type of chromosomal abnormality would develop familial AD. Since they have the defect systemically, early diagnosis should be feasible, perhaps even at a prenatal stage. The detection of an increased amount of the DNA of chromosome 21 in both the brains and blood of sporadic AD cases suggests that the causative event could occur either in the germ line or in somatic tissue very early in development. This finding could also be adduced as an argument in favor of the concept that most AD is really genetically based and familial.

Part of the extraordinary difficulty with early diagnosis of AD is due to its wide range of symptoms and manifestations. Rates of misdiagnosis have been estimated at 20-50% (103-107). Currently, the only definitive diagnostic criteria is provided by autopsy. Increased understanding of the causes of AD should permit increased delineation of the mechanisms of AD effects; improved treatments could result. Clarification of the relationship of AD and DS should provide a new range of insights into the causes and classification of both conditions, and could have relevance for improved understanding of the normal processes of aging. For instance, it may be inappropriate to refer to an "AD gene" at present for the location discussed here. We use "DS DNA" for the genetic effects involved in DS because the pattern of control includes regulatory effects on genes located on chromosomes other than 21 as well as gene dosage effects of chromosome 21 loci (29,108). The multiple biochemical and anatomical effects of AD may involve similar regulatory phenomena (74). The implication of the ETS-2 site on chromosome 21 seems suggestive in this regard. Investigation of such possibilities might produce new, and it is hoped, more effective therapeutic strategies for AD.

The method of controlled quantification of Southern blots described here requires only a single tracing of a single gel lane containing the DNA of a single individual on a single Southern blot to produce meaningful results. Because of its possible applicability to all categories of AD, this method may provide a means for improved clinical diagnosis. This could permit early clinical intervention. It will take a great deal of effort to ascertain the possibilities, including that of predictive, presymptomatic diagnosis.

At present, various ethical and social issues center around persons with DS and AD; many of these issues have public health implications. The development of effective, early diagnostic procedures may raise additional new sets of considerations. The hope is that such issues can be successfully confronted; the assumption is that increased understanding and knowledge can someday be beneficial.

ACKNOWLEDGMENTS

The research described here was supported by a grant from the Retirement Research Foundation and an Allied Corporation/Alzheimer Disease and Related Disorders Foundation Faculty Scholar Award. Assistance in these studies was provided by Drs. R. Shiloh and Z. Ben-Neriah, and Ms. Clare Tuson and Francine Dzialo. Statistical assistance was provided by Dr. L. Adrienne Cupples, Karen Fung, and especially Dr. James Crow. Dr. Nick Proudfoot, Oxford University, England, kindly supplied the ϵ-globin probe. Special thanks are due to Dr. Yoram Groner, Weizmann Institute, Israel, who provided the SOD-1 subclone. The sources listed in Table 1 all generously supplied tissue samples; special cooperation came from Dr. Florence Lai, who provided blood samples from the Shriver Institute, Waltham, MA.

REFERENCES

1. Watson, J. (1986). Foreword. In: *Molecular Biology of Homo sapiens*, CSHSQB LI, New York, Cold Spring Harbor Laboratory Press, pp. XV-XVI.
2. Kurnit, D., and Hoehn, H. (1979). Prenatal diagnosis of human genome variation. *Annu. Rev. Genet.* 13: 235-258.
3. Antonarakis, S.E., Kazazian, H.H., and Orkin, S.H. (1985). DNA polymorphism and the molecular pathology of the human globin gene cluster. *Hum. Genet.* 69: 1-14.
4. Chang, J.C., and Kan, Y.W. (1982). A sensitive new prenatal test for sickle cell anemia. *N. Engl. J. Med.* 307: 30-32.
5. Orkin, S.H., Little, P.F., Kazazian, H.H., and Boehm, C.D. (1982). Improved detection of the sickle mutation by DNA analysis. *N. Engl. J. Med.* 307: 32-36.
6. Myers, R.M., and Maniatis, T. (1986). Recent advances in the development of methods for detecting single-base substitutions associated with human genetic diseases. In: *Molecular Biology of Homo sapiens*, CSHSQB LI, New York, Cold Spring Harbor Laboratory Press, pp. 275-284.
7. de Martinville, B., Wyman, A., White, R., and Francke, U. (1982). Assignment of the first random RFLP locus (RRO1) to a region of human chromosome 14. *Am. J. Hum. Genet.* 34: 216-226.
8. See *Molecular Biology of Homo sapiens*, CSHSQB LI, New York, Cold Spring Harbor Laboratory Press, 1986, pp. 309-410.
9. St. George-Hyslop, P.H., et al., Chapter 8, this volume.
10. Caskey, C.T. (1987). Disease diagnosis by recombinant DNA methods. *Science* 236: 1223-1229.

11. Patterson, D., and Schandle, V. (1982). A comparison of Chinese hamster/human hybrid cells containing different fragments of chromosome 21 using cytogenetic, biochemical, and molecular approaches. In: *Recombinant DNA Applications to Human Disease.* Banbury Report #14, C. Caskey and R. White (Eds.) New York, Cold Spring Harbor Laboratory Press, pp. 215-223.
12. Summit, R. (1982). Chromosome 21; specific segments that cause the phenotype of Down syndrome. In: *Trisomy 21 (Down Syndrome) Research Perspectives.* National Institute of Child Health, Developmental Mental Retardation Research Center Series, F. de la Cruz and P. Gerald (Eds.) Baltimore, University Park Press, pp. 225-236.
13. Mitchell, A. (1876). With notes on sixty-two cases. Appended to M. Fraser, Kalmyc idiocy: Report of a case with autopsy. *Mental Sci.* 22: 174-179.
14. Struwe, W. (1929). Histopathologische untersucheungen uber entstehung und wesen der senilen plaques. *Acta Neurol. Psychiatry* 122: 299-306.
15. Oliver, C., and Holland, A. J. (1986). Down's syndrome and Alzheimer's disease: A review. *Psychol. Med.* 16: 307-322.
16. Schweber, M. (1989). Alzheimer's Disease and Down Syndrome. In: *Alzheimer's Disease and Related Disorders,* K. Iqbal, H. Wisniewski, and B. Winblad (Eds.) New York, Alan Liss Publishers, in press.
17. Wisniewski, Wisniewski, H., and Wen, G.Y. (1985). Occurrence of neuropathological changes and dementia of Alzheimer's disease in Down's syndrome. *Ann. Neurol.* 17: 278-282.
18. Coyle, J.T., Oster-Granite, M.L., and Gearhart, J.D. (1986). The neurobiologic consequences of Down syndrome. *Brain Res. Bull.* 16: 773-787.
19. Woodard, J. (1966). Alzheimer's disease in late adult life. *Am. J. Pathol.* 49: 1157-1169.
20. Balzas, R., and Brookbanks, B.W. (1985). Neurochemical approaches to the pathogenesis of Down's syndrome. *J. Ment. Defic. Res.* 29: 1-14.
21. Heston, L., Mastri, A., Anderson, E., and White, J. (1981). Dementia of the Alzheimer type. Clinical genetics, natural history, and associated conditions. *Arch. Gen. Psychiatry* 38: 1085-1090.
22. Heston, L. (1982). Alzheimer's dementia and Down's syndrome; genetic evidence suggesting an association. *Ann. N.Y. Acad. Sci.* 450: 29-38.
23. Heston, L. (1983). Dementia of the Alzheimer type. In: *Biological Aspects of Alzheimer's Disease,* Banbury Report #15, R. Katzman (Ed.) New York, Cold Spring Harbor Laboratory Press, pp. 183-192.
24. Heyman, A., Wilkinson, W., Hurwitz, B., Schmechel, D., Sigmon, A., Weinberg, T., Helms, M., and Swift, M. (1983). Alzheimer's disease: Genetic aspects and associated clinical disorders. *Ann. Neurol.* 14: 507-515.
25. Sinex, F.M., and Merril, C. (Eds.) (1982). *Alzheimer's Disease, Down's Syndrome, and Aging. Ann. N.Y. Acad. Sci.* 396.
26. Whalley, L. (1982). The dementia of Down's syndrome and its relevance to aetiological studies of Alzheimer's disease. *Ann. N.Y. Acad. Sci.* 396: 39-54.
27. Whalley, L., Carothes, A., Collyer, S., de Mey, R., and Frackiewicz, A. (1982). A study of familial factors in Alzheimer's disease. *Br. J. Psychiatry* 140: 249-256.

28. Wright, A., and Whalley, L. (1984). Genetics, ageing and dementia. *Br. J. Psychiatry* 145: 20-38.
29. Epstein, C. (1983). Down's syndrome and Alzheimer's disease: Implications and approaches. In: *Biological Aspects of Alzheimer's Disease*, Banbury Report #15, R. Katzman (Ed.) New York, Cold Spring Harbor Laboratory Press, pp. 169-182.
30. Ingrahm, V. (1984). The relationship between Down's syndrome and Alzheimer's Disease. In: *Alzheimer's Disease: Advances in Basic Research and Therapies*, R. Wurtman, S. Corkin, and J. Growdon (Eds.) Proceedings, 3d Meeting of the International Study Group on Treatment of Memory Disorders Associated with Aging, Zurich, Switzerland, pp. 449-452.
31. Ropper, A., and Williams, R. (1980). Relationship between plaques, tangles, and dementia in Down syndrome. *Neurology* 30: 639-678.
32. Wisniewski, K., and Wisniewski, H. (1983). Age-associated changes and dementia in Down's syndrome. In: *Alzheimer's Disease*, B. Reisberg (Ed.) New York, Free Press, pp. 319-326.
33. Wisniewski, H., and Rabe, A. (1986). Discrepancy between Alzheimer-type neuropathology and dementia in people with Down syndrome. *Ann. N.Y. Acad. Sci.* 477: 247-260.
34. Ellis, W., McCulloch, J., and Corley, C. (1974). Presenile dementia in Down's syndrome. *Neurology* 24: 101-106.
35. Bundey, S. (1985). *Genetics and Neurology*. New York, Churchill Livingstone.
36. Jervis, G. (1970). Premature senility in Down's syndrome. *Ann. N.Y. Acad. Sci.* 171: 559-561.
37. Martin, G. (1977). Genetic syndromes in man with potential relevance to the pathology of aging. *Birth Defects* 14: 5-39.
38. Wisniewski, K., Howe, J., Williams, D., and Wisniewski, H. (1978). Precocious aging and dementia in patients with Down's syndrome. *Biol. Psychiatry* 13: 619-626.
39. Hirabayashi, K., Ideda, K., Shimokawa, K., and Orthner, H. (1979). Vorzetiges gehirnaltern bei Down-syndrom. *Folia Psychiatr. Neurol. Jpn.* 33: 81-96.
40. Wisniewski, K., French, J., Rosen, J., Kozlowski, P., Tenner, M., and Wisniewski, H. (1982). Basal ganglia calcification in Down's syndrome—another manifestation of premature aging. *Ann. N.Y. Acad. Sci.* 396: 179-190.
41. Scroggins, C., and Patterson, D. (1982). Down's syndrome as a model disease. *Arch. Intern. Med.* 142: 462-464.
42. Editorial. (1985). Aging in Down's syndrome. *Lancet* 1: 855-856.
43. Fishman, M. (1986). Will the study of Down syndrome solve the riddle of Alzheimer disease? *J. Pediatr.* 108: 627-629.
44. Hurley, A., and Sovner, R. (1986). Dementia, mental retardation and Down's syndrome. *Psychiatr. Aspects Ment. Retard. Rev.* 5: 39-43.
45. Rowe, J.W., and Kahn, R.L. (1987). Human aging: Usual and successful. *Science* 237: 143-149.
46. Villee, D. (1983). Progeric syndrome. In: *Intervention in the Aging Process. Part A. Quantitation, Epidemiology and Clinical Research*, W. Regelson and F.M. Sinex (Eds.) New York, Alan R. Liss, pp. 151-168.

47. Mann, D., Yates, P., and Stamp, J. (1978). Relationship of lipofucsin pigment to ageing in the human nervous system. *J. Neurol. Sci.* 35: 83-93.
48. Mann, D., Yates, P., and Marcyniuk, B. (1984). Relationship between pigment accumulation and age in Alzheimer's disease and Downs syndrome. *Acta Neuropathol.* (*Berl.*) 63: 72-77.
49. Owens, D., Dawson, J., and Losin, S. (1971). Alzheimer's disease in Down's syndrome. *Am. J. Ment. Defic.* 75: 606-612.
50. Dalton, A., Crapper, D., and Schlotterer, E. (1974). Alzheimer's disease in Down's syndrome; visual retention deficits. *Cortex* 10: 366-377.
51. Miniszek, N. (1983). Development of Alzheimer disease in Down syndrome individuals. *Am. J. Ment. Defic.* 87: 177-185.
52. Thase, M., Tigner, R., Smeltzer, D., and Liss, L. (1984). Age-related neuropsychological deficits in Down's syndrome. *Biol. Psychiatry* 19: 571-585.
53. Dalton, A., and Crapper-MacLachlan, D. (1984). Incidence of memory deterioration in aging persons with Down's syndrome. In: *Perspectives and Progress in Mental Retardation. Vol. II. Biomedical Aspects*, J. Berg (Ed.) Baltimore, University Park Press, pp. 55-62.
54. Hewitt, K., Carter, G., and Jancar, J. (1985). Ageing in Down's syndrome. *Br. J. Psychiatry* 147: 58-62.
55. Wisniewski, K., Dalton, A., Crapper-McLachlan, M., Wen, G., and Wisniewski, H. (1985). Alzheimer disease in Down syndrome: Clinico-pathological studies. *Neurology* 35: 957-961.
56. Wisniewski, K., and Hill, A. (1985). Clinical aspects of dementia in mental retardation and developmental disabilities. In: *Aging and Developmental Disabilities: Issues and Approaches*, M. Janicki and H. Wisniewski (Eds.) Baltimore, Paul Brookes, pp. 195-210.
57. Adams, M., Erickson, J., Layde, P., and Oakley, G. (1981). Down syndrome. Recent trends in the United States. *JAMA* 246: 758-760.
58. Hook, E. (1981). Down syndrome: Its frequency in human populations and some factors pertinent to variation in rates. In: *Trisomy 21 (Down Syndrome) Research Perspectives.* National Institute of Child Health, Developmental Mental Retardation Research Center Series, F. de la Cruz and P. Gerald (Eds.) Baltimore, University Park, pp. 3-68.
59. Mikkelsen, M. (1982). Down syndrome; current stage of cytogenetic epidemiology. In: *Human Genetics, Part B; Medical Aspects.* New York. Alan R. Liss, pp. 297-309.
60. Nee, L., Polinsky, R., Eldridge, R., Weingartner, H., Smallberg, S., and Ebert, M. (1983). A family with histologically confirmed Alzheimer's disease. *Arch. Neurol.* 40: 203-208.
61. Amaducci, L.A., Fratiglioni, L., Rocca, W.A., Fieschi, C., Livrea, P., Pedone, D., Bracco, L., Lippi, A., Gandolfo, C., Bino, G., Prencipe, M., Bonatti, M., Girotti, F., Carella, F., Tabolato, B., Ferla, S., Lenzi, G., Carolei, A., Gambi, A., Grigoletto, F., and Schoenberg, B. (1986). Risk factors for clinically diagnosed Alzheimer's disease: A case controlled study of an Italian population. *Neurology* 36: 1922-1931.

62. Cohen, D., Eisdorfer, C., and Leverenz, J. (1982). Alzheimer's disease and maternal age. *J. Am. Gerontol. Soc.* 10: 656-659.
63. Knesevich, J., LaBarge, E., Martin, R., Danziger, W., and Berg, L. (1982). Birth order and maternal age effect in dementia of the Alzheimer type. *Psychiatry Res.* 7: 345-350.
64. Growdon, J., and Rasmussen, S. (1983). Parental age as a risk factor in Alzheimer's disease. *Ann. Neurol.* 13: 674-676.
65. Cohen, D., and English, D. (1985). A case controlled study of maternal age in Alzheimer's disease. *J. Am. Geriatr. Soc.* 33: 167-169.
66. White, J., McGue, M., and Heston, L. (1986). Fertility and parental age in Alzheimer's disease. *J. Gerontol.* 41: 40-43.
67. Hook, E.B. (1985). Maternal age, paternal age, and human chromosome abnormality; nature, magnitude, etiology, and mechanisms of effects. *Basic Life Sci.* 36: 117-132.
68. Carothers, A. (1987). Down syndrome and maternal age: The effect of erroneous assignment of parental origin. *Am. J. Hum. Genet.* 40: 147-150.
69. Hook, E. (1984). Parental age and unbalanced Robertsoninan translocations associated with Down syndrome and Patau syndrome; comparison with maternal and paternal age effects for 47, +21 and 47, +13. *Ann. Hum. Genet.* 48: 313-325.
70. Hamerton, J. (1981). Frequency of mosaicism, translocation, and other variants of Trisomy 21. In: *Trisomy 21 (Down Syndrome) Research Perspectives*, National Institute of Child Health, Developmental Mental Retardation Research Center Series, F. de la Cruz and P. Gerald (Eds.) Baltimore, University Park Press, pp. 99-110.
71. St. George-Hyslop, P.H., Tanzi, R., Polinsky, R., Haines, J.L., Nee, L., Watkins, P.C., Myers, R.H., Feldman, R.G., Pollen, D., Drachman, D., Growdon, J., Bruni, A., Foncin, J.-F., Salmon, D., Frommelt, P., Amaducci, L., Sorbi, S., Piacentini, S., Stewart, G., Hobbs, W., Conneally, P.M., and Gusella, J.F. (1987). The genetic defect causing familial Alzheimer's disease maps on chromosome 21. *Science* 235: 885-890.
72. Heston, L. (1977). Alzheimer's disease, trisomy 21 and myeloproliferative disorders: Associations suggesting a genetic diathesis. *Science* 196: 322-323.
73. Mozar, H.N., Bal, D.G., and Howard, J.T. (1987). Perspectives in the etiology of Alzheimer's disease. *JAMA* 257: 1503-1507.
74. Schweber, M. (1985). A possible unitary hypothesis for Alzheimer's disease and Down syndrome. *Ann. N.Y. Acad. Sci.* 450: 223-238.
75. Schweber, M. (1986). Interrelation of Alzheimer disease and Down syndrome. In: *New Perspectives on Down Syndrome*, S. Pueschel, C. Tingey, J. Rynders, A. Crocker, and D. Crutcher (Eds.) Baltimore, Paul Brookes, pp. 136-146.
76. Schweber, M., Tuson, C., Shiloh, R., and Ben-Neriah, Z. (1989). Increased chromosome 21 DNA in early, late, familial, and sporadic Alzheimer's Disease. In Press.
77. Schweber, M. (1986). Improved quantification of Southerns applied to Down syndrome and Alzheimer's disease. *J. Cell Biol.* 103: 517 A.

78. Campbell, N., and Pless, I. (1956). Optical system to simplify analysis of bubble chamber photographs. *Rev. Sci. Instr.* 27: 875.
79. Pless, I. (1961). Bubble chambers. In: *Techniques of High Energy Physics, Vol. V*, D. Ritson (Ed.) New York, Interscience, pp. 87-113.
80. Barelle, F., Shoulders, C., and Proudfoot, N. (1980). The primary structure of the human ϵ-globin gene. *Cell* 221: 621-626.
81. Lieman-Hurwitz, J., Dafni, N., Larie, V., and Groner, Y. (1982). Human cytoplasic superoxide dismutase cDNA clone; a probe for studying the molecular biology of Down syndrome. *Proc. Natl. Acad. Sci. USA* 79: 2808-2811.
82. Sherman, L., Dafni, N., Lieman-Hurwitz, J., and Groner, Y. (1983). Nucleotide sequence and expression of human chromosome 21-encoded superoxide dismutase mRNA. *Proc. Natl. Acad. Sci. USA* 80: 5465-5469.
83. Schweber, M., Tuson, C., and Shiloh, R. (1987). Triplication of chromosome 21 material in Alzheimer's disease. *Neurology* 37: 222.
84. Weinreb, H. (1985). Fingerprint patterns in Alzheimer's disease. *Arch. Neurol.* 42: 50-54.
85. Weinreb, H. (1986). Dermatoglyphic patterns in Alzheimer's disease. *J. Neurogenet.* 3: 233-246.
86. Selzer, B., and Sherwin, I. (1986). Fingerprint pattern differences in early- and late-on-set primary degenerative dementia. *Arch. Neurol.* 43: 665-668.
87. Sinet, P., Couturier, J., Dutrillaux, B., Possonier, M., Raoul, O., Rethore, M.-O., Allard, D., Lejeune, J., and Jerome, H. (1976). Trisome 21 et superoxide dismutase-1. Tentative localisation sur la sous bande 21q22.2. *Exp. Cell Res.* 97: 47-55.
88. Phillips, T., Fraisse, J., Sinet, P., Lauras, B., Robers, J., and Freycon, F. (1978). Confirmation of the assignment of the human SOD gene to chromosome 21q22. *Cytogenet. Cell. Genet.* 22: 521-523.
89. Wulfsberg, E., Carrel, R., Ivana, J., O'Brien, T., Sykes, J., and Sparkes, R. (1983). Normal superoxide dismutase-1 (SOD-1) activity with deletion of chromosome band 21q22 supports localization of SOD-1 locus to 21q22. *Hum. Genet.* 64: 271-272.
90. Delabar, J.-M., Goldgaber, D., Lamour, Y., Nicole, A., Huret, J.-L., de Grouchy, J., Brown, P., Gajdusek, D., and Sinet, P.-M. (1987). Amyloid gene duplication in Alzheimer's Disease and karyotypically normal Down syndrome. *Science* 235: 1390-1394.
91. St. George-Hyslop, P., Tanzi, R., Polinsky, R., Neve, R., Pollen, D., Drachman, D., Growdon, J., Cupples, L.A., Nee, L., Myers, R.H., O'Sullivan, D., Watkins, P., Amos, J., Deutsch, C., Bodfish, J., Kinsbourne, M., Feldman, R., Bruni, A., Amaducci, L., Foncin, J.-F., and Gusella, J.F. (1987). Absence of duplication of chromosome 21 genes in familial and sporadic Alzheimer's disease. *Science* 238: 664-666.
92. Levanon, D., Lieman-Hurwitz, J., Dafni, N., Wigderson, M., Sherman, L., Bernstein, Y., Laver-Rudick, Z., Danciger, E., Stein, O., and Groner, Y. (1985). Architecture and anatomy of the chromosomal locus in human chromosome 21 encoding the Cu/Zn superoxide dismutase. *EMBO J.* 4: 77-84.

93. Danciger, E., Dafni, N., Bernstein, Y., Laver-Rudich, Z., Neer, A., and Groner, Y. (1986). Human Cu/Zn superoxide dismutase gene family: Molecular structure and characterization of four Cu/Zn superoxide dismutase-related pseudogenes. *Proc. Natl. Acad. Sci. USA* 83: 3619-3623.
94. Marklund, S., Adolfsson, R., Gottfries, C., and Winblad, B. (1985). Superoxide dismutase isoenzymes in normal brains and in brains from patients with dementia of Alzheimer type. *J. Neurol. Sci.* 67: 319-325.
95. Goldgaber, D., Lerman, M., McBride, O.W., Saffiotti, U., and Gajdusek, D.C. (1987). Characterization and chromosomal localization of a cDNA encoding brain amyloid of Alzheimer's disease. *Science* 235: 877-880.
96. Tanzi, R., Gusella, J., Watkins, P., Bruns, G., St. George-Hyslop, P., Van Keuren, M.L., Patterson, D., Pagan, S., Kurnit, D., and Neve, R.L. (1987). Amyloid protein gene: cDNA, mRNA distribution, and genetic linkage near the Alzheimer locus. *Science* 235: 880-884.
97. Kang, J., Lemaire, H.-G., Unterbeck, A., Salbaum, J.M., Masters, C.L., Grzeschik, K.-H., Multhaup, G., Beyreuther, K., and Muller-Hill, B. (1987). The precursor of Alzheimer's disease amyloid A4 protein resembles a cell-surface receptor. *Nature (London)* 325: 733-736.
98. Robakis, N., Wisniewski, H., Jenkins, E., Devine-Gage, E., Houck, G., Yao, X.-L., Ramakrishna, N., Wolfe, G., Silverman, W., and Brown, W. (1987). Chromosome 21q21 sublocalisation of gene encoding beta-amyloid peptide in cerebral vessels and neuritic (senile) plaques of people with Alzheimer's disease and Down syndrome. *Lancet* 1: 384-385.
99. Podlisny, M., Lee, G., and Selkoe, D. (1987). Gene dosage of the β-amyloid precursor protein in Alzheimer's disease. *Science* 238: 669-671.
100. Tanzi, R., Bird, E., Latt, S., and Neve, R. (1987). The amyloid β-protein gene is not duplicated in Alzheimer's disease brain. *Science* 238: 666-669.
101. Van Broeckhoven, C., Genthe, A.M., Vandenberghe, A., Horsthemke, B., Backhovens, H., Raeymaekers, P., Van Hul, W., Wehnert, A., Gheuens, J., Cras, P., Bruyland, M., Martin, J.J., Salbaum, M., Multhaup, G., Masters, C.L., Beyreuther, K., Gurling, H.M., Mullan, M.J., Holland, A., Barton, A., Irving, N., Williamson, R., Richards, S.J., and Hardy, J.A. (1987). Failure of familial Alzheimer's disease to segregate with the A4-amyloid gene in several European families. *Nature* 329: 153-155.
102. Tanzi, R., St. George-Hyslop, P., Haines, J.L., Polinsky, R.J., Nee, L., Foncin, J.-F., Veve, R., McClatchey, A., Conneally, P.M., and Gusella, J.F. (1987). The genetic defect in familial Alzheimer's disease is not tightly linked to the amyloid β-protein gene. *Nature* 329: 156-157.
103. Nott, P., and Pleminger, J. (1975). Presenile dementia: The difficulties of early diagnosis. *Acta Psychiatr. Scand.* 51: 210-217.
104. Garcia, C., Reding, M.J., and Blass, J. (1981). Overdiagnosis of dementia. *J. Am. Geriatr. Soc.* 29: 407-410.
105. Ron, M.A., Toone, B.K., Garralda, M.E., and Lishman, W.A. (1979). Diagnostic accuracy in presenile dementia. *Br. J. Psychiatry* 134: 161-168.

106. Sulkava, R., Haltia, M., Paetau, A., Wikstrom, J., and Palo, J. (1983). Accuracy of clinical diagnosis in primary degenerative dementia: Correlation with neuropathological findings. *J. Neurol. Neurosurg. Psychiatry* 46: 9-13.
107. Wade, J., Mirsen, T., Hachinski, V., Fisman, M., Lau, C., and Merskey, H. (1987). The clinical diagnosis of Alzheimer's disease. *Arch. Neurol.* 44: 24-29.
108. Franke, U. (1981). Gene dosage studies in Down syndrome. A review. In: *Trisomy 21 (Down Syndrome) Research Perspectives.* National Institute of Child Health, Developmental Mental Retardation Research Center Series, F. de al Cruz and P. Gerald (Eds.) Baltimore, University Park Press, pp. 237-251.

10

Molecular Pathology of Intra- and Extraneuronal Filaments in Brain Aging and Alzheimer's Disease

DENNIS J. SELKOE, LAWRENCE K. DUFFY, NOBUYUKI NUKINA, MARCIA B. PODLISNY, CARMELA ABRAHAM, and KENNETH S. KOSIK / *Brigham and Women's Hospital, Boston, Massachusetts*

INTRODUCTION

Recent progress in the macromolecular analysis of abnormal filaments in Alzheimer's disease is the latest extension of work that derives from the seminal ultrastructural descriptions of neurofibrillary tangles and neuritic plaques made independently by Robert Terry and by Michael Kidd in 1963. Following their initial findings, numerous investigators have attempted to characterize the composition and cellular origin of the filamentous protein polymers that accumulate progressively in the brain tissue of patients with Alzheimer's disease. Despite doubts expressed over the years about the utility of analyzing the plaques and tangles, it appears increasingly likely that molecular studies of these fibrous lesions can provide important insights into the pathogenesis of progressive cortical degeneration in Alzheimer's disease. Skepticism about the study of plaques and tangles has now given way to almost the opposite: the notion, probably premature, that protein chemical and molecular genetic studies of amyloid deposition could provide a complete understanding of the pathogenesis of Alzheimer's disease. The understandable enthusiasm that recent discoveries have generated should be tempered by the realization that the chemistry and cell biology of amyloidogenesis appears to be highly complex and the control of this process is not yet understood. The role of endogenous and/or environmental factors in precipitating the process remains unknown. Most importantly, evidence that the amyloid filaments directly cause microvascular and cortical injury is lacking.

Despite these caveats, a detailed understanding of the expression and processing of amyloidogenic protein(s) in Alzheimer's disease appears to be one of the most attractive ways to discover further clues about causation. Moreover, such studies will probably provide important information about one mechanism of brain aging in normal humans and lower mammals. This conclusion arises from the fact that the complex structural alterations that characterize Alzheimer's disease are qualitatively indistinguishable from lesions that accumulate progressively in the brains of virtually all aged humans. In addition, recent evidence suggests that the neuritic plaques in aged primates and other mammals have striking similarity to those in aged humans and patients with Alzheimer's disease, particularly their amyloid protein. At this juncture, one reasonable view of the Alzheimer's disease problem is that it represents a quantitative acceleration of an involutional process in the cerebral cortex that occurs normally in at least some mammals during aging. The relationship of the prevalence of Alzheimer's disease to age is striking. This virtually linear relationship must be taken into account by any hypothesis that seeks to explain the pathogenesis of Alzheimer's disease.

This chapter reviews the complex, sometimes conflicting, information currently available about the intraneuronal filaments making up neurofibrillary tangles and the extracellular filaments making up amyloid deposits in senile plaques and cerebral microvessels. It should be emphasized at the outset that neurofibrillary tangles, with their characteristic paired helical filaments (PHF), are a much less specific lesion for Alzheimer's disease than is the neuritic plaque with its associated amyloid deposit. Neurofibrillary tangles occur in a wide variety of brain disorders due to diverse causes, including metabolic, viral, traumatic, and perhaps toxic insults. In contrast, the amyloid-bearing neuritic plaques that occur invariably in patients with Alzheimer's disease (AD) are otherwise found only in aged normal individuals and in patients with Down's syndrome (trisomy 21). Thus, studies of the genesis of neuritic plaques and the role of amyloidogenic proteins in that process appear more likely to provide clues about seminal events in Alzheimer's disease than does the analysis of neurofibrillary tangles.

INTRANEURONAL FILAMENTS AND THE PROTEINS THAT CONTRIBUTE TO THEM

The major ultrastructural components of the neurofibrillary tangles are the PHF. However, tangles in many patients with AD (both familial and sporadic cases) contain straight filaments that vary in diameter from 10 to 20 nm and are intermixed with PHF. The PHF and/or pathological straight filaments can be found in some of the dystrophic axonal terminals and dendrites that contribute to neuritic plaques in the cerebral cortex of aged normals and AD patients. Numerous immunocytochemical studies have shown that the straight filaments seen in AD neurons, as well as those found in patients with other degenerative disorders such as progressive supranuclear palsy or Pick's disease, have a close antigenic relationship to PHF. Whether such straight filaments are derived from the same protein precursors as

PHF is not yet known; their distinct fine structures suggest that some protein chemical differences will be found.

It is now well recognized that two related problems have hampered the characterization of PHF: their insolubility and the consequent difficulty in purifying them and isolating their subunit proteins. To date, a method for the rigorous, high-grade purification of PHF from brain tissue has not been achieved, although methods that lead to considerable enrichment of the filaments are available (1-3). Investigators have been forced to rely on immunocytochemistry to delineate some of the proteins contributing to PHF.

Both polyclonal (1,4) and monoclonal (5-7) antibodies raised directly to partially purified PHF have generally failed to recognize normal cellular structures or specific fibrous proteins in adult brain tissue. This paradox was resolved in part by the independent discovery in several laboratories that brain fractions highly enriched in the microtubule-associated phosphoprotein, tau, reacted strongly with PHF polyclonal antibodies and also some monoclonal PHF antibodies (8-12). Conversely, polyclonal and monoclonal antibodies raised against normal tau from various mammalian brains, including human, almost always recognize neurofibrillary tangles and altered neurites in AD and normal aged cortex (8-12). It is reasonable to conclude that tau, which is actually a heterogeneous family of phosphoproteins ranging in molecular weight from ~50 to ~65 kDa, is a principal antigenic constituent of PHF and also of related straight filaments that are seen in patients with progressive supranuclear palsy (PSP), Pick's disease, and certain other degenerations. However, it is not known to what extent tau contributes to the composition of PHF, since stiochiometry is precluded by the insolubility and lack of purity of the fibers. It is apparent that other neuronal proteins distinct from tau must contribute to or at least be closely associated with, PHF. One piece of evidence supporting this conclusion is the fact that extensive absorption of polyclonal PHF antibodies with normal tau (to the point that tau is no longer recognized by the antibodies on Western blots) still allows the antisera to recognize tangles and neurites in AD cortex. This result can be interpreted to mean that polyclonal antisera to PHF contain antibodies directed either against highly altered forms of tau or distinct proteins. One such distinct protein has recently been identified by the elegant studies of Mori and colleagues (13). These investigators used a monoclonal antibody to PHF and peptide mixtures cleaved proteolytically from PHF-enriched and control brain fractions to identify the protein ubiquitin as an additional component of the pathological fibers. Subsequent immunocytochemical studies with antibodies to native ubiquitin have confirmed the association of ubiquitin, not only with AD tangles but also with Pick bodies, Lewy bodies in parkinsonian brains, and tangles in PSP (14,15). One of the functions of ubiquitin is to bind to certain altered or short-lived cellular proteins prior to their ATP-dependent proteolysis. Whether this mechanism occurs unsuccessfully in Alzheimer neurons remains to be determined.

Accumulating evidence indicates that the tau proteins associated with PHF have properties distinct from those of normal brain tau. Tau epitopes in PHF are highly resistant to postmortem effects and formalin fixation, in contrast to tau in normal axons, which is difficult to demonstrate in human brain sections. The tau in AD lesions is present in a highly insoluble form, in contrast to the marked solubility of tau prepared from normal mammalian brain. Tau peptides associated with PHF are resistant to proteolytic degradation by enzymes such as proteinase K, which completely degrades normal tau (16). Preliminary evidence for the preferential presence of phosphorylated forms of tau in AD fibrous lesions has also been reported (12,17,18). Tau, like other microtubule-associated proteins (MAPs), can promote tubulin assembly into microtubules in vitro, although its functions in vivo remain unknown. It is not yet clear whether the various alterations in tau just reviewed could lead to abnormalities of microtubule polymerization in AD neurons (19).

The fact that virtually all tau antibodies tested to date react with tangles and neurites in AD brain has led to a reexamination of the small subset of neurofilament monoclonal antibodies that also recognize these lesions (20,21). Several laboratories had previously described neurofilament antibodies that recognized neurofibrillary tangles and some plaque neurites in AD and aged normal brain (see, for example, 22-27). A number of these antibodies have now been shown to recognize phosphorylated forms of tau (20,21). In vitro dephosphorylation of tau or neurofilament proteins decreases or abolishes their reactivity with such neurofilament antibodies. In similar fashion, dephosphorylation of tangles in brain sections also diminishes or removes their immunoreactivity. Conversely, certain neurofilament monoclonal antibodies tested to date that do not recognize AD tangles do not cross-react with tau (20). These recent studies indicate that there is currently much stronger evidence implicating tau as an antigenic component of PHF than there is for neurofilament proteins. Nonetheless, further studies are needed to demonstrate whether neurofilament proteins and another microtubule-associated protein, MAP 2 (28), are constituents of the fibers.

Finally, current information about PHF antigenic structures leaves open the possibility that an as yet undefined protein forms the "central core" of the PHF and related straight filaments. The fact that apparently extracellular ("ghost") tangles are usually not recognized by antibodies to tau or other cytoskeletal proteins suggests that they could be composed of a highly inert "core" protein, distinct from the currently known components. Alternatively, this filamentous residue could be derived from neuronal cytoskeletal proteins (e.g., tau) that have undergone marked conformational modifications. Whether the amyloid β-protein now receiving intensive study could be the "core protein" of PHF, as has been hypothesized (29), remains a subject of debate (30).

The various results summarized in this section are generally applicable to proteinaceous filaments accumulating pathologically in Pick bodies and in tangles found in a variety of other disorders, including Guam Parkinson-dementia complex, variants of Hallervorden-Spatz disease, PSP, normal aging, and other conditions (15,31). This fact underscores the relative nonspecificity of the protein alterations leading to PHF deposition in Alzheimer's disease neurons. It is reasonable to speculate at present that fibrous alterations occurring both in cell bodies (i.e., tangles) and in cortical neurites within and outside of senile plaques represent a secondary neuronal alteration that can arise as a result of a variety of primary insults.

COMPLEXITY OF AMYLOID PROTEINS IN PLAQUES AND MICROVESSELS

It has been known for several decades, although not always emphasized, that amyloid filaments are deposited in the cerebral mocrivasculature in addition to the centers of neuritic plaques. These filaments appear to be 5-10 nm in diameter, often measuring around 8 nm, and are unpaired. The filaments are therefore slightly less than the diameter of each member of the PHF found intraneuronally. The fine structure of amyloid filaments in AD and normal aged brain tissue is essentially indistinguishable from amyloid filaments in a wide range of other human amyloidoses affecting nonneural organs. Like other amyloids, AD amyloid deposits have the tinctorial property of staining with Congo red and thioflavin and are found extracellularly. With very few exceptions, human amyloidoses are marked by the extracellular accumulation of amyloid filaments. This localization and the distinct ultrastructure of the filaments suggests that their chemical composition may turn out to be different than the intraneuronal PHF. Indeed, all antibodies raised to AD amyloid filaments and their constituent proteins (i.e., the β-protein and additional associated proteins) have failed to recognize the intraneuronal bundles of PHF immunocytochemically. There have been descriptions of close association of amyloid filaments with the plasma membrane of microglial cells, in that they may lie within deep invaginations of the cytoplasm but are still extracellular. Amyloid filaments have also been observed within certain microglial cells associated with plaques in AD, but the interpretation of this finding has favored the possibility that they were phagocytosed after formation (32) The precise cellular origin of the amyloid filaments forming the vascular deposits on plaques of Alzheimer's disease is a major area of inquiry at present.

It is well known that amyloid filaments in various human systemic diseases are composed of distinct gene products (proteins) that may be incorporated in toto into filamentous polymers or, more commonly, are first proteolytically cleaved and a portion of the precursor protein aggregated as amyloid. Recent data about the presumed precusor of AD-type amyloid, the β-protein, suggest that the latter mechanism may be operative in AD, but the details are entirely unknown.

As we review the available information about amyloid proteins and the genes encoding them, it is worth bearing in mind that microvascular amyloid deposition is very common, if not always present, in Alzheimer's disease. A recent analysis of 100 consecutive cases of pathologically diagnosed Alzheimer's disease by Joachim et al. (33) demonstrated that all 100 cases showed one or more microvessels in the cerebral cortex or meningeal space that had focal amyloid deposits as identified by Congo red staining. The latter technique is a less sensitive detector of amyloid than thioflavin or, perhaps, immunostaining with amyloid antibodies. Therefore, it is likely that virtually all cases of AD show some microvascular amyloidosis. On the other hand, it is equally clear that many such cases show only trace amounts of amyloid in scattered microvessels, giving rise to a major discrepancy between the number of amyloid-bearing neuritic plaques and the degree of cerebrovascular amyloidosis. The explanation for this often striking discrepancy is not available.

Protein Chemical Studies of Plaque and Vascular Amyloid

In contrast to the situation with PHF, it has been possible to prepare the compacted amyloid cores of senile plaques to a relatively high grade of purity. Several methods have been published (34-36). In the author's laboratory, fluorescence-activated cell sorting (FACS) has been used to prepare amyloid core fractions that are 90-95% amyloid cores and 5-10% lipofuscin granules according to light or electron microscopic particle counting. Amino acid analyses of such highly purified core fractions demonstrated a composition that includes approximately 50% nonpolar residues with abundant glycine and no proline (35,37). When we obtained this composition for cores, we realized that it was highly similar to the composition of a meningeal vessel amyloid protein described by Glenner and Wong (38). Moreover, antibodies we raised against a hydrophobic low-molecular-weight (4-7 kDa) protein released by formic acid or guanidine thiocyanate from our FACS-purified amyloid cores stained both plaque cores and amyloid in meningeal and cortical microvessels (35). This result was also obtained by Wong et al. (39), using antibodies not to the native amyloid protein but to a synthetic beta-amyloid peptide.

Despite this immunochemical cross-reaction, we have clearly observed differences between plaque and vascular amyloid in AD brain. First, compacted amyloid cores are insoluble in 6 molar guanidine hydrochloride, the reagent used by Glenner and Wong to solubilize and isolate the meningovascular beta amyloid protein. Second, it has not been possible to sequence the core-derived low-molecular-weight protein, either in our hands (35) or in other laboratories (40, 41), whereas we are able to obtain unambiguous β-protein sequence (through residue 40) from meningovascular amyloid prepared by a sodium dodecyl sulfate (SDS) isolation method (42), which confirms the seminal sequence data provided by Glenner and Wong (38). Thus, the amyloid deposits found in the centers of neuritic plaques, while related by antigenicity and amino acid composition to microvascular amyloid, have an apparently blocked amino terminus and are insoluble in guanidine hydrochloride. These properties suggest a further processing, in the case of the plaque core, of a common precursor protein.

The antisera we have raised directly against intact amyloid filaments or the low-molecular-weight protein solubilized from them have not shown reactions with intra- or extracellular neurofibrillary tangles or the neurites of plaques under any circumstances. This fact does not yet preclude the possibility of an amyloid protein in the PHF whose epitopes are completely modified or buried.

The availability of a partial protein sequence for AD amyloid deposits, provided by Glenner and Wong (38) and confirmed by other laboratories (34,40,41, 42), has allowed research on AD amyloid to advance much more rapidly. We have synthesized several peptides having the sequence of portions of the β-amyloid protein. A synthetic peptide of residues 1-28 readily comes out of the solution after brief storage in the cold and forms abundant filaments of approximately 8-10 nm diameter that in sectioned or negatively stained specimens bear a striking resemblance to amyloid filaments in situ (43). We have substituted an alanine for a lysine at position 16 of this peptide and found that the mutant peptide has a much lower propensity to form amyloid filaments in vitro and that the resultant filaments do not have the fine structure of those derived from the correct sequence. Moreover, only the correct β-peptide 1-28 filaments aggregate in vitro into large bundles that closely resemble portions of amyloid plaque cores (43). X-ray diffraction analysis (43) clearly demonstrates the cross β-pleated sheet confirmation expected for all amyloid filaments and previously demonstrated by us in AD amyloid cores (44). The studies just summarized suggest that a peptide having residues 1-28 of the β-amyloid protein has many of the properties attributed to amyloid filaments in AD brain. However, this peptide probably does not include the full sequence of the native amyloid filament, which may end around residue 40 (40, 42). The precise carboxy-terminal residue is not yet pinpointed and could turn out to be variable.

The availability of protein sequence data has allowed several laboratories (45-48) to use oligonucleotides to isolate cDNAs from human brain libraries that encode all or part of the β-protein precursor. Among the first developments that arose from the isolation of such cDNAs was the report that three patients with apparently sporadic AD had a 50% increased gene dosage of the beta amyloid gene on chromosome 21, similar to the elevation of dosage found in patients with trisomy 21 (49). This initial finding was interpreted by the authors to indicate a microduplication occurring during meiosis of a subsegment of chromosome 21 in the region of the beta amyloid gene, that is around 21q21 (49). Because of the potential importance of this observation for understanding the pathogenesis of AD and for diagnosis of the disease, we undertook a larger study of 14 patients with clinically diagnosed AD and 10 patients with trisomy 21 in comparison with 12 aged control subjects (50). We carried out densitometric analyses of Southern blots probed with a cDNA for the beta protein to determine the relative dosage of this gene in genomic DNA from these 35 individuals. Whereas the nine patients with trisomy 21 showed the expected 1.5-fold increase in dosage of this gene, none of the 14 AD patients had a gene dosage higher than that of the normal controls. These results were highly significant statistically ($p < 0.001$). Our results do not support the recent reports of microduplication of a segment of chromosome 21 as the genetic basis for AD (49,51). Alternative mechanisms for the brain-specific increase in β-protein deposition in AD compared to aged normal humans should be sought.

Identification of Native β-Protein Precursor Polypeptides in Brain

While we were unable to document increased gene dosage for the β-amyloid precursor protein in AD, we have recently used a series of antibodies against synthetic peptides from amyloid and nonamyloid regions of the β-protein precursor to document a group of specifically cross-reactive proteins in AD cerebral cortex (52). An antibody to the C-terminus recognizes proteins at approximately 110-135 kDa at equal levels in AD and control cortex on Western blots. These several proteins also appear to be detected by two other amyloid protein antibodies: one to a synthetic peptide of residues 1-45 (amyloid region) and another to the 15 residues making up the C-terminus of the precursor, which is well outside the amyloidogenic region (52). An analysis of different brain regions of AD and controls showed relatively equal amounts of these polypeptides in brain regions that include neocortex from the four main lobes, hippocampus, striatum, subcortical white matter, thalamus, pons, and cerebellum. Additional studies with the antibodies to β-protein precursor peptides outside of the amyloid region show that senile plaques are selectively immuno-labeled, suggesting that much or all of the precursor molecule accumulates locally in cortical regions undergoing amyloidosis. The results to date suggest that the β-protein precursor found normally in human brain occurs as 110-135 kDa membrane-associated proteins in mammalian neural and non-neural tissues (52). Our findings suggest either enhanced expression of the precursor or alterations in its normal catabolism, resulting in local increases in the entire precursor followed by abnormal proteolytic processing that could lead to cleavage of the amyloidogenic region and subsequent filament formation.

Complexity of Amyloid-Associated Proteins in AD

The availability of a panel of polyclonal antibodies to amyloid filaments and their constituent proteins has enabled us to demonstrate the apparent complexity of

AD amyloid antigens. We classify our current antibodies into three groups: I, antibodies raised to intact amyloid filaments, partially purified from AD cortex; II, antibodies raised to the low-molecular-weight (4-5 kDa) β-protein solubilized by formic acid from amyloid filaments; and III, antibodies raised to synthetic β-protein peptides. The latter two groups react strongly with synthetic β-protein and recognize both microvascular and plaque amyloid in tissue sections, particularly the former. In contrast, antibodies of category I recognize the synthetic β-protein very weakly if at all and yet have strong immunoreactivity with both in situ and SDS-isolated amyloid deposits. The antibodies represented by group I are not absorbed out by excess synthetic β-peptide. Instead, they cross-react with several discrete proteins found in normal human plasma (53). Affinity purification of antibodies from such antisera on the cross-reactive plasma proteins (immobilized on nitrocellulose membrane) shows that the purified antibodies specifically react with core and vascular amyloid in AD brain sections (53). Certain of these cross-reactive plasma proteins have been partially purified and further characterized, but their exact identity is not fully known.

In view of this class of amyloid antibodies that reacts with certain plasma proteins but not with the β-protein, Abraham and colleagues (54) screened several systemic tissues using such an antiserum and detected specific reactivity only in liver. Subsequent use of the antibodies to screen a human liver expression library led to the isolation of three cDNAs that all encoded the serine-protease inhibitor, α-1-antichymotrypsin (54). Several antibodies to this protein were in turn found to label virtually all senile plaque cores and many meningeal vascular deposits in AD brain sections (54). Even isolated amyloid cores prepared by vigorous SDS extraction retained their reactivity with α-1 antichymotrypsin antibodies. In contrast, antibodies to several other normal plasma proteins (including IgG prealbumin, transferrin, α1-antitrypsin, etc.) did not label in situ or in isolated amyloid cores.

These data indicate that α1-antichymotrypsin is strongly and selectively associated with β-amyloid deposits in AD. However, no conclusions can be drawn about any potential role of this protease inhibitor in the local processing of the β-protein. A search for specific proteases associated with the β-protein and α1-antichymotrypsin in AD amyloid deposits is underway. This work provides evidence of protein components in addition to the β-protein in AD amyloid.

Conservation of AD-Type Amyloid Proteins in the Cerebral Amyloid of Other Aged Mammals

The lack of a naturally occurring analogue of AD in animals has been a major obstacle to our study of the pathogenesis of the disease. An animal model that shows cortical neuritic degeneration and deposition of amyloid fibers that are biochemically closely related to or the same as those in aged humans could facilitate understanding of the genesis of neuritic plaques and microvascular amyloidosis. Aged monkeys and dogs are known to develop plaques in the cerebral cortex composed of neurites from multiple neurotransmitter systems surrounding deposits of amyloid. We have now shown that the amyloid in senile plaques and cerebral vessels of three species of aged nonhuman primates, of dogs, and of a polar bear cross-react with a panel of antibodies raised against human senile plaque amyloid and its constituent proteins (55). All three classes (I-III) of amyloid antibodies referred to in the previous section cross-react with both microvascular and plaque amyloid in the aged mammals studied. Antibodies to a β-protein 1-28 synthetic peptide recognized the animal amyloid deposits, and absorption of the antibodies with this peptide abolished amyloid staining in both humans and animals. It is interesting that antibodies to human paired helical filaments or to tau failed to label plaque neurites in these amyloid-bearing animals; this is in contrast to the situation in AD and aged normal brains in humans. The plaque neurites in monkeys were, however, recognized by monoclonal antibodies to phosphorylated neurofilament proteins. Our study shows that the β-amyloid protein associated with progressive cortical degeneration in AD are also deposited in the brains of other mammals with age. Aged primates can provide biochemically relevant models for a principal feature of Alzheimer's disease: cerebrovascular amyloidosis and neuritic plaque formation. The absence of neurofibrillary tangles in aged mammals does not necessarily lessen the usefulness of such animals for studying aspects of brain amyloidosis in AD.

CONCLUSION

The information about intraneuronal and extracellular protein filaments in AD brain tissue summarized here appears to apply to both familial (autosomal dominant) and apparently sporadic cases of the disease. Although familial forms of AD (FAD) often show even more marked neuropathological changes (including abundant amyloid-bearing senile plaques and vessels) than so-called sporadic AD cases, there is no known qualitative difference at the protein chemical or immunochemical level between these two forms of the disease. Since it is often observed that familial Alzheimer's disease may occur at an earlier age than most sporadic cases, it is possible that an autosomal dominant mutation(s) alters normal control mechanisms for β-protein cerebral amyloidosis. The linkage of the beta-protein amyloid locus to anonymous DNA markers in the vicinity of the FAD gene suggests, but by no means proves, that an alteration in DNA somehow controlling the expression of processing of β-amyloid precursor protein could be operative in familial AD.

From several perspectives, it seems likely that studies of regionally selective cerebral amyloidosis in Down's syndrome and familial Alzheimer's disease will provide major insights into the pathogenesis of apparently sporadic cases of Alzheimer's disease. Nonetheless, the low concordance rate for Alzheimer's disease in monozygotic twins (approximately 0.4 in several studies) suggests that there are as yet undefined environmental factors that can promote or perhaps retard a genetic predisposition to widespread cortical amyloidosis of the Alzheimer type. While the unfolding story of the role of amyloid proteins and the genes that encode them in the pathogenesis of AD will progress rapidly, it is also important to identify the role of aging and putative environmental factors in promoting the formation of structural lesions in the cerebral cortex of AD patients.

REFERENCES

1. Ihara, Y., Abraham, C., and Selkoe, D.J. (1983). Antibodies to paired helical filaments in Alzheimer's disease do not recognize normal brain proteins. *Nature* 304: 727-730.
2. Iqbal, K., Zaidi, T., Thompson, C.H., Merz, P.A., and Visniewski, H.M. (1984). Alzheimer paired helical filaments: Bulk isolation, solubility and protein composition. *Acta Neuropathol. (Berl.)* 62: 167-177.
3. Selkoe, D.J., and Abraham, C.R. Isolation of paired helical filaments and amyloid fibers from human brain. In: *Methods in Enzymology*, vol. 134, R. Vallee (Ed.).
4. Grundke-Iqbal, I., Johnson, A.B., Terry, R.D., Visniewski, H.M., and Iqbal, K. (1979). Alzheimer neurofibrillary tangles: Antiserum and immunohistochemical staining. *Ann. Neurol.* 6: 532-537.
5. Wang, G.P., Grundke-Iqbal, I., Kascsak, R.J., Iqbal, K., and Visniewski, H.M. (1984). Alzheimer neurofibrillary tangles: Monoclonal antibodies to inherent antigen(s). *Acta Neuropathol. (Berl.)* 62: 268-275.
6. Yen, S.-H., Crowe, A., and Dickson, D.V. (1985). Monoclonal antibodies to Alzheimer's neurofibrillary tangles. I. Identification of polypeptides. *Am. J. Pathol.* 120: 282-291.
7. Selkoe, D.J., Abraham, C., Rasool, C.G., McCluskey, A., and Duffy, L.K. (1985). Production and characterization of monoclonal antibodies to Alzheimer paired helical filaments. *Ann. N.Y. Acad. Sci.* 455: 774-778.
8. Brion, J.P., van Den Bosch de Aguilar, P., and Flament-Durand, J. (1985). In: *Advances in Applied Neurological Science: Senile Dementia of the Alzheimer Type.* J. Traber and W.H. Gispens (Eds.), Berlin, Springer, pp. 164-174.
9. Nukina, N., and Ihara, Y. (1986). One of the antigenic determinants of paired helical filaments is related to tau protein. *J. Biochem.* 99: 1541-1544.
10. Grundke-Iqbal, I., Iqbal, K., Ouinlan, M., Turg, Y.-C., Zaidi, M.S., and Visniewski, H.M. (1986). Microtubule-associated protein tau: A component of Alzheimer paired helical filaments. *J. Biol. Chem.* 261: 6084-6089.
11. Kosik, K., Joachim, C.L., and Selkoe, D.J. (1986). The microtubule-associated protein, tau, is a major antigenic component of paired helical filaments in Alzheimer's disease. *Proc. Natl. Acad. Sci. USA* 83: 4044-4048.

12. Wood, J.G., Mirra, S.S., Pollock, N.J., and Binder, L.I. (1986). Neurofibrillary tangles of Alzheimer's disease share antigenic determinants with the axonal microtubule-associated protein tau. *Proc. Natl. Acad. Sci. USA* 83: 4040-4043.
13. Mori, H., Kondu, J., and Ihara, Y. (1987). Ubiquitin is a component of paired helical filaments in Alzheimer's disease. *Science* 235: 1641-1644.
14. Perry, G., Friedman, R., Shaw, G., and Chau, V. (1987). Ubiquitin is detected in neurofibrillary tangles and senile plaque neurites of Alzheimer disease brains. *Proc. Natl. Acad. Sci. USA* 84: 3033-3036.
15. Kuzuhara, S., Mori, H., Izumiyama, N., Yoshimura, M., and Ihara, Y. (1988). Lewy bodies are ubiquinated. A light- and electron-microscopic immunocytochemical study. *Acta Neuropathol.* (Berl) 75: 345-353.
15a. Kuzuhara, S., Mori, H., Izumiyama, N., Yoshimura, M., and Ihara, Y. Lewy bodies are ubiquinated. A light- and electron-microscopic immunocytochemical study. *Acta Neuropathol.* (in press).
16. Nukina, N., and Ihara, Y. (1985). Proteolytic fragments of Alzheimer's paired helical filaments. *J. Biochem.* 98: 1715-1718.
17. Grundke-Iqbal, I., Iqbal, K., Turg, Y.-C., Ouinlan, M., Visniewski, H.M., and Binder, L.I. (1986). Abnormal phosphorylation of the microtubule-associated protein tau in Alzheimer cytoskeletal pathology. *Proc. Natl. Acad. Sci. USA* 83: 4913-4917.
18. Ihara, Y., Nukina, N., Miura, R., and Ogawarra, H. (1986). Phosphorylated tau protein is integrated into paired helical filaments in Alzheimer's disease. *J. Biochem.* 99: 1807-1810.
19. Iqbal, K., Grundke-Iqbal, I., Zaida, T., Merz, P.A., Wen, G.Y., Shaikh, S.S., Wiesniewski, H.M., Alafvzoff, I., and Winblad, B. (1986). Defective brain microtubule assembly in Alzheimer's disease. *Lancet* 2: 421-426.
20. Nukina, N., Kosik, K.S., and Selkoe, D.J. (1987). Recognition of Alzheimer paired helical filaments by monoclonal antibodies is due to crossreaction with tau protein. *Proc. Natl. Acad. Sci. USA* 84: 3415-3419.
21. Ksiezak-Reding, H., Dickson, D.V., Davies, P., and Yen, S.-H. (1987). Recognition of tau epitopes by anti-neurofilament antibodies that bind to Alzheimer neurofibrillary tangles. *Proc. Natl. Acad. Sci. USA* 84: 3410-3414.
22. Ihara, Y., Nukina, N., Sugita, H., and Toyokura, V. (1981). Staining of Alzheimer's neurofibrillary tangles with antiserum against 200K component of neurofilament. *Proc. Jpn. Acad. Sci.* 57: 152-156.
23. Anderton, B.H., Breinburg, D., Dovnes, M.J., Green, P.J., Tomlinson, B.E., Ulrich, J., Vood, J.N., and Kahn, J. (1982). Monoclonal antibodies show that neurofibrillary tangles and neurofilaments share antigenic determinants. *Nature* 298: 84-86.
24. Rasool, C.G., Abraham, C., Anderton, B.H., Haugh, M.C., Kahn, J., and Selkoe, D.J. (1984). Alzheimer's disease: Immunoreactivity of neurofibrillary tangles with antineurofilament and anti-paired helical filament antibodies. *Brain Res.* 310: 249-260.
25. Perry, G., Rizzuto, N., Autilio-Gambetti, L., and Gambetti, P. (1985). Alzheimer's paired helical filaments contain cytoskeletal components. *Proc. Natl. Acad. Sci. USA* 82: 3916-3920.

26. Sternberg, N.H., Sternberg, L.A., and Ulrich, J. (1985). Aberrant neurofilament phosphorylation in Alzheimer's disease. *Proc. Natl. Acad. Sci. USA* 82: 4274-4276.
27. Cork, L.C., Sternberger, N.H., Sternberger, C.A., Casanova, M.F. Struble, R.G., and Price, D.C. (1986). Phosphorylated neurofilament antigens in neurofibrillary tangles in Alzheimer's disease. *J. Neuropathol. Exp. Neurol.* 455: 56-64.
28. Kosik, K.S., Duffy, L.K., Dowling, M.M., Abraham, C., McCluskey, A., and Selkoe, D.J. (1984). Microtubule-associated protein 2: Monoclonal antibodies demonstrate the selective incorporation of certain epitopes into Alzheimer neurofibrillary tangles. *Proc. Natl. Acad. Sci. USA* 81: 7941-7945.
29. Masters, C.L., Multhaup, G., Simms, G., Pottigiesser, J., Martins, R.N., and Beyreuther, K. (1985). Neuronal origin of a cerebral amyloid: Neurofibrillary tangles of Alzheimer's disease contain the same protein as the amyloid of plaque cores and blood vessels. *EMBO J.* 4: 2757-2763.
30. Selkoe, D.J. (1986). Altered structural proteins in plaques and tangles: What do they tell us about the biology of Alzheimer's disease? *Neurobiol. Aging* 7: 425-432.
31. Joachim, C.L., Morris, J.H., Kosik, K.S., and Selkoe, D.J. (1987). Tau antisera recognize neurofibrillay tangles in a range of neurodegenerative disorders. *Ann. Neurol.* 22 (4): 514-520.
32. Mirra, S.S., and Austin, G.E. (1985). Neuritic plaque amyloid in Alzheimer's disease is ingested by receptor-mediated endocytosis (abstract). *J. Neuropathol. Exp. Neurol.* 44: 365.
33. Joachim, C.L., Morris, J.H., and Selkoe, D.J. (1987). Amyloid angiopathy in 100 cases of Alzheimer's disease (abstract). *Neurology* 37 (Suppl. 1): 225.
34. Masters, C.L., Simms, G., Veinman, N.A., Multhaup, G., McDonald, B.L., and Beyreuther, K. (1985). Amyloid plaque protein in Alzheimer's disease and Down's syndrome. *Proc. Natl. Acad. Sci. USA* 82: 4245-4249.
35. Selkoe, D.J., Abraham, C.R., Podlisny, M.B., and Duffy, L.K. (1986). Isolation of low-molecular-weight proteins from amyloid plaque fibers in Alzheimer's disease. *J. Neurochem.* 146: 1820-1834.
36. Roher, A., Volfe, D., Palutke, M., and KuKuruga, D. (1986). Purification, ultrastructure, and chemical analysis of Alzheimer disease amyloid plaque core protein. *Proc. Natl. Acad. Sci. USA* 83: 2662-2666.
37. Selkoe, D.J., and Abraham, C. (1985). Plaque amyloid in Alzheimer's disease (AD): Purification by flow cytometry and protein characterization (abstract). *Neurology* 35 (Suppl. 1). 217.
38. Glenner, G.G., and Wong, C.W. (1984). Alzheimer's disease: Initial report of the purification and characterization of a novel cerebrovascular amyloid protein. *Biochem. Biophys. Res. Commun.* 120: 885-890.
39. Wong, C.V., Ouaranta, V., and Glenner, G.G. (1985). Neuritic plaques and cerebrovascular amyloid in Alzheimer disease are antigenically related. *Proc. Natl. Acad. Sci. USA* 82: 8729-8732.

40. Bobin, S.A., Currie, J.R., Chen, M.-C., Iqbal, K., Miller, D.L., Styles, J.J., and Visniewski, H.M. (1987). Comparisons between the structures of cerebral vascular amyloid (CVA) and senile plaque core amyloid (SPCA) peptides found in Alzheimer's disease (abstract). *Proc. Fed. Am. Soc. Exp. Biol.* 46: 2137.
41. Gorevic, P., Goni, F., Pons-Estel, B., Alvarez, F., Peress, R., and Frangione, B. (1985). Isolation and partial characterization of neurofibrillary tangles and amyloid plaque core in Alzheimer's disease: Immunohistochemical studies. *J. Neuropathol. Exp. Neurol.* 45: 647-664.
42. Joachim, C.L., Duffy, L.K., Morris, J.H., and Selkoe, D.J. (1987). Protein chemical and immunocytochemical studies of meningovascular beta-amyloid protein in Alzheimer's disease and normal aging. *Brain Research* (in press).
43. Kirschner, D.A., Inouye, H., Duffy, L.K., Sinclair, A., Lind, M., and Selkoe, D.J. (1987). Synthetic β-peptide of Alzheimer disease forms amyloid-like fibrils *in vitro*. *Proc. Natl. Acad. Sci. USA* 84: 6953-6957.
44. Kirschner, D.A., Abraham, C., and Selkoe, D.J. (1986). X-ray diffraction from intraneuronal paired helical filaments and extraneuronal amyloid fibers in Alzheimer disease indicates cross-β conformation. *Proc. Natl. Acad. Sci. USA* 83: 503-507.
45. Kang, J., Lemaire, H.-G., Unterbeck, A., Salbaum, J.M., Masters, C.L., Grzeschik, K.H., Multhaup, G., Keyreuther, K., and Muller-Hill, B. (1987). The precursor of Alzheimer's disease amyloid A4 protein resembles a cell-surface receptor. *Nature* 325: 733-736.
46. Goldgaber, D., Lerman, M.I., McBride, O.W., Saffiotti, U., and Gajdusek, D.C. (1987). Characterization and chromosomal localization of a cDNA encoding brain amyloid of Alzheimer's disease. *Science* 235: 877-880.
47. Robakis, N.K., Wisniewski, H.M., Jenkins, E.C., Devine-Gage, E.A., Houck, G.E., Yao, X.-L., Ramakrishna, N., Wolfe, G., Silverman, W.P., and Brown, W.T. (1987). Chromosome 21q21 sublocalisation of gene encoding beta-amyloid peptide in cerebral vessels and neuritic (senile) plaques of people with Alzheimer disease and Down syndrome. *Lancet* 1: 385.
48. Tanzi, R.E., Gusella, J.F., Watkins, P.C., Bruns, G.A.P., St. George-Hyslop, P., van Keuren, M.L., Patterson, D., Pagan, S., Kurnit, D.M., and Neve, R.L. (1987). Amyloid β protein gene: cDNA, mRNA distribution, and genetic linkage near the Alzheimer locus. *Science* 235: 880-884.
49. Delabar, J.-M., Goldgaber, D., Lamour, Y., Nicole, A., Huret, J.-L., de Grouchy, J., Brown, P., Gajdusek, D.C., and Sinet, P.-M. (1987). β amyloid gene duplication in Alzheimer's disease and karyotypically normal Down syndrome. *Science* 235: 1390-1392.
50. Podlisny, M.B., Lee, G., and Selkoe, D.J. Gene dosage of the β-amyloid precursor protein in Alzheimer's disease. *Science* 238: 669-671.
51. Schweber, M., Tuson, C., Shiloh, R., and Ben-Neriah, Z. (1987). Triplication of chromosome 21 material in Alzheimer's disease (abstract). *Neurology* 37 (Suppl. 1): 222.
52. Selkoe, D.J., Podlisny, M.B., Joachim, C.L., Vickers, E.A., Lee, G., Fritz, L. C., and Oltersdorf, T. (1988). β-Amyloid precursor protein of Alzheimer disease occurs as 110- to 135-kilodalton membrane-associated proteins in neural and nonneural tissues. *Proc. Natl. Acad. Sci. USA* 85 (in press).

53. Selkoe, D.J., Galibert, L., Podlisny, M., and Duffy, L.K. (1986). Normal human plasma proteins share antigenic determinants with CNS amyloid fibrils in Alzheimer's disease (AD) (abstract). *Soc. Neurosci. Abstr.* 12 (1): 35.
54. Abraham, C.R., Selkoe, D.J., and Potter, H. (1988). Immunochemical identification of the serine protease inhibitor α_1-antichymotrypsin in the brain amyloid deposits of Alzheimer's disease. *Cell* 52: 487-501.
55. Selkoe, D.J., Bell, D., Podlisny, M.B., Cork, L.C., and Price, D.L. (1987). Conservation of brain amyloid proteins in aged mammals and humans with Alzheimer's disease. *Science* 235: 873-877.

11

Molecular Cloning of Amyloid cDNA from Alzheimer's Brain Messenger RNA: Correlative Neuroimmunological and *in Situ* Hybridization Studies

M. SALIM[a], SAYEEDA B. ZAIN[a], WEN-GANG CHOU[a,c], ELIZABETH M. SAJDEL-SULKOWSKA[b,c,d], RONALD E. MAJOCHA[b,c,d], S. REHMAN[a], FRANCINE M. BENES[b,c], and CHARLES A. MAROTTA[b,c,d] / [a]*University of Rochester, Medical School, Rochester, New York*; [b]*Harvard Medical School, Boston, Massachusetts*; [c]*McLean Hospital, Belmont, Massachusetts*; [d]*Massachusetts General Hospital, Boston, Massachusetts*

The presence of amyloid in senile plaques of the brains of patients with Alzheimer's disease (AD) was noted over 60 years ago (1). However, molecular mechanisms involved in the production and increased accumulation of this fibrous material in the aged human brain and in AD remain unknown. The present studies were carried out to examine processes that may contribute to amyloid formation in the AD cortex. Our research has focused on the application of antibodies to a known amyloid polypeptide and, concurrently, on the detailed molecular analysis of amyloid cDNA cloned directly from AD brain mRNA. Molecular cloning of the amyloid precursor cDNA from AD brain mRNA appeared to be essential since previous studies of this type made use of brain mRNA derived exclusively from non-AD sources (2-5). The combined neuroimmunological and molecular approaches allowed us to correlate certain morphological analyses of amyloid protein deposits with the cellular localization of amyloid mRNA.

To facilitate studies on molecular mechanisms involved in fibrous protein accumulation in the brains of aged and demented persons, we prepared monoclonal antibodies (Mabs) to a synthetic amyloid polypeptide with a sequence of

28 amino acids (6) that was designated the A4 amyloid polypeptide. The latter was derived from amyloid plaque cores of the AD brain (6). The peptide sequence shares strong homology with the earlier described β-amyloid polypeptide obtained from blood vessels of AD and Down's syndrome brains (7,8). Three Mabs were extensively characterized and used to obtain information on detailed morphological features of plaque amyloid in the AD cortex as revealed by the distribution of individual target epitopes. When combined with oligonucleotide probes, the Mabs allowed us to screen cDNA libraries prepared from AD brain mRNA for the purpose of isolating AD amyloid cDNA.

The synthetic amyloid 28-mer polypeptide (6) was analyzed by polyacrylamide gel electrophoresis (PAGE) procedures (9) before immunological studies were undertaken. The peptide was dissolved in a PAGE sample buffer containing SDS and urea and was electrophoresed on a 10% gel containing SDS (Fig. 1). After being stained with Coomassie blue, the peptide appeared as a broad band at approximately 23-25 kd and a narrow band that migrated at the gel front during electrophoresis (Fig. 1). The higher-molecular-weight species appeared to be an aggregate since it was eliminated by the addition of urea to the separating gel and, subsequently, a 3-4 kd band was obtained (not shown). Polyclonal antiserum to the 28-mer was prepared and applied to nitrocellulose blots of an overloaded gel. The latter contained a series of aggregated peptides of various apparent molecular weights, all of which reacted with the antiserum. Thus, the synthetic 28-mer had aggregational properties not unlike the naturally occurring A4 amyloid protein of 4 kd (6).

Monoclonal antibodies were prepared to the 28-mer peptide by established procedures (10) and the supernatants of three hybridomas were used in further studies. Dot blots demonstrated that the Mabs, designated 4E12, 5E2, and 10H3, were at least as potent as the polyclonal antisera (11).

The Mabs were used to characterize the detailed distribution of individual epitopic sites of neuritic plaque amyloid. Observations on numerous plaques stained with the three Mabs indicated that these antibodies provided more detailed architectonic information than was observable with polyclonal antisera or Thioflavin S (11). For example, Mab 10H3 defined the nonrandom distribution of an epitope exposed primarily in the outer rim of a plaque core in the AD prefrontal cortex (Fig. 2a). Mab 4E12, applied to AD hippocampus, demonstrated that its target epitope occurred in plaques of different sizes and at least three different distributions: homogeneously within the plaque core (Fig. 2b, upper left), primarily in the periphery (Fig. 2b, central), or in the plaque core plus periphery (Fig. 2b, lower left and right). Thus, a single Mab was able to differentiate among morphologically distinct types of senile plaques of the AD brain. Control brains without evidence of senile plaques were unreactive with the Mabs except for light background staining. In double labeling experiments it was shown that senile plaques stained with Thioflavin S were also labeled with the Mabs.

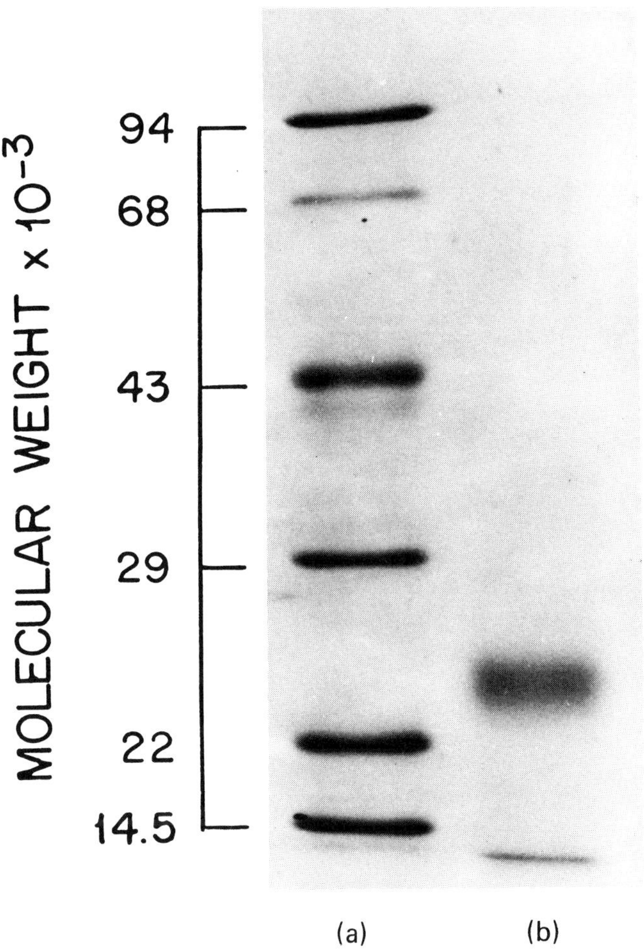

FIGURE 1 PAGE of the synthetic amyloid peptide in an SDS gel. The amyloid peptide (10 μg) was suspended in sample buffer containing 2% SDS and 9.5 M urea. Electrophoresis was carried out on a uniform 10% gel containing 0.1% SDS. (a) Molecular weight markers: phosphorylase B (94 kd), bovine serum albumin (68 kd), ovalbumin (43 kd), carbonic anhydrase (29 kd), trypsin inhibitor (22 kd), lysozyme (14.5 kd). (b) The synthetic amyloid peptide ran as a sharp band at the front of the gel and as an aggregated form of higher molecular weight.

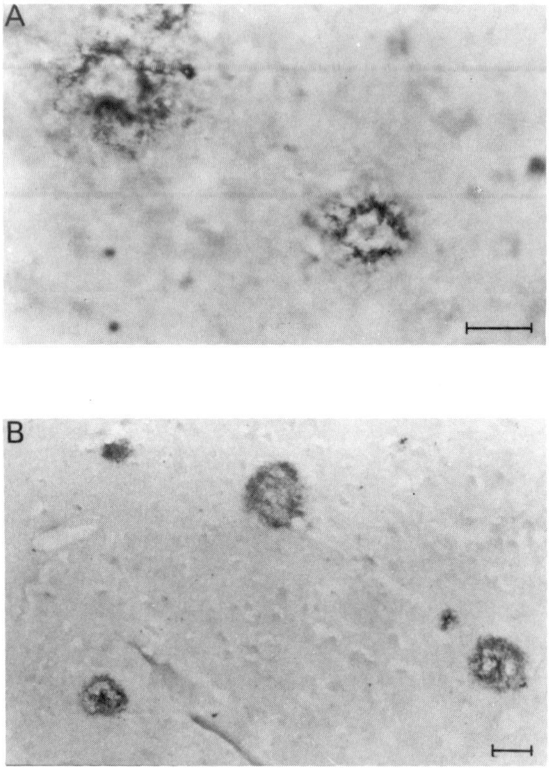

FIGURE 2 Immunostaining of AD brain with Mabs. Formalin-fixed human postmortem brain tissue was cut on a vibratome at 50 μm thickness. The general procedure is described elsewhere (11). Biotin-conjugated antimouse IgG was applied to tissues for 1 hr. The final step used an avidin-biotin horseradish peroxidase complex with 3,3'-diaminobenzidine hydrochloride and H_2O_2. In these figures, the Mab culture supernatants were applied undiluted. Detailed procedures are presented elsewhere (11). (A) The prefrontal cortex of a patient with AD was immunostained with Mab 10H3 to reveal the amyloid of senile plaques. (B) The hippocampus of a patient with AD was immunostained with Mab 4E12. (C) The prefrontal cortex of a patient with AD was immunostained with Mab 4E12 to reveal an amyloid-containing blood vessel. (D) Amyloid of a hippocampus vessel was visualized after immunostaining with a mixture of equal parts of Mabs 4E12, 5E2, and 10H3. In all cases the bar represents 20 μm.

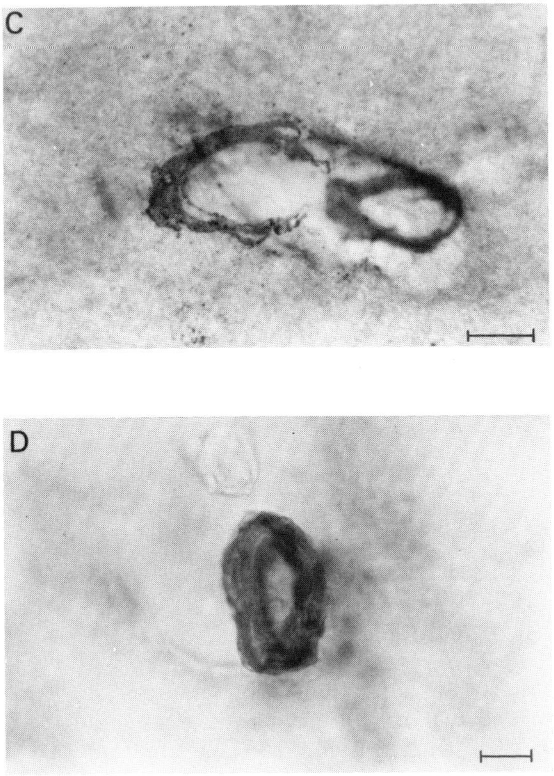

These studies were expanded upon elsewhere (11). Amyloid-containing blood vessels of the AD brain were stained by all three Mabs (e.g., Fig. 2c, d), indicating that individual epitopes are shared between vascular amyloid and senile plaques. A previous investigation demonstrated shared antigenic determinants in vascular and senile plaque amyloid using polyclonal antiserum to a synthetic peptide, corresponding to the first 10 amino acids of β-amyloid (12).

With the availability of Mabs that were highly specific towards AD brain amyloid, the means became available to address questions concerning mechanisms involved in amyloid deposition. Thus, immunostained areas were recognized and measured with relative ease by computer-assisted densitometric procedures; these studies served as a prelude to molecular investigations aimed at defining the site of origin of amyloid in the AD brain. Although numerous factors may regulate the increase in plaque size during aging and in dementia, the rate of deposition of amyloid may be particularly significant. Computer-assisted densitometry of immunostained amyloid deposits measured the numbers of pixels corresponding to immunoperoxidase reaction product within each plaque and expressed these values in relation to plaque size (Fig. 3). For all brains examined, the pixel count increased linearly in relation to the area of the plaque ($r = 0.94$). Thus, plaque size exhibited a direct linear relationship to the concentration of amyloid. The

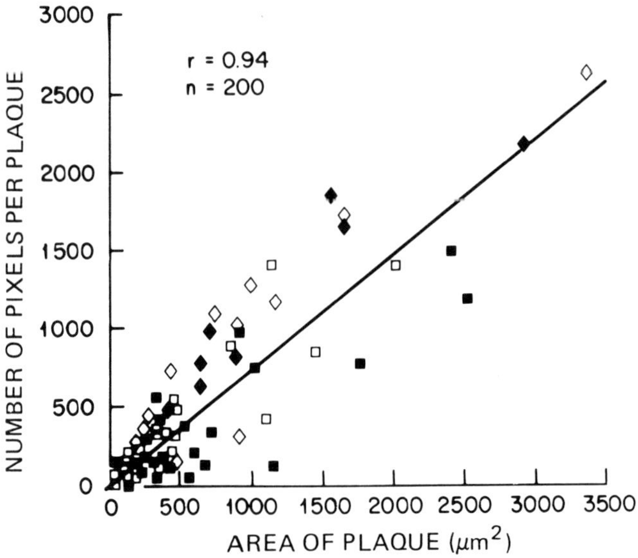

FIGURE 3 Regression analysis of the amyloid content of neuritic plaques relative to plaque size. The amyloid content of individual plaques was quantitated using video-counting software (Bioquant, Nashville, TN) compatible with an Apple IIE computer. The number of pixel units corresponding to immunoperoxidase reaction product within each plaque was measured. The first 50 plaques consecutively encountered in a field were assayed. The data were expressed as a mean and standard error of the mean for both pixel counts per plaque and plaque size (μm^2). In addition, the data were subjected to bivariate analysis, with pixel count treated as the dependent variable and plaque size as the covariate. Linear regression analysis was used to assess the significant of the relationship between pixel counts per plaque and plaque size. The data are expressed as the numbers of pixels corresponding to amyloid immunoperoxidase reaction product in each plaque (y axis) charted against the area of the plaque (x axis). A scattergram plot of the data points (n = 200) was derived from four separate AD cases.

data are consistent with the accumulation of amyloid from a focal source. Molecular genetic investigations were initiated to identify the source.

In early studies, we first demonstrated that human postmorten brain tissue exposed to long postmortem intervals retained functionally intact polysomes and mRNA (13-15). Subsequent investigations indicated that although the yields of postmortem AD brain mRNA were often lower than those from controls (16), sufficient amounts of mRNA could be extracted to analyze the more abundant

```
GAT GCA GAA TTC CGA CAT GAC TCA GGA TAT GAA GTT CAT CAT CAA AAA TTG GTG
Asp Ala Glu Phe Arg His Asp Ser Gly Tyr Glu Val His His Gln Lys Leu Val

TTC TTT GCA GAA GAT GTG GGT TCA AAC AAA GGT GCA ATC ATT GGA CTC ATG GTG
Phe Phe Ala Glu Asp Val Gly Ser Asn Lys Gly Ala Ile Ile Gly Leu Met Val

GGC GGT GTT GTC ATA GCG
Gly Gly Val Val Ile Ala
```

FIGURE 4 The A4 region of cloned cDNA insert amy37. The amy37 insert, derived from a recombinant cDNA library made from AD brain mRNA, was isolated and subjected to sequence analysis. The cDNA sequence is shown on the upper line and the predicted amino acids on the lower line. The nucleotide sequence exactly matches the corresponding region of amyloid cDNA from nondemented sources (2-5).

translation products (17) and for the preparation of recombinant cDNA libraries (18,19). Our early observations concerning the reduced levels of AD brain RNA were subsequently confirmed by molecular hybridization analyses (20) and by direct measurements of neuronal RNA in histological sections (21). Davison and co-workers (22) obtained similar results with biopsied cortical tissues from patients with AD.

We prepared AD poly(A+) RNA for the construction of two separate λgt11 recombinant cDNA libraries using the general methods previously described (18, 23). Two cases of sporadic AD were diagnosed by rigorous neuropathological criteria. In the first instance, poly(A+) RNA from a 67-year-old postmortem AD brain was prepared and the resulting cDNA library was screened with the aforementioned Mabs, as well as with synthetic oligonucleotides corresponding to the A4 amyloid polypeptide sequence reported by Masters and co-workers (6). A small insert, of approximately 200 nucleotides, was positive with both types of reagents. After being subcloned and sequenced, the insert and a synthetic oligonucleotide based upon the sequence data were used to screen a second cDNA library. The latter was prepared from poly(A+) RNA derived from a 77-year-old AD brain. Numerous positive recombinants were obtained that yielded inserts in the size range of 1-1.5 kb (24,25).

One insert, designated amy37, was subcloned into PGEM vectors and sequenced by the chemical modification method (26). In addition, the complete sequence analysis was carried out by the chain termination method (27). The structure of the 1564 nucleotide insert was reported elsewhere (25). For the present purposes it was of interest to focus on the A4 (or β-polypeptide) domain that corresponds to the amyloid protein extracted from senile plaques and blood vessels (6-8,2). Figure 4 shows the Alzheimer cDNA sequence corresponding to 42 amino acids of the A4 region. With respect to this region of the amyloid precursor cloned from AD cDNA, the derived sequence exactly matches the similar region of fetal and nondemented adult amyloid cDNAs (2-4). However, these results do not rule out the possibility that sequence variants of the amyloid cDNA will be found as additional cloned inserts are analyzed from other sporadic AD cases, and, in particular, from familial cases.

FIGURE 5 In situ hybridization. Amy37 cDNA was subcloned into the PGEM vector system and riboprobes were prepared. In situ hybridization was carried out in which the tritium-labeled probes were applied to 5 μm thick sections of AD brains and counterstained with hematoxylin and eosin. Detailed procedures will be presented elsewhere. The silver grains were apparent over large pyramidal neurons in layers 3 and 5 of cortex. Smaller neurons and other cortical layers had lower grain densities. Shown in the figure is layer 3 of an AD frontal cortex; the bar represents 20 μm.

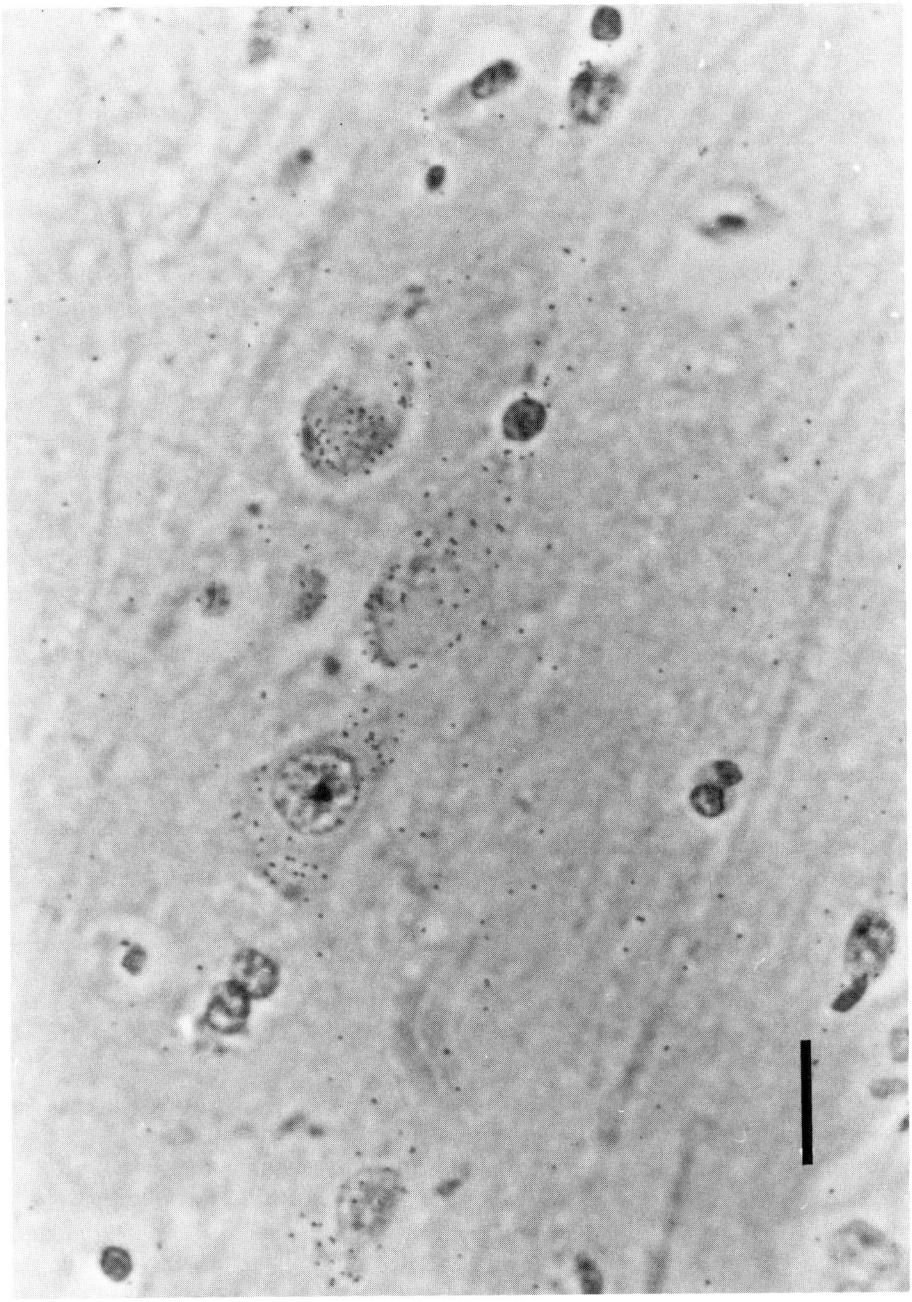

FIGURE 5

From the first AD cDNA library described above we also isolated an insert corresponding to glial fibrillary acidic protein (GFAP). Molecular cloning of human GFAP cDNA is described elsewhere (24,28,29). Thus Northern blot hybridization analyses using the amyloid cDNA as a probe could be compared with data derived from a glial-specific probe. Analysis of both control and AD cortical poly(A+) RNAs revealed that the level of amyloid mRNA was variable in different cases and did not correspond uniformly to the levels of GFAP mRNA (24, 25).

In situ hybridization studies were carried out to establish the cellular localization of amyloid mRNA in the AD cortex. Probes were derived from cloned amy37 cDNA after being digested with Eco RI restriction endonuclease and subcloned into PGEM vectors; the latter were transcribed in vitro in the presence of tritiated ribonucleotides. The riboprobes were applied to formalin-fixed sections of AD cortex using the general hybridization and autoradiography conditions described by Angerer and co-workers (30). Detailed methods will be presented elsewhere. Figure 5 shows an example of an antisense probe, containing the A4 domain, that specifically labeled large pyramidal neurons of an Alzheimer cortex. Similar results were also obtained by Bahmanyar et al. (31). However, these studies do not rule out the possibility that other cell types within the brain also produce amyloid mRNA. Indeed, amyloid mRNA appears to be present in a variety of tissues and may be an intracellular and/or membrane constituent that is common to variety of cells (2-4).

The combined use of neuroimmunological approaches, molecular cloning, Northern blot analyses, and in situ hybridization procedures led to the conclusion that the amyloid gene is expressed within neurons of the AD cortex as a high-molecular-weight precursor mRNA that contains an A4 domain identical to the brain gene product from nondemented cases. With respect to the common sequence, the results suggest that transcriptional and/or cytoplasmic factors, rather than a unique primary structure of the AD A4 mRNA domain, may be associated with the increased deposition of the corresponding amyloid protein in the cortex of a case of sporadic AD.

ACKNOWLEDGMENTS

The authors are grateful to Kathleen Moore, Anne Rodenrys, Jennifer Reifel, Montserrat Michelman, S. Hussain, and Thomas Webb for excellent technical assistance. We thank Dr. M. Stoler for his helpful suggestions during the early phases of hybridization studies. This research was supported by the following grants: AG 02126, AG 04522, AG 05134, CA 11198, and CA 36432 from the National Institutes of Health, the Katherine Smith Bolt Fund, the Axelrod Family Fund; and awards from the American Health Assistance Foundation and the

McKnight Foundation. F.M.B. was the recipient of National Institute of Mental Health Research Scientist Development Award MH00423.

REFERENCES

1. Divry, P. (1927). Etude histo-chimique des plaques seniles. *J. Neurol. Psychiatry* 27: 643-657.
2. Kang, J., Lemaire, J.-G., Unterbeck, A., Salbaum, J.M., Masters, C.L., Grzeschik, K.H., Multhaup, G., Beyreuther, K., and Muller-Hill, B. (1987). The precursor of Alzheimer's disease amyloid A4 protein resembles a cell-surface receptor. *Nature* 325: 733-736.
3. Goldgaber, D., Lerman, M.I., McBride, O.W., Saffiotti, U., and Gajdusek, D. C. (1987). Characterization and chromosomal localization of a cDNA encoding brain amyloid of Alzheimer's disease. *Science* 235: 877-880.
4. Tanzi, R.E., Gusella, J.F., Watkins, P.C., Gruns, G.A.P., Hyslop, P., VanKeuren, M.L., Patterson, D., Pagan, S., Kurnit, D.M., and Neve, R.L. (1987). Amyloid β protein gene: cDNA, mRNA distribution and genetic linkage near the Alzheimer locus. *Science* 235: 880-884.
5. Robakis, N.K., Ramakrishna, N., Wolfe, G., and Wisniewski, H.M. (1987). Molecular cloning and characterization of a cDNA encoding the cerebrovascular and neuritic plaque amyloid peptides. *Proc. Natl. Acad. Sci. U.S.A.* 84: 4190-4194.
6. Masters, C.L., Simms, G., Weinman, N.A., Multhaup, G., McDonald, B.L., and Beyreuther, I. (1985). Amyloid plaque core protein in Alzheimer's disease and Down syndrome. *Proc. Natl. Acad. Sci. U.S.A.* 82: 4245-4249.
7. Glenner, G.G., and Wong, C.W. (1984). Alzheimer's disease: Initial report of the purification and characterization of a novel cerebrovascular amyloid protein. *Biochem. Biophys. Res. Commun.* 120: 885-890.
8. Glenner, G.G., and Wong, C.W. (1984). Alzheimer's disease and Down's syndrome: Sharing of a unique cerebrovascular amyloid fibril protein. *Biochem. Biophys. Res. Commun.* 122: 1131-1135.
9. Brown, B.A., Majocha, R.E., Staton, D.M., and Marotta, C.A. (1983). Axonal polypeptides cross-reactive with antibodies to neurofilament proteins. *J. Neurochem.* 40: 299-308.
10. Galfre, G., Howe, S., Milstein, C., Butcher, G.W., and Howard, J.C. (1977). Antibodies to major histocompatibility antigens produced by hybrid cell lines. *Nature* 266: 550-552.
11. Majocha, R.E., Benes, F.M., Reifel, J.L., and Marotta, C.A. (1988). Laminar-specific distribution and infrastructural detail of amyloid in the Alzheimer disease cortex demonstrated by computer-enhanced imaging of unique epitopes recognized by monoclonal antibodies. *Proc. Natl. Acad. Sci. USA* 85: 6182-6186.
12. Wong, C.W., Quaranta, V., and Glenner, G.G. (1985). Neuritic plaques and cerebrovascular amyloid in Alzheimer disease are antigenically related. *Proc. Natl. Acad. Sci. U.S.A.* 82: 8729-8732.

13. Marotta, C.A., Strocchi, P., Brown, B.A., Bonventre, J.A., and Gilbert, J.M. (1981). Gel electrophoresis methods for the examination of human and rat brain fibrous proteins. Application to studies of human brain proteins from postmortem tissue. In: *Genetic Research Strategies for Psychobiology and Psychiatry (American College of Neuropsychopharmacology Satellite Meeting, December 10, 1979)*, E.S. Gershon, S. Matthysse, X.O. Breakefield and R.D. Ciarancllo (Eds.). Pqcific Grovc, CA, Boxwood Prcss, pp. 39-57.
14. Marotta, C.A., Brown, B.A., Strocchi, P., Bird, E.D., and Gilbert, J.M. (1981). In vitro synthesis of human brain proteins including tubulin and actin by purified postmortem polysomes. *J. Neurochem.* 36: 976-984.
15. Sajdel-Sulkowska, E.M., Coughlin, J.F., and Marotta, C.A. (1983). *In vitro* synthesis of polypeptides of moderately large size by poly(A) containing messenger RNA from postmortem human brain and mouse brain. *J. Neurochem.* 40: 670-680.
16. Sajdel-Sulkowska, E.M., and Marotta, C.A. (1984). Alzheimer's disease brain: Alterations in RNA levels and in a ribonuclease inhibitor complex. *Science* 225: 947-949.
17. Sajdel-Sulkowska, E.M., Coughlin, J.F., Staton, D.M., and Marotta, C.A. (1983). *In vitro* synthesis by messenger RNA from the Alzheimer's disease brain. In: *Banbury Report 15: Biological Aspects of Alzheimer's Disease*, R. Katzman (Ed.). New York, Cold Spring Harbor Press, pp. 193-200.
18. Marotta, C.A., Majocha, R.E., Coughlin, J.F., Manz, H.J., Davies, P., Ventosa-Micelman, M., Chou, W.-G., Zain, S.B., and Sajdel-Sulkowska, E.M. (1986). Transcriptional and translational regulatory mechanisms during normal aging of the mammalian brain and in Alzheimer's disease. *Prog. Brain Res.* 70: 303-320.
19. Marotta, C.A. (1987). Postmortem human brain: Functional messenger RNA. In: *Encyclopedia of Neuroscience*, G. Adelman (Ed.). Boston, p. 148.
20. Taylor, G.R., Carter, G.I., Crow, T.J., Johnson, J.A., Fairbairn, A.F., Perry, E.K., and Perry, R.H. (1987). Recovery and measurement of RNA in Alzheimer's disease by molecular hybridisation. *J. Neurol. Neurosurg. Psychiatry* 50: 356.
21. Doebler, J.A., Markkesbery, W.R., Anthony, A., and Rhoads, R.E. (1987). Neuronal RNA in relation to neuronal loss and neurofibrillary pathology in the hippocampus in Alzheimer's disease. *J. Neuropathol. Exp. Neurol.* 46: 28-39.
22. Neary, D., Snowden, J.S., Mann, D.N.A., Bowen, D.N., Sims, N.R., Northen, B., Yates, P.O., and Davison, A.N. (1986). Alzheimer's disease. A correlative study. *J. Neurol. Neurosurg. Psychiatry* 49: 229-237.
23. Young, R., and Davis, R. (1983). Efficient isolation of genes using antibody probes. *Proc. Natl. Acad. Sci. U.S.A.* 80: 1194-1198.
24. Zain, S.B., Salim, M., Rehman, S., Sajdel-Sulkowska, E.M., Chou, W.-G., Majocha, R.E., Moore, K., and Marotta, C.A. (1987). Molecular cloning of cDNA transcribed from messenger RNA of the Alzheimer brain. Identification of cDNA for amyloid and glial fibrillary acidic protein. *Soc. Neurosci.* (abstracts), 13: 558.

25. Zain, S.B., Salim, M., Chou, W.-G., Sajdel-Sulkowska, E.M., Majocha, R.E., and Marotta, C.A. (1988). Molecular cloning of amyloid cDNA derived from mRNA of the Alzheimer brain. Coding and non-coding regions of the fetal precursor mRNA are expressed in the Alzheimer cortex. *Proc. Natl. Acad. Sci. USA* 85: 929-933.
26. Maxam, A.M., and Gilbert, W. (1980). Sequencing end-labeled DNA with base specific chemical cleavages. *Methods Enzymol.* 65: 499-560.
27. Sanger, F., Nicklen, S., and Coulson, A.R. (1977). DNA sequencing with chain-terminating inhibitors. *Proc. Natl. Acad. Sci. U.S.A.* 74: 5463-5467.
28. Zain, S.B., Rehman, S., Sajdel-Sulkowska, E.M., Salim, M., Majocha, R., Chou, W., and Marotta, C.A. (1987). Molecular cloning and *in vitro* translation studies of GFAP mRNA from normal and Alzheimer disease brain tissue. *J. Cell. Biochem.* (Suppl. 11D, UCLA Symposia on Molecular and Cellular Biology) 198.
29. Salim, M., Rehman, S., Sajdel-Sulkowska, E.M., Chou, W.-G., Majocha, R.E., Marotta, C.A., and Zain, S.B. (1988). Preparation of a recombinant cDNA library from poly(A+) RNA of the Alzheimer brain. Identification and partial characterization of a cDNA copy encoding a glial-specific protein. *Neurobiol. Aging* 9: 163-171.
30. Angerer, R., Cox, K., and Angerer, L. (1985). *In situ* hybridization to cellular RNAs. *Genet. Eng. Principles Methods* 7: 43-65.
31. Bahmanyar, S., Higgins, G.A., Goldgaber, D., Lewis, D.A., Morrison, J.H., Wilson, M.C., Shankar, S.K., and Gujdusek, D.C. (1987). Localization of amyloid β protein messenger RNA in brains from patients with Alzheimer's disease. *Science* 327: 77-80.
32. Merrifield, R.B. (1963). Solid phase peptide synthesis. I. The synthesis of a tetrapeptide. *J. Am. Chem. Soc.* 85: 2149-2154.

12

On the Discovery of the Amyloid ß Protein in Alzheimer's Disease and Down's Syndrome

GEORGE G. GLENNER / *University of California, San Diego, School of Medicine, La Jolla, California*

While I was writing a review on amyloidosis (1), examination of the literature on the histopathological findings in Alzheimer's disease revealed considerable conflicting evidence as to the relation, if any, of cerebrovascular amyloidosis (CVA) to the presence of "senile" plaques and tangles. Nonetheless, the data available appeared to suggest the possibility of a coherent theory explaining the pathogenesis of the pathognomonic lesions of Alzheimer's disease (2). Salient to this theory was the almost invariable presence of CVA in patients with Alzheimer's disease.

The discovery of the amyloid β protein derived from the results of careful pathological examination of cerebral tissues of patients with Alzheimer's disease. Surveys of Alzheimer's disease showed an incidence of CVA of up to 92% (3,4) while further examination has now revealed that up to 100% (5) of cerebral tissue in Alzheimer's disease is involved by CVA. Age-matched controls with and without other cerebral pathological changes failed to reveal CVA. Since adult individuals over age 40 with Down's syndrome invariably were reported to have "senile" plaques and tangles (6), the incidence of CVA in these individuals was pertinent to us. A microscopic survey showed 100% of these adults with Down's syndrome had CVA (4). Since CVA is not a benign process, has been frequently documented to lead to cerebral hemorrhage (7), and produces, at the least, local, if not extensive, compromise of the blood-brain barrier by disrupting tight-junction endothelia (2), the impetus to determine the nature of the amyloid fibril protein of CVA was established. In addition, it had been predicted that the plaques and tangles of Alzheimer's disease also were composed of β-pleated sheet twisted fibrils (i.e., amyloid), based on their polarization characteristics after Congo red staining (8,9). This had been previously suggested by Divry (10).

In 1984 the cerebral vascular amyloid fibril protein, β protein, was isolated and its amino acid sequence and molecular weight (4.2 kD) determined (11).

The CVA fibril protein of adults with Down's syndrome was isolated next and was found to be essentially identical to the CVA β protein of Alzheimer's disease (12). This protein had no homology to any protein sequenced as of that date. Since this protein appeared to be a chemical phenotype in adult Down's syndrome, appearing in 100% of cases, it was predicted that, in logical fashion, it would be encoded by a gene present on chromosome 21 (12). Thus, for the first time by chemical analysis the cerebral amyloidosis of Down's syndrome and Alzheimer's disease were inextricably joined.

Antibodies to the β protein of Alzheimer's disease localized to all CVA in both Alzheimer's disease and Down's syndrome as well as to all "senile" plaques in these conditions (13). A biochemical study by others (14) revealed that isolated amyloid plaque cores were composed of unresolved peptides that were incorporated in a high-performance liquid chromatography peak that could be aligned on amino acid sequence analysis to correspond to the then known sequence of β protein. These immunohistochemical and biochemical data placed β protein in the plaque cores and by so doing linked irrevocably the β protein of CVA not only to plaques but more significantly to Alzheimer's disease. Electron microscopic evidence using an immunogold technique indicated that antibodies to β protein localized selectively to the amyloid fibers of both CVA and plaques (15), further substantiating the fact that β protein is an intrinsic protein of the amyloid fibril.

Using antibodies to β protein, we have demonstrated in the serum of a patient with familial Alzheimer's disease the presence of two immunologically reactive serum proteins of approximately 54 kD (16). Based on precedent in other types of amyloidosis affecting cerebral or peripheral vasculature (1), one or both of these proteins may be the precursor to the amyloid β protein of plaques and CVA. Since we and others have failed to demonstrate immunohistochemically the presence of β protein in tangles, even under denaturing conditions, we do not consider that CVA or plaque amyloid derives from a neural source, although biochemical evidence purporting to demonstrate the presence of β protein in neurofibrillary tangles has been reported (17). We believe instead that the amyloid fibrils of plaques and CVA derive from a serum protein precursor of peripheral tissue origin, hematogenously disseminated to be processed selectively by cerebrovascular endothelia to form vascular amyloid fibrils and intracortically by neuroglia to form plaques (18).

The discovery of the gene on chromosome 21 coding for the amyloid β protein in Alzheimer's disease and Down's syndrome (19-22) substantiated our earlier prediction (12) and further linked β protein to these two conditions. If it is confirmed that a double gene dosage effect is found in Alzheimer's disease and Down's syndrome (23), a diagnostic genomic test will potentially be available. It may also be possible to create an animal model of Alzheimer's disease by producing transgenic mice with the amyloid β protein gene.

Several major questions remain unanswered. What is the physiological function of β protein precursor? It has been suggested, based on sequence analysis, that it is a receptor protein (21). If so, what is the compound liganded? Since 100% of all patients with Down's syndrome eventually have Alzheimer's disease lesions, is the fact that the amyloid β protein gene is located on chromosome 21 indicative of some direct or indirect causal effect of this gene on chromosome 21 nondisjunction? A murine model of Down's syndrome (trisomy 16) with the amyloid β protein gene localized to chromosome 16 (24) may provide an answer. Which mechanisms are the most likely to explain amyloid fibril formation? One of the two alleles may be coding for an abnormal isotypic, "amyloidogenic" protein, as in familial amyloidotic polyneuropathy (25), or an excess of β protein precursor may saturate available proteolytic systems leading to amyloid formation (26). Alternative pathological mechanisms, including abnormalities in proteolysis (27,28), may be invoked to explain the pathogenesis of amyloid formation in Alzheimer's disease.

It would appear that the discovery of β protein has modified many concepts of the pathogenesis of Alzheimer's disease, has given it new dimensions and direction, and perhaps eventually will allow us to diagnose and treat this devastating condition specifically.

REFERENCES

1. Glenner, G.G. (1980). Amyloid deposits and amyloidosis: The β-fibrilloses (medical progress report). *N. Engl. J. Med.* 302: 1283-1292.
2. Glenner, G.G. (1979). Congophilic microangiopathy in the pathogenesis of Alzheimer's syndrome (presenile dementia). *Med. Hypotheses* 5: 1231-1236.
3. Glenner, G.G., Henry, J.R., and Fujihara, S. (1981). Congophilic angiopathy in the pathogenesis of Alzheimer's degeneration. *Ann. Pathol.* 1: 120-129.
4. Glenner, G.G. (1983). Alzheimer's disease: Multiple cerebral amyloidosis. In: *Banbury Recort 15:Biological Aspects of Alzheimer's Disease*, R. Katzman (Ed.) New York, Cold Spring Harbor Laboratory, pp. 137-144.
5. Selkoe, D.J. (1987). In: *Banbury Report: The Neurochemistry of Aging*, P. Finch and P. Davies (Eds.) New York, Cold Spring Harbor Laboratory (in press).
6. Ellis, W.G., McCulloch, J.R., and Coley, C.L. (1974). Presenile dementia in Down's syndrome. *Neurology* 24: 101-106.
7. Vinters, H.V. (1987). Cerebral amyloid angiopathy, a critical review. *Stroke* 18: 311-324.
8. Glenner, G.G., Eanes, E.D., Bladen, H.A., Linke, R.P., and Termine, J.D. (1974). β-pleated sheet fibrils: A comparison of native amyloid with synthetic protein fibrils. *J. Histochem. Cytochem.* 22: 1141-1158.
9. Glenner, G.G. (1983). Alzheimer's disease: The commonest form of amyloidosis (editorial). *Arch. Pathol. Lab. Med.* 107: 218-282.

10. Divry, P., and Florkin, M. (1927). Sur les propriétés optiques de l'amyloid. *C.R. Soc. Biol.* 97: 1808-1810.
11. Glenner, G.G., and Wong, C.W. (1984). Alzheimer's disease: Initial report of the purification and characterization of a novel cerebrovascular amyloid protein. *Biochem. Biophys. Res. Commun.* 120: 885-890.
12. Glenner, G.G., and Wong, C.W. (1984). Alzheimer's disease and Down's syndrome: Sharing of a unique cerebrovascular amyloid fibril protein. *Biochem. Biophys. Res. Commun.* 122: 1131-1135.
13. Wong, C.W., Quaranta, W.V., and Glenner, G.G. (1985). Neuritic plaques and cerebrovascular amyloid in Alzheimer's disease are antigenically related. *Proc. Natl. Acad. Sci. USA* 82: 8729-8732.
14. Masters, C.L., Simms, G., Weinman, N.A., Multhaup, G., McDonald, B.L., and Beyreuther, K. (1985). Amyloid plaque core protein in Alzheimer's disease and Down's syndrome. *Proc. Natl. Acad. Sci. USA* 82: 4245-4249.
15. Ikeda, S., Wong, C.W., Allsop, D., Landon, M., Kidd, M., and Glenner, G.G. (1987). Immunogold labeling of cerebrovascular and neuritic plaque amyloid fibrils in Alzheimer's disease with an anti β-protein monoclonal antibody. *Lab Investig.* 57: 446-449.
16. Glenner, G.G. (1987). Amyloid β protein a marker protein for Alzheimer's disease. *Clin. Res.* (abstr.) 35: 456A.
17. Guiroy, D.C., Miyazaki, M., Multhaup, G., Fischer, P., Garruto, R.M., Beyreuther, K., Masters, C.L., Simms, G., Gibbs, C.J., and Gajdusek, D.C. (1987). Amyloid of neurofibrillary tangles of Guamanian parkinsonism-dementia and Alzheimer disease share identical amino acid sequence. *Proc. Natl. Acad. Sci. USA* 84: 2073-2077.
18. Glenner, G.G., Wong, C.W., Quaranta, V., and Eanes, E.D. (1984). The amyloid deposits in Alzheimer's disease: Their nature and pathogenesis. *Appl. Pathol.* 2: 357-369.
19. Goldgaber, D., Lerman, M.I., McBride, O.W., Saffiotti, U., and Gajdusek, D.C. (1987). Characterization and chromosomal localization of a cDNA encoding brain amyloid of Alzheimer's disease. *Science* 23: 877-880.
20. Robakis, M.K., Wisniewski, H.M., Jenkins, E.C., Devine-Gage, E.A., Houck, G.E., Yao, X.L., Ramakrishma, N., Wolfe, G., Silverman, W.P., and Brown, W.T. (1987). Chromosome 21q21 sublocalization of gene encoding beta-amyloid peptide in cerebral vessels and neuritic (senile) plaques of people with Alzheimer disease and Down syndrome. *Lancet* 1: 384-385.
21. Kang, J., Lemaire, H.G., Unterbeck, A., Salbaum, J.M., Masters, C.L., Grzeschik, K.H., Multhaup, G., Beyreuther, K., and Muller-Hill, B. (1987). The precursor of Alzheimer's disease amyloid A4 protein resembles a cell-surface receptor. *Nature* 325: 733-736.
22. Tanzi, R.E., Gusella, J.F., Walkins, P.C., Bruns, G.A.P., St. George-Hyslop, P., Van Keuren, M.L., Patterson, D., Pagan, S., Kurnit, D.M., and Neve, R.L. (1987). Amyloid protein gene: cDNA, mRNA distribution, and genetic linkage near the Alzheimer locus. *Science* 235: 880-884.
23. Delabar, J.M., Goldgaber, D., Lamour, Y., Nicole, A., Huret, J.L., De Groughy, J., Brown, P., Gajdusek, D.C., and Sinet, P.M. (1987). β Amyloid gene dupli-

cation in Alzheimer's disease and karyotypically normal Down syndrome. *Science* 235: 1390-1391.

24. Lovett, M., Goldgaber, D., Ashley, P., Cox, D.R., Gajdusek, D.C., and Epstein, C.J. (1987). The mouse homolog of the human amyloid β protein (AD-AP) gene is located on the distal end of mouse chromosome 16: further extension of the homology between human chromosome 21 and mouse chromosome 16. *Biochem. Biophys. Res. Commun.* 14: 1069-1075.
25. Dwulet, F.E., and Benson, M.D. (1984). Primary structure of an amyloid prealbumin and its plasma precursor in a heredofamilial polyneuropathy of Swedish origin. *Proc. Natl. Acad. Sci. USA* 81: 694-698.
26. Gorevic, P.D., Munoz, P.C., Casey, T.T., DiRaimondo, C.R., Stone, W.J., Prelli, F.C., Rodriquez, M.M., Poulik, M.D., and Frangione, B. (1986). Polymerization of intact β_2-microglobulin in tissue causes amyloidosis in patients on chronic hemodialysis. *Proc. Natl. Acad. Sci. USA* 83: 7908-7912.
27. Glenner, G.G. (1978). The hereditary amyloidoses. In: *Metabolic Basis of Inherited Diseases*, ed. 4, J.B. Stanbury, J.B. Wyngaarden, and D.S. Fredrickson (Eds.) New York, McGraw-Hill, pp. 1308-1339.
28. Glenner, G.G. (1986). Future directions in amyloid research. In: *Amyloidosis*, J. Marrink and M.H. Van Rijswijk (Eds.) Dordrecht, M. Nijhoff, pp. 237-367.

13

The Molecular Basis of Amyloid Protein Deposition in Alzheimer's Disease and the Unconventional Virus Diseases

C. L. MASTERS, R. MARTINS, G. SIMMS, B. RUMBLE, and S. FULLER / *Department of Pathology, University of Western Australia, Perth, Australia*

J. BEER, C. HILBICH, T. DYRKS, P. FISCHER, A. WEIDEMANN, U. MÖNNING, G. MULTHAUP, M. CRAMER, J. M. SALBAUM, S. WEHR, and K. BEYREUTHER / *Center for Molecular Biology, University of Heidelberg, Heidelberg, Federal Republic of Germany*

The recent advances in the molecular biology and genetics of Alzheimer's disease (AD) stem from an understanding of the importance of the amyloid fibril in this disease process.

Pathognomonic amyloid deposition in AD is restricted to certain areas of the central nervous system, and then occurs within two clearly definable compartments.

Intracellularly, the polymerization of fibrils form neurofibrillary tangles (NFT) and "dystrophic" neurites, composed of characteristic paired helical filaments (PHF) and single "straight" filaments; NFT occur in the soma of pyramidal cells and the "dystrophic" neurites accumulate around the periphery of the extracellular amyloid deposits.

Extracellularly, amyloid fibrils first polymerize and then condense in a spherical fashion in the neuropil, and finally crystallize into an amyloid plaque core (APC). At the same time, and to a variable degree, the same molecular species polymerizes into amyloid fibrils around the walls of selected blood vessels to form an amyloid congophilic angiopathy (ACA).

The relationship of the amyloid plaque to the neuronal cell body is best illustrated by the Golgi impregnation studies of Probst, which in turn highlight the perspicaciousness of Cajal when he described the neurites around the extracellular amyloid as "reactive."

The poineering electron microscopic studies of Kidd, Terry, Wisniewski, and Gonatas demonstrated the differences in the amyloid filaments that form the NFT and APC, but we are still left with many unanswered questions on the fine structural analysis. All filaments, whether of intracellular or extracellular origin, appear to have a protofilamentous substructure with a paired or quadrupled helical arrangement.

The topographic distribution of the amyloid deposits (NFT, APC, ACA) within the brain are yielding important information (1,2). In neocortical areas, NFT/APC have laminar distribution, with the NFT principally in layers III and V while the APC tend to be accentuated in layers II and III and, to a lesser degree, in layers V and VI. There is no correlation of the distribution of lesions with any known neurotransmitter or neuropeptide system, nor with any pattern of vascular distribution or vascular innervation. The lesions are more severe in association cortex and are less pronounced in the primary sensorimotor cortices, which are involved only in the more severe cases. The only clear systematic distribution of lesions lies in the olfactory pathway/hippocampus/amygdala and basal forebrain nuclei.

Although the proportion of the population with neuropathologically confirmed AD increases exponentially with age (from 50 years onwards), nevertheless AD is not an invariable component of the aging process. There are clearly genetic, epigenetic, and probably environmental factors that operate to induce the deposition of amyloid fibrils as the major structural anomaly in AD. The neuropathological diagnosis of AD has been difficult with the use of conventional histologic techniques, but with more sensitive immunocytochemical screening procedures for the deposition of the A4 amyloid protein, a clearer picture is emerging (3).

Many authors have drawn attention to the autosomal dominantly inherited forms of AD (familial Alzheimer's disease; FAD) (4). It is probable that many cases of FAD go unrecognized and that the proportion of all cases of AD that are familial exceeds 50%.

The association of AD with Down's syndrome (DS) elucidates one of a number of possible pathways in the molecular pathogenesis of AD. Although conventional histological examination shows that all patients with DS have cerebral amyloid deposits by the age of 40 years, the more sensitive immunocytochemical techniques now show that the amyloidogenic process begins much earlier.

Our strategy over the last few years has been to purify and characterize biochemically the amyloid deposits. A similar line of investigation was also pursued by groups in San Diego (Glenner), Nottingham (Kidd, Allsop, Landon), Boston (Selkoe), Detroit (Wolfe, Roher), New York (Frangione), Staten Island (Bobin, Iqbal, Wisniewski), and Tokyo (Ihara).

Glenner (5,6) was the first to purify and sequence the ACA material. We purified the APC from both AD and DS, and showed that the principal subunit (termed A4) was a small protein (mass 4.5 kD), which was similar if not identical to the β-protein of Glenner (7). The A4 protein had a great tendency to aggregate and form dimers, tetramers, and higher oligomeric species.

When we next purified an NFT preparation from AD and DS (8), we found that the amyloid material in these preparations had a very similar biochemical profile to the APC preparations (similar in amino acid composition, SDS-gel electrophoresis, HPLC gel chromatography, and N-terminal amino acid sequence). We concluded that the A4 subunit was also the principal component of the NFT. Many investigators could not accept this result because of the clear structural and immunochemical differences between NFT and APC/ACA. They attributed our results to the presence of contaminating APC/ACA within the NFT preparations (9). Accordingly, we next showed that the NFT in the Guam parkinsonism-amyotrophic lateral sclerosis complex (PD-ALS) was also composed of the A4 subunit (10). In the Guam AD-ALS complex, APC/ACA does not occur to any appreciable degree.

The N-terminal sequences of the NFT and APC showed considerable heterogeneity; the NFT more so than APC, and both more than ACA (7,8,11). This suggested to us that *in situ* processing was occurring, and possibly that the degree of heterogeneity was a direct reflection of the age of the deposits.

The full length of the A4 molecule has now been sequenced, and shown to consist of 42-43 residues (12). One remarkable feature is the hydrophobic C terminus (residues 30-42).

As soon as the partial sequence of the A4 protein was determined, many groups around the world set about gene cloning experiments to determine the structure of the precursor protein (the A4 product as such is small and unlikely to be derived as a primary translational product). At the same time, knowing the amino acid sequence permitted the construction of synthetic peptides that could then be used for studies of the biophysical nature of the A4 molecule, and also for raising antibodies of predetermined specifity.

The synthetic A4 material clearly showed that there are two regions in the molecule responsible for fibril formation. The synthetic fibrils closely match the native amyloid fibrils (13,14). X-ray diffraction studies by Kirschner et al. (14,15) and infrared spectroscopy by our group showed that the basic packing of the subunit is as an antiparallel, β-pleated sheet. This type of subunit orientation is similar to that found in other forms of amyloid fibrils (prealbumin, light chains of immunoglobulin, etc.).

Monoclonal and polyclonal antisera raised against the A4 synthetic peptides and the native molecule are now proving to be most useful in the immunocytochemical demonstration of amyloid deposits in the AD brain, in the DS brain, and in the studies of amyloid deposits of aged normal animals such as the polar bear, rhesus monkey, and dog (3,8,13,16-19).

The A4 protein epitopes are not usually demonstrable on NFT, although some antisera to the N-terminal region of the A4 molecule do recognize a subpopulation of NFT (8). Most antisera or histochemical reactions demonstrate a variety of adventitial molecules that may only be coating the surface of the PHF. These include neurofilament triplet protein (20,21), ubiquitin (22), microtubule-associated protein 2 (23), tau protein (24), ganglioside GQ1c (25), and sulfated glycosaminoglycans (26). Epitopes unique to NFT/PHF are also claimed (27). In contrast, the A4 epitopes are readily demonstrable in situ in both APC and ACA, but even these structures also have adventitial molecules incorporated (28).

The gene (cDNA) coding for the A4 protein was partially sequenced by a number of workers (29-31) and fully sequenced by Kang et al. (12). The precursor protein (PreA4) has a predicted length of 695 residues, and has the structural domains typical of an integral membrane glycoprotein. PreA4 is not homologous with any other known protein. The A4 fragment is derived from a region of the molecule that encompasses part of the extracellular domain and part of the transmembrane region (thereby explaining its hydrophobic C-terminal region).

The A4 precursor gene is highly conserved, being present in all vertebrate species so far examined. The gene is expressed in most mammalian tissues (human, rodent) (12,29-31) but expression in neurons is particularly evident from in situ hybridization studies (32,33).

The A4 precursor gene is located in chromosome 21 (12,29-31), at the junction of band q21.3 and q22.1. This is very close, if not actually within, the region of chromosome 21 that must be duplicated for the phenotypic expression of DS. The gene is also present on the homologous mouse chromosome 16 (34, 35).

St. George-Hyslop et al. (36) found linkage between the gene locus of FAD (early-onset cases) and anonymous probes for the long arm of chromosome 21. Using restriction fragment length polymorphism analysis of FAD, Van Broekhoven et al. (37) and Tanzi et al. (38) have now shown that the FAD gene is distinct from the PreA4 gene. More than one gene for FAD may exist.

Initially it was thought that the PreA4 gene may be duplicated in AD (39). We and others find no evidence for any form of duplication of the A4 precursor gene in sporadic and familial AD (37,40-42). The gene is duplicated in DS, and we now have biochemical evidence for the overexpression of this gene in DS but not in AD (Rumble et al., manuscript in preparation).

The normal function and metabolism of the A4 precursor is now our primary target for research. The PreA4 has a molecular mass of 90-110 kD and is very labile. Its transmembrane orientation has been confirmed from in vitro translation experiments (43). The normal cellular location of the PreA4 is now being visualized using antisera to synthetic peptides corresponding to regions of the PreA4 molecule. In muscle, it is principally located at the perinuclear region of differentiated myofibres (44).

We speculate that there are two distinct pathways involved in the pathogenesis of AD. The intracellular processing of PreA4 gives rise to A4 aggregates, which form NFT. The extracellular processing of PreA4 gives rise to either APC or ACA.

It is most likely that the main origin of the extracellular material is neuronal. In situ hybridization for mRNA shows a principally neuronal origin (32,33), and we are now awaiting the results of immunocytochemical studies.

Some investigators (5,6,45) argue strongly for the hematogenous origin of the APC and ACA. We would argue equally strongly against this proposition on the following grounds:

1. The topographic distribution of APC/ACA does not correlate with any vascular territory or supply.
2. Deposition of ACA occurs in the outer walls of arterioles, less in capillaries, and least in venules.
3. There is often a demarcation of the deposition at the intima/media boundary in arterioles.
4. There is a preferential deposition in the Virchow-Robin space and overlying leptomeningeal arteries.
5. PreA4 has been localized to neurons by in situ hybridization and immunocytochemistry.
6. There is a relative lack of PreA4 in the liver and blood by Northern blots and radioimmunoassay.
7. Analogy to the neuronal PrP, which polymerizes into APC/ACA in the unconventional virus diseases, may be applicable.

Is there one gene for AD? Given our present knowledge of the multiple steps likely to occur in the processing of PreA4, this now seems unlikely. Even if we can rule out overproduction of the A4 precursor, we are now faced with the prospect of multiple forms of the precursor, the mechanisms by which it is inserted and released from the cell membrane, and the processes that allow its degradative processing and the aggregation of the A4 subunit. A simple gene mutation or epimutation (46) may be involved at any step in this complicated pathway, but it is more likely that two or more errors combine to contribute to the formation of NFT/APC/ACA.

AD shares a number of clinical and pathological features with Creutzfeldt-Jakob disease (CJD), the human counterpart of scrapie in animals (4). Not least is the familial (autosomal dominant) inheritance of CJD and the occurrence of amyloid plaques and amyloid filaments (47). The amyloid plaques occur as nonneuritic APC/ACA in all forms of the unconventional virus diseases, and are best seen in the Gerstmann-Sträussler syndrome (GSS) (47). The amyloid filaments, as in AD, occur in two forms: a distinctive scrapie-associated filament (SAF) (48) that bears some resemblance to the PHF, and a more typical amyloid filament with its presumed origin in the APC/ACA (49).

The principal protein component of the SAF is the PrP protein (50,51) with a mass of 33-35 kD. The gene for this protein is linked to genes that control the incubation period of scrapie (52). The predicted structure of the PrP shows that it too is a membrane glycoprotein (53) and in situ hybridization and immunochemical studies show that it is probably a neuronal membrane protein. Antisera to PrP and the direct biochemical analysis of the GSS-APC show that the APC in these virus diseases is composed of PrP molecules. Since it appears that PrP plays an important role in the replication cycle of the infectious agent, it is logical to question whether PreA4 may also participate in a similar process.

Many other causative hypotheses for AD exist, some of which can be easily woven into the background of the studies now emerging on the A4 molecule and its role in amyloidogenesis. For example, if PreA4 requires membrane damage before it is released and becomes susceptible to amyloidogenic proteolytic cleavage, theories and data that deal with lipid peroxidation, free radical attack, and oxidative stress should be investigated (54). Do aluminosilicates play a role in the proteolytic degradation of PreA4 (8,55)? These and other interesting theories (46) will form the basis for research into the cause of AD and its relationship to normal aging of the brain.

REFERENCES

1. Pearson, R.C.A., Esiri, M.M., Hiorns, R.W., Wilcock, G.K., and Powell, T.P.S. (1985). Anatomical correlates of the distribution of the pathological changes in neocortex in Alzheimer disease. *Proc. Natl. Acad. Sci. USA* 82: 4531-4535.
2. Rogers, J., and Morrison, J.H. (1985). Quantitative morphology and regional and laminar distributions of senile plaques in Alzheimer's disease. *J. Neurosci.* 5: 2801-2808.
3. Davies, L., Wolska, B., Hilbich, C., Multhaup, G., Martins, R., Simms, G., Beyreuther, K., and Masters, C.L. (1988). A4 amyloid protein deposition and the diagnosis of Alzheimer's disease: prevalence in aged brains determined by immunocytochemistry compared with conventional neuropathologic techniques. *Neurology* (In Press).
4. Masters, C.L., Gajdusek, D.C., and Gibbs, C.J., Jr. (1981). The familial occurrence of Cretuzfeldt-Jakob and Alzheimer's disease. *Brain* 104: 535-558.
5. Glenner, G.G., and Wong, C.W. (1984). Alzheimer's disease: Initial report of the purification and characterization of a novel cerebrovascular amyloid protein. *Biochem. Biophys. Res. Commun.* 120: 885-890.
6. Glenner, G.G., and Wong, C.W. (1984). Alzheimer's disease and Down's syndrome: Sharing of a unique cerebrovascular amyloid fibril protein. *Biochem. Biophys. Res. Commun.* 122: 1131-1135.
7. Masters, C.L., Simms, G., Weinman, N.A., Multhaup, G., McDonald, B.L., and Beyreuther, K. (1985). Amyloid plaque core protein in Alzheimer disease and Down syndrome. *Proc. Natl. Acad. Sci. USA* 82: 4245-4249.
8. Masters, C.L., Multhaup, G., Simms, G., Pottgiesser, J., Martins, R.N., and Beyreuther, K. (1985). Neuronal origin of a cerebral amyloid: Neurofibrillary tangles of Alzheimer's disease contain the same protein as the amyloid of plaque cores and blood vessels. *EMBO J.* 4: 2757-2763.

9. Gorevic, P.D., Goñi, F., Pons-Estel, B., Alvarez, F., Peress, N.S., and Frangione, B. (1986). Isolation and partial characterization of neurofibrillary tangles and amyloid plaque core in Alzheimer's disease: Immunohistological studies. *J. Neuropathol. Exp. Neurol.* 45: 647-664.
10. Guiroy, D.C., Miyazaki, M., Multhaup, G. Fischer, P., Garruto, R.M., Beyreuther, K., Masters, C.L., Simms, G., Gibbs, C.J., Jr., and Gajdusek, D.C. (1987). Amyloid of neurofibrillary tangles of Guamanian parkinsonism-dementia and Alzheimer disease share identical amino acid sequence. *Proc. Natl. Acad. Sci. USA* 84: 2073-2077.
11. Pardridge, W.M., Winters, H.V., Yang, J., Eisenberg, J., Choi, T.B., Tourtellotte, W.W., Huebner, V., and Shively, J.E. (1987). Amyloid angiopathy of Alzheimer's disease: Amino acid composition and partial sequence of a 4,200-Dalton peptide isolated from cortical microvessels. *J. Neurochem.* 49: 1394-1401.
12. Kang, J., Lemaire, H.-G., Unterbeck, A., Salbaum, J.M., Masters, C.L., Grzeschik, K.-H., Multhaup, G., Beyreuther, K., and Müller-Hill, B. (1987). The precursor of Alzheimer's disease amyloid A4 protein resembles a cell-surface receptor. *Nature* 325: 733-736.
13. Castaño, E.M., Ghiso, J., Prelli, F., Gorevic, P.D., Migheli, A., and Frangione, B. (1986). In vitro formation of amyloid fibrils from two synthetic peptides of different lengths homologous to Alzheimer's disease β-protein. *Biochem. Biophys. Res. Commun.* 141: 782-789.
14. Kirschner, D.A., Abraham, C., and Selkoe, D.J. (1986). X-ray diffraction from intraneuronal paired helical filaments and extraneuronal amyloid fibers in Alzheimer's disease indicates cross-β conformation. *Proc. Natl. Acad. Sci. USA* 83: 503-507.
15. Kirschner, D.A., Inouye, H., Duffy, L.K., Sinclair, A., Lind, M., and Selkoe, D.J. (1987). Synthetic peptide homologous to β-protein from Alzheimer disease forms amyloid-like fibrils *in vitro*. *Proc. Natl. Acad. Sci. USA* 84: 6953-6957.
16. Allsop, D., Landon, M., Kidd, M., Lowe, J.S., Reynolds, G.P., and Gardner, A. (1986). Monoclonal antibodies raised against a subsequence of senile plaque core protein react with plaque cores, plaque periphery and cerebrovascular amyloid in Alzheimer's disease. *Neurosci. Lett.* 68: 252-256.
17. Bobin, S.A., Currie, J.R., Merz, P.A., Miller, D.L., Styles, J., Walker, W.A., Wen, G.Y., and Wisniewski, H.M. (1987). The comparative immunoreactivities of brain amyloids in Alzheimer's disease and scrapie. *Acta Neuropathol.* 74: 313-323.
18. Selkoe, D.J., Bell, D.S., Podlisny, M.B., Price, D.L., and Cork, L.C. (1987). Conservation of brain amyloid proteins in aged mammals and humans with Alzheimer's disease. *Science* 235: 873-877.
19. Wong, C.W., Quaranta, V., and Glenner, G.G. (1985). Neuritic plaques and cerebrovascular amyloid in Alzheimer disease are antigenically related. *Proc. Natl. Acad. Sci. USA* 82: 8729-8732.
20. Anderton, B.H., Breinburg, D., Downes, M.J., Green, P.J., Tomlinson, B.E., Ulrich, J., Wood, J.N., and Kahn, J. (1982). Monoclonal antibodies show

that neurofibrillary tangles and neurofilaments share antigenic determinants. *Nature* 298: 84-86.

21. Sternberger, N.H., Sternberger, L.A., and Ulrich, J. (1985). Aberrant neurofilament phosphorylation in Alzheimer disease. *Proc. Natl. Acad. Sci. USA* 82: 4274-4276.
22. Mori, H., Kondo, J., and Ihara, Y. (1987). Ubiquitin is a component of paired helical filaments in Alzheimer's disease. *Science* 235: 1641-1644.
23. Kosik, K.S., Duffy, L.K., Dowling, M.M., Abraham, C., McCluskey, A., and Selkoe, D.J. (1984). Microtubule-associated protein 2: Monoclonal antibodies demonstrate the selective incorporation of certain epitopes into Alzheimer neurofibrillary tangles. *Proc. Natl. Acad. Sci. USA* 81: 7941-7945.
24. Brion, J.P., van den Bosch de Aguilar, P., and Flament-Durand, J. (1985). Senile dementia of the Alzheimer type: Morphological and immunocytochemical studies. In: *Senile Dementia of the Alzheimer Type. Early Diagnosis, Neuropathology and Animal Models*, J. Traber and W.H. Gispen (Eds.) Berlin, Springer Verlag, pp. 164-174.
25. Emory, C.R., Ala, T.A., and Frey, W.H. (1987). Ganglioside monoclonal antibody (A2B5) labels Alzheimer's neurofibrillary tangles. *Neurology* 37: 768-772.
26. Snow, A.D., Willmer, J.P., and Kisilevsky, R. (1987). Sulfated glycosaminoglycans in Alzheimer's disease. *Hum. Pathol.* 18: 506-510.
27. Ihara, Y., Abraham, C., and Selkoe, D.J. (1983). Antibodies to paired helical filaments in Alzheimer's disease do not recognize normal brain proteins. *Nature* 304: 727-730.
28. Eikelenboom, P., and Stam, F.C. (1982). Immunoglobulins and complement factors in senile plaques. *Acta Neuropathol.* 57: 239-242.
29. Goldgaber, D., Lerman, M.I., McBride, O.W., Saffiotti, U., and Gajdusek, D.C. (1987). Characterization and chromosomal localization of a cDNA encoding brain amyloid of Alzheimer's disease. *Science* 235: 877-880.
30. Tanzi, R.E., Gusella, J.F., Watkins, P.L., Bruns, G.A.P., St. George-Hyslop, P., van Keuren, M.L., Patterson, D., Pagan, S., Kurnit, D.M., and Neve, R.L. (1987). Amyloid β-protein gene: cDNA, mRNA distribution, and genetic linkage near the Alzheimer locus. *Science* 235: 880-884.
31. Robakis, N.K., Ramakrishna, N., Wolfe, G., and Wisniewski, H.M. (1987). Molecular cloning and characterization of a cDNA encoding the cerebrovascular and neuritic plaque amyloid peptides. *Proc. Natl. Acad. Sci. USA* 84: 4190-4194.
32. Bahmanyar, S., Higgins, G.A., Goldgaber, D., Lewis, D.A., Morrison, J.H., Wilson, M.C., Shankar, S.K., and Gajdusek, D.C. (1987). Localization of amyloid β-protein messenger RNA in brains from Alzheimer's disease patients. *Science* 237: 77-80.
33. Goedert, M. (1987). Neuronal localization of amyloid beta protein precursor mRNA in normal human brain and in Alzheimer's disease. *EMBO J.* 6: 3627-3632.
34. Lovett, M., Goldgaber, D., Ashley, P., Cox, D.R., Gajdusek, D.C., and Epstein, C.J. (1987). The mouse homolog of the human amyloid β-protein

(AD-AP) gene is located on the distal end of mouse chromosome 16: Further extension of the homology between human chromosome 21 and mouse chromosome 16. *Biochem. Biophys. Res. Commun.* 144: 1069-1075.
35. Reeves, R.H., Robakis, N.K., Oster-Granite, M.L., Wisniewski, H.M., Coyle, J.T., and Gearhart, J.D. (1987). Genetic linkage in the mouse of genes involved in Down syndrome and Alzheimer's disease in man. *Mol. Brain Res.* 2: 215-221.
36. St. George-Hyslop, P.H., Tanzi, R.E., Polinsky, R.J., Haines, J.L., Nee, L., Watkins, P.C., Myers, R.H., Feldman, R.G., Pollen, D., Drachman, D., Growdon, J., Bruni, A., Foncin, J.-F., Salmon, D., Frommelt, P., Amaducci, L., Sorbi, S., Piacentini, S., Stewart, G.D., Hobbs, W.J., Conneally, P.M., and Gusella, J.F. (1987). The genetic defect causing familial Alzheimer's disease maps on chromosome 21. *Science* 235: 885-890.
37. Van Broeckhoven, C., Genthe, A.M., Vandenberghe, A., Horsthemke, B., Backhovens, H., Raeymaekers, P., Van Hul, W., Wehnert, A., Gheuens, J., Cras, P., Bruyland, M., Martin, J.J., Salbaum, M., Multhaup, G., Masters, C.L., Beyreuther, K., Gurling, H.M.D., Mullan, M.J., Holland, A., Barton, A., Irving, N., Williamson, R., Richards, S.J., and Hardy, J.A. (1987). Failure of familial Alzheimer's disease to segregate with the A4-amyloid gene in several European families. *Nature* 329: 153-155.
38. Tanzi, R.E., St. George-Hyslop, P.H., Haines, J.L., Polinsky, R.J., Nee, L., Foncin, J.-F., Neve, R.L., McClatchey, A.I., Conneally, P.M., and Gusella, J.F. (1987). The genetic defect in familial Alzheimer's disease is not tightly linked to the amyloid β-protein gene. *Nature* 329: 156-157.
39. Delabar, J.-M., Goldgaber, D., Lamour, Y., Nicole, A., Huret, J.-L., de Grouchy, J., Brown, P., Gajdusek, D.C., and Sinet, P.-M. (1987). β-Amyloid gene duplication in Alzheimer's disease and karyotypically normal Down syndrome. *Science* 235: 1390-1392.
40. Podlisny, M.B., Lee, G., and Selkoe, D.J. (1987). Gene dosage of the amyloid-β precursor protein in Alzheimer's disease. *Science* 238: 669-671.
41. St. George-Hyslop, P.H., Tanzi, R.E., Polinsky, R.J., Neve, R.L., Pollen, D., Drachman, D., Growdon, J., Cupples, L.A., Nee, L., Myers, R.H., O'Sullivan, D., Watkins, P.C., Amos, J.A., Deutsch, C.K., Bodfish, J.W., Kinsbourne, M., Feldman, R.G., Bruni, A., Amaducci, L., Foncin, J.-F., and Gusella, J.F. (1987). Absence of duplication of chromosome 21 genes in familial and sporadic Alzheimer's disease. *Science* 238: 664-666.
42. Tanzi, R.E., Bird, E.D., Latt, S.A., and Neve, R.L. (1987). The amyloid β-protein gene is not duplicated in brains from patients with Alzheimer's disease. *Science* 238: 666-669.
43. Dyrks, T., Weidemann, A., Multhaup, G., Salbaum, J.M., Lemaire, H.-G., Kang, J., Müller-Hill, B., Masters, C.L., and Beyreuther, K. (1988). Identification, transmembrane orientation and biogenesis of the amyloid A4 precursor of Alzheimer's disease. *EMBO J.* 7: 949-957.
44. Zimmermann, K., Herget, T., Salbaum, J.M., Schubert, W., Hilbich, C., Cramer, M., Masters, C.L., Multhaup, G., Kang, J., Lemaire, H.-G., Beyreuther, K., and Starzinski-Powitz, A. (1988). Localization of the putative precursor of Alz-

heimer's disease specific amyloid at nuclear envelopes of adult human muscle. *EMBO J.* 7: 367-372.
45. Selkoe, D.J., Abraham, C.R., Podlisny, M.B., and Duffy, L.K. (1986). Isolation of low-molecular-weight proteins from amyloid plaque fibers in Alzheimer's disease. *J. Neurochem.* 46: 1820-1834.
46. Holliday, R. (1987). The inheritance of epigenetic defects. *Science* 238: 163-170.
47. Masters, C.L., Gajdusek, D.C., and Gibbs, C.J., Jr. (1981). Creutzfeldt-Jakob disease virus isolation from the Gerstmann-Sträussler syndrome. With an analysis of the various forms of amyloid plaque deposition in the virus-induced spongiform encephalopathies. *Brain* 104: 559-587.
48. Merz, P.A., Somerville, R.A., Wisniewski, H.M., and Iqbal, K. (1981). Abnormal fibrils from scrapie-infected brain. *Acta Neuropathol.* 54: 63-74.
49. Merz, P.A., Wisniewski, H.M., Somerville, R.A., Bobin, S.A., Masters, C.L., and Iqbal, K. (1983). Ultrastructural morphology of amyloid fibrils from neuritic and amyloid plaques. *Acta Neuropathol.* 60: 113-124.
50. Bolton, D.C., McKinley, M.P., and Prusiner, S.B. (1984). Molecular characteristics of the major scrapie prion protein. *Biochemistry* 23: 5898-5906.
51. Prusiner, S.B., McKinley, M.P., Bowman, K.A., Bolton, D.C., Bendheim, P.E., Groth, D.F., and Glenner, G.G. (1983). Scrapie prions aggregate to form amyloid-like birefringent rods. *Cell* 35: 349-358.
52. Carlson, G.A., Kingsbury, D.T., Goodman, P.A., Coleman, S., Marshall, S.T., DeArmond, S., Westaway, D., and Prusiner, S.B. (1986). Linkage of prion protein and scrapie incubation time genes. *Cell* 46: 503-511.
53. Oesch, B., Westaway, D., Wälchli, M., McKinley, M.P., Kent, S.B.H., Aebersold, R., Barry, R.A., Tempst, P., Teplow, D.B., Hood, L.E., Prusiner, S.B., and Weissman, C. (1985). A cellular gene encodes scrapie PrP 27-30 protein. *Cell* 40: 735-746.
54. Martins, R.N., Harper, C.G., Stokes, G.B., and Masters, C.L. (1986). Increased cerebral glucose-6-phosphate dehydrogenase activity in Alzheimer's disease may reflect oxidative stress. *J. Neurochem.* 46: 1042-1045.
55. Candy, J.M., Oakley, A.E., Klinowski, J., Carpenter, T.A., Perry, R.H., Atack, J.R., Perry, E.K., Blessed, G., Fairbairn, A., and Edwardson, J.A. (1986). Aluminosilicates and senile plaque formation in Alzheimer's disease. *Lancet* 1: 354-357.

Invited Editorial Comments for Part II

Problems in Detecting Heterogeneity by Linkage Studies

JONATHAN L. HAINES, RUDOLPH E. TANZI, and PETER ST. GEORGE-HYSLOP / *Harvard Medical School, Massachusetts General Hospital, Boston, Massachusetts*

Alzheimer's disease (AD) is a neurodegenerative disorder affecting millions of individuals worldwide. It has long been noted that AD may "run in families," which implies that at least some cases may have an underlying genetic cause. Recently, linkage of a familial AD gene to markers on chromosome 21 has been found, confirming the role of genetics in these families. The logical question arises: Is this gene responsible for all AD or only a portion? If only a portion, what percentage is caused by this gene? Given a detectable defect in a known gene, these are straightforward questions to answer. However, since we have not yet isolated the gene responsible for familial AD, we must rely on the more indirect method of linkage analysis to answer these questions of heterogeneity. The ability to detect heterogeneity is influenced by two factors. First, it is crucial to generate individual family scores of the logarithm base 10 of the odds favoring linkage (LOD scores) between the disease and a marker as accurately as possible. Linkage analysis is an exercise in probability and many potential problems must be overcome to calculate accurate LOD scores. Such problems include the actual calculation of the LOD scores and the pedigrees on which they are calculated. Second, the power of the particular statistical test(s) being used (given the particular data set at hand) must be considered. Each of these factors has its own peculiarities, and each will be discussed below.

LOD SCORE CALCULATION

Linkage analysis can be a powerful tool for localizing a disease gene, particularly when the underlying biological abnormality is not known (1). Linkage analysis depends solely on the cosegregation of closely linked markers for this localization. The probability of cosegregation is captured by a statistic called the LOD score. A LOD score of +3 is generally taken as significant evidence of linkage, while a LOD score of −2 is taken as significant evidence against linkage. LOD score calculation is a massive task best left to computers, and many programs have been written for this purpose (2,3). However, the calculation of LOD scores depends critically on the assumptions made before the score is generated. These assumptions make up the genetic model and include such things as disease and marker allele frequencies, disease gene penetrance, and mutation. Errors in defining the genetic model can drastically alter the resulting LOD scores, and hence the conclusions drawn from them.

Allele Frequencies

In general, allele frequencies for marker loci are easy to determine by examining either the unrelated married-in individuals in the families segregating AD, or 50 or so random unrelated individuals. For the latter it is important to check the allele frequencies in the married-in individuals as well because allele frequencies can vary dramatically due to ethnic background or population isolates. The effects of specifying the wrong allele frequencies can be devastating, particularly when an infrequent allele is incorrectly specified as frequent. For example, in our large FAD1 pedigree, we examined an infrequent polymorphism in which virutally every person was homozygous for the common allele. By incorrectly specifying the uncommon allele as common, we could generate a LOD score well above 3 at 0 centiMorgans (CM). Correct specification of allele frequencies generated a much smaller LOD score (less than 1) at 0 CM (this is shown graphically in Fig. 1). Thus we went from confirmed linkage to a mere suggestion of linkage, all with one simple transposition of allele frequencies. A similar effect can be obtained if restriction fragment length polymorphisms (RFLPs) of the same locus are in linkage disequilibrium. In this case it is very important to generate the haplotype frequencies accurately and not just the individual RFLP allele frequencies. In the families segregating AD, this can be a difficult proposition because parental information (often missing due to death) is necessary to determine which alleles at different loci travel together on the same chromosome ("set phase"), and thus correctly determine the actual haplotypes of the children and spouses.

The allele frequencies for a disease such as AD are more difficult to determine. They depend on the accuracy of estimates of prevalence and incidence of the disease and how it is inherited. For rare diseases with clear diagnostic criteria, these factors are relatively easy to determine. However, as is succinctly pointed out elsewhere in this volume (4,5), AD is not rare, nor is the mode of inheritance clear in most families. Specifying a frequent AD allele increases the chance that affected individuals receive the AD gene from outside the main line of descent, thus reducing the probability that such a person will be considered a recombinant

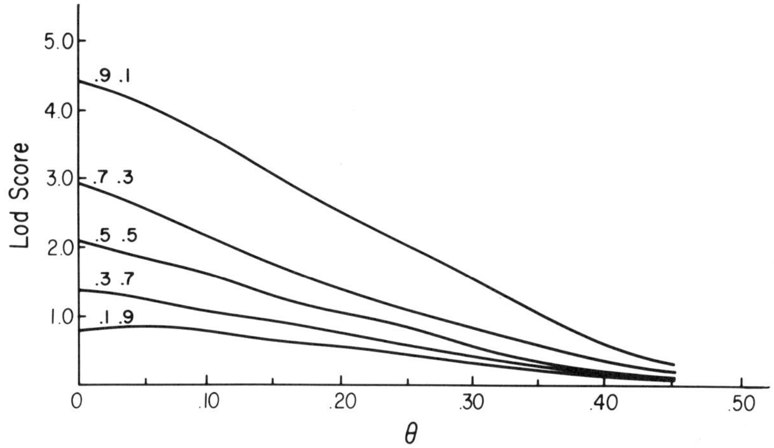

FIGURE 1 LOD score curves for a test marker vs. Alzheimer's disease in FAD1. Numbers indicate the allele frequencies for allele 1 and allele 2, respectively.

with any marker. In similar fashion, if a smaller AD gene frequency is specified, the effects of potentially recombinant individuals increase.

Penetrance of the AD Gene

Penetrance is a measure of how often persons with the putative AD gene actually develop AD. This may be dependant on many factors including age and sex of the individuals, environmental exposures, and true nonpenetrance of the trait. Thus in AD, where onset is generally in the 50s-80s, individuals at risk but below age 50 could very well be gene carriers, yet are not old enough to express the trait. Thus these individuals provide little information. At full penetrance, an elderly individual carrying the putative affected marker genotype becomes an obligate recombinant. If we drop the penetrance to 95%, however, the individual is no longer an obligate recombinant, and the amount of information from him or her is diminished. In fact, most of the information from unaffected individuals is lost once penetrance drops below 80-90%. When a large number of such individuals are included in an analysis, changes in the calculated age-at-onset curve can have dramatic effects on the resulting LOD score. Figure 2 presents some LOD score curves at differing penetrance levels using the large FAD1 pedigree. The resulting LOD scores are substantially reduced when penetrance drops below 80%.

Data on age at onset and penetrance are difficult to collect, particularly since age at onset is a somewhat arbitrary breakpoint in a continuum of decline. It is also dependent on reports from relatives, particularly spouses and children, who

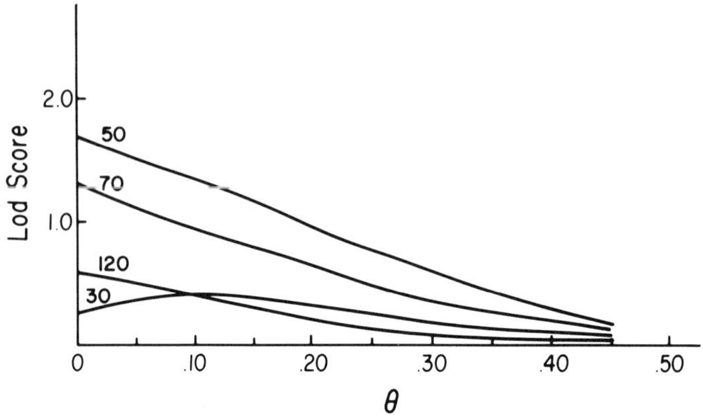

FIGURE 2 LOD score curves for a test marker vs. Alzheimer's disease in a simulated large pedigree. Numbers indicate the average age at onset of the penetrance function used.

are not schooled about what to look for, and are wholly dependent on their own memory for critical events indicating impairment of the patient. There is also a tendency by the relatives to report a round number, usually a multiple of five, for age at onset, a tendency we have clearly observed in patients with Huntington's disease (6).

Mutation Rate

In general, the mutation rate has little effect on the calculation of LOD scores, unless an absurdly high rate (on the order of 1/100) is used. In most pedigrees, the chances of a new mutation giving rise to AD are minuscule compared to those of inheriting an existing AD gene from one or the other parent.

PEDIGREE STRUCTURE

One given of linkage analysis is that the larger the family studied, the better. Big families have the advantage of an easily traceable disease gene inheritance, many potentially informative meioses, and good information about possible family specific traits such as age at onset or clinical course. In adult-onset diseases such as Huntington's disease or AD, this predictably leads to the examination of families with an earlier than average age at onset, since these families have more living affected and unaffected individuals from whom linkage information may be gained. The elderly unaffected individuals not only provide very useful linkage information but also serve as a valuable source of genealogical and clinical information, thus ensuring the ability to enlarge and expand the pedigree. This is not to say that later-onset pedigrees cannot be collected or studied, but they are usually restricted to sibships, or perhaps cousins, with, at most, one living parent.

Unfortunately there are at least two major potential practical disadvantages to large pedigrees in examining diseases such as AD. First, these pedigrees will, almost of necessity, have many generations of deceased individuals who are required to link up the various branches of living, studied individuals. Marker genotypes will be unknown for these individuals, and the disease phenotype may be in question. The maximum likelihood method for the calculation of LOD scores must consider, for each unknown individual, every possible genotype at every locus. For a two-point analysis, the time required is usually trivial. Unfortunately, the computer time necessary for analysis increases at least exponentially with the number of markers (and the number of possible alleles per marker), leading to unmanageably long computing times. The results also become more and more

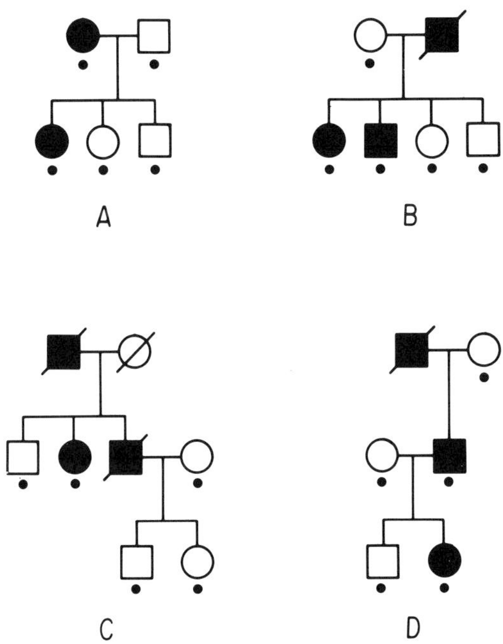

FIGURE 3 Four examples of minimal pedigree structures necessary to observe meiotic events. Dots indicate availability for testing.

dependent on the initial allele frequencies specified in the model (see above). Thus there is a practical limit to the size of a pedigree that can be considered. Second, relatives in distant pedigree branches are usually spread over widely varying geographical locations, making sample collection difficult.

On the other hand, small pedigrees are easier to collect since they require little genealogical information and members generally are living in the same geographical location. These pedigrees are much more limited in the amount of linkage information available, however, because they have only a small number of potentially informative meioses. It is often much more difficult to determine "phase," that is, which alleles of the various loci are traveling together. The information gained from these pedigrees is most often solely dependent on the allele frequencies specified in the genetic model rather than on observable cosegregation or recombination. Figure 3 presents several different pedigree structures that allow the observation of at least one cosegregating event. the basic requirement is two living affected individuals and two generations of data to allow some inference of phase. Pedigrees not meeting these minimal criteria will not be helpful in linkage analysis.

HETEROGENEITY

There are several types of heterogeneity. Allelic heterogeneity occurs when there are different mutations at the same locus causing a disease, as has been described for familial amyloidosis (7). This type of heterogeneity may only be detectable once the actual disease locus is discerned. Nonallelic heterogeneity arises when mutations at different loci give rise to the same disease phenotype. Finally, nongenetic heterogeneity may arise when nongenetic factors, such as environmental exposures, can also generate the disease phenotype.

Linkage analysis may be used to detect nonallelic and nongenetic heterogeneity once a disease linkage is found. The theory is straightforward. One merely hypothesizes that a certain portion of families (α) is of the linked variety, and the remainder are of an unlinked variety (either caused by another locus or by nongenetic factors). We use as the test data the LOD scores in each family generated over a variety of recombination fractions. Thus the linked families should produce positive LOD scores, and those not linked should generate negative LOD scores. From these individual pedigree LOD scores, the overall α and recombination fraction can be estimated and the possibility of heterogeneity may be tested using a chi square statistic. There are many practical issues that make this test difficult to implement, however.

First, the informativeness of the pedigrees studied has enormous impact. The more information (positive or negative) a single pedigree contains, the more definitively a peak recombination fraction or exclusion can be estimated in that family, and the more statistical power it holds. Thus families with only two or three potentially informative meioses will provide little or no evidence for or against heterogeneity. Thus, by their very nature, late-onset pedigrees, already limited in size, can provide little in the way of information on heterogeneity.

Second, the recombination fraction at which the disease and the marker are linked can have a profound effect on our ability to detect linkage heterogeneity. At a very small recombination fraction (less than a few cM), the discriminatory power of heterogeneity tests is fairly good. However, when the recombination fraction is beyond 10 cM, it will be very difficult to detect heterogeneity with small families, as has been pointed out (8,9). The reason for this is straightforward. At small recombination fractions, even a single recombination event argues strongly against linkage in that family and will produce negative LOD scores at that recombination fraction. However, at larger recombination fractions, the probability that a recombination is observed, even if the disease is linked in that family, is reasonably high and thus the LOD score is not very negative and results in little discriminatory power. In the case of AD, where the estimated recombination fraction with D21S1/D21S11 for the whole sample is approximately 20 cM, only very large families are going to provide enough individual information to allow us to test for linkage heterogeneity. Unfortunately, there are not yet enough of these pedigrees available for study.

Finally, the actual proportion of linked families (α) can affect the power of these statistical tests as well. If α is quite high (>90%), that is, most families are of the linked type, the power of these tests is quite good. However, as α decreases to values below 0.70, the power of these tests also decreases. This is because the overall LOD score will be a mixture of large portions of positive and negative family-specific LOD scores, and the overall result may not reach the critical value of +3 necessary to conclude that linkage exists.

CONCLUSIONS

Heterogeneity in AD is a difficult hypothesis to test. The actual calculation of the LOD scores is fraught with practical problems that can produce misleading results. Most families available for study are small and will provide little linkage information if the marker is not tightly linked to AD, as is the current situation. In addition, the power of the statistical tests themselves is sensitive to both the recombination fraction between the marker and AD and the proportion of linked families. It will take a closely linked marker and numerous large families before linkage heterogeneity, if it exists, can be proven.

REFERENCES

1. Gusella, J.F. (1986). DNA polymorphism and human disease. *Annu. Rev. Biochem.* 55: 831-854.

2. Ott, J. (1976). A computer program for linkage analysis of general human pedigrees. *Am. J. Hum. Genet.* 28: 528-529.
3. Lathrop, G.M., Lalouel, J.M., Julier, C., and Ott, J. (1984). Strategies for multilocus linkage analysis in humans. *Proc. Natl. Acad. Sci. USA* 81: 3443-3446.
4. Folstein, M., and Powell, D. (1989). Why search for the Alzheimer's disease gene?
5. Bird, T.D., and Lampe, T.H. (1989). Neurogenetics and familial Alzheimer's disease: A review.
6. Haines, J.L. Unpublished results.
7. Wallace, M.R., Conneally, P.M., Long, G.L., and Benson, M.D. (1986). Molecular detection of carriers of hereditary amyloidosis in a Swedish-American family. *Am. J. Med. Genet.* 25: 335-341.
8. Cavalli-Sforza, L.L., and King, M.C. (1986). Detecting linkage for genetically heterogeneous diseases and detecting heterogeneity with linkage data. *Am. J. Hum. Genet.* 38: 599-616.
9. Ott, J. (1985). *Analysis of Human Genetic Linkage.* Baltimore, Johns Hopkins University Press.

Part III
Promising New Avenues of Research

14

Family and Genetic Studies of Platelet Membrane Fluidity in Alzheimer's Disease

GEORGE S. ZUBENKO / *Western Psychiatric Institute and Clinic, University of Pittsburgh, Pittsburgh, Pennsylvania*

Mounting evidence suggests that Alzheimer's disease is associated with pathological changes in cells outside the central nervous system (1,2). Several of the abnormalities described in nonneural cells reflect an alteration in cell membrane structure or function. Among these is an increase in platelet membrane fluidity, as revealed by a reduction in the fluorescence anisotropy of 1,6-diphenyl-1,3,5-hexatriene (DPH) in labeled membranes (3-8). At the cellular level, several lines of evidence suggest that the increase in platelet membrane fluidity associated with Alzheimer's disease results from an accumulation of internal membranes rather than a generalized abnormality of cell membranes (6-9). Alterations in cell membrane composition and structure have also been found in brain tissue obtained at autopsy from patients who died with confirmed Alzheimer's disease. These include changes in brain phospholipid metabolism as revealed by nuclear magnetic resonance spectroscopy (10,11), disordering of cortical myelin as indicated by x-ray diffraction (12), and an alteration in the molecular dynamics of hippocampal membranes as documented by fluorescence spectroscopy (13).

Initial assessments of the stability and specificity of this platelet membrane alteration have been promising. Platelet membrane fluidity, as reflected by DPH anisotropy, is stable over a period of at least 1 year in patients with Alzheimer's disease as well as in neurologically healthy elderly controls (14). Furthermore, the increase in platelet membrane fluidity associated with Alzheimer's disease was not found in platelets from patients with depression (7), mania (15), multi-infarct dementia (8), or in cognitively intact patients with Parkinson's disease (unpublished results).

A cutoff point for DPH anisotropy of 0.1920 at 37°C (90th percentile for healthy elderly controls) (Fig. 1) segregates patients with Alzheimer's disease into

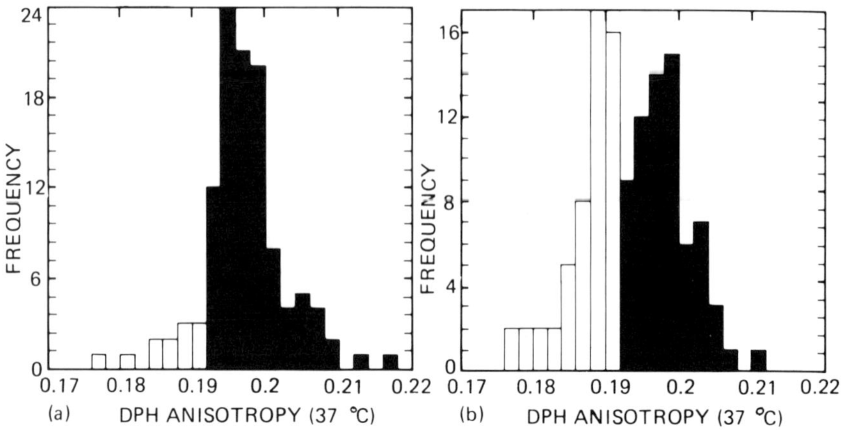

FIGURE 1 Distribution of fluorescence anisotropy for DPH-labeled platelet membranes from (a) 123 age- and sex-matched demented patients with probable Alzheimer's disease and (b) 114 neurologically healthy controls (21). The mean DPH value and associated variance for the group of subjects with Alzheimer's disease, 0.1933 (±0.0070), were significantly different than the respective values for the control group, 0.1972 (±0.0057) (comparison of means, $p=1.3 \times 10^{-5}$, comparison of variances, $p<5 \times 10^{-2}$). The cutoff point for normal fluidity, 0.1920, was based on the lowest 90th percentile of anisotropy values in the control group. (From Ref. 19.)

two clinical subtypes. As a group, patients with increased platelet membrane fluidity (DPH anisotropy less than 0.1920) show an earlier onset of symptoms (7), have a more rapidly progressive course (7), are more likely to manifest left-right dissociations in cognitive functions (16), and are less likely to exhibit focal electroencephalographic (EEG) slowing (17) and risk factors for stroke (unpublished results). A family history of dementia, especially early-onset dementia, also appears to be a more common feature of patients in this group (18).

A family study was conducted to determine whether increased platelet membrane fluidity aggregates in the families of patients with Alzheimer's disease and, if so, whether this platelet abnormality selectively runs in the families of probands who themselves exhibit the abnormality (19). A series of 23 patients with probable Alzheimer's disease who had at least one available first-degree relative living in the Pittsburgh area were chosen as probands from the large cohort of patients described in Figure 1. The diagnosis of probable Alzheimer's disease was made according to currently accepted clinical criteria as applied conjointly by board-certified neurologists and psychiatrists (20). An additional 15 patients with Alzheimer's disease that had been confirmed by autopsy (21), from whom platelet membranes could not be obtained but who had at least one available first-degree

TABLE 1 Platelet Membrane Fluidity in Asymptomatic First-Degree Relatives of Probands with Autopsy-Proven or "Probable" Alzheimer's Disease

	n	Sibs/Offspring	M/F	Age (years)	DPH Anisotropy	DPH Anisotropy <0.1920 (Total)	DPH Anisotropy <0.1920 (%)
Probands							
Autopsy-Proven	15	3/29	8/24	49.1 (9.5)	0.1952 (0.0068)	10/32	31.3
Probable AD	23	10/33	19/24	50.0 (12.0)	0.1948 (0.0075)	15/43	34.9
Total	38	13/62	27/48	49.6 (10.9)	0.1950 (0.0071)[a]	25/75[c]	33.3
Controls	34	–	13/21	51.0 (7.5)	0.1976 (0.0037)[b]	1/34[d]	2.9

The probands with probable Alzheimer's disease consisted of 1 male and 22 females with a mean age of 73.3 years (± 6.2 [SD]). Their mean age of symptomatic onset was 69.1 years (± 7.6) with a mean duration of illness of 4.4 years (± 2.3). The group was moderately to severely demented as reflected by a mean MMS score of 12.7 (± 4.6) and a DRS score of 10.9 (± 5.8). Because gender does not affect platelet membrane fluidity for subjects over the age of 40 years, the excess of females in the proband group was not expected to affect the results. The mean DPH anisotropy value and standard deviation for this group, 0.1925 (± 0.0081) were similar to the respective values for the larger demeted cohort from which they were recruited: 0.1933 (± 0.0070). Forty-eight percent of the proband group exhibited increased platelet membrane fluidity (DPH anisotropy less than 0.1920), similar to the respective proportion of the larger demented cohort, 44%. Means for subject age and DPH anisotropy for labeled platelet membranes are presented with standard deviations in parentheses (19).

[a] vs. [b]: For comparison of means; $p = 1.7 \times 10^{-2}$, one-tailed Mann-Whitney-Wilcoxon test; for comparison of variances; $p < 5.0 \times 10^{-3}$, one-tailed F test.

[c] vs. [d]: $p = 2.0 \times 10^{-3}$, one-tailed Fisher's exact test.

relative, also served as probands. The participation of all neurologically healthy first-degree relatives of the 38 probands was solicited and an age- and sex-matched cohort of neurologically healthy controls, chosen without regard to family history of dementia, was recruited. all asymptomatic relatives and controls had mini-mental state (MMS) scores (22) that were greater than or equal to 26 and dementia rating scale (DRS) scores (23) less than or equal to 4. Disorders that affect blood cell membrane lipid composition or serum lipid profiles, restrictive diets, and exposure to medications that affect platelet membrane fluidity in vitro or in vivo served as additional exclusion criteria (6,9,24). Fasting blood samples were collected and platelet isolation was performed in plasticware at room temperature according to a minor modification (9) of the method of Corash and co-workers (25). Laboratory analyses were carried out by staff who were blind to the subjects' demographic status and clinical histories (6,7,9).

Data for the high-risk cohort of asymptomatic, first-degree relatives of demented probands along with the neurologically healthy controls are presented in Table 1. Platelet membrane fluidity was not significantly correlated with subject age between 35 years and 90 years in previous studies (6,7) or in any of the subject groups described in this study. Therefore, age adjustment of the cutoff for increased platelet membrane fluidity was not used. Both groups of relatives as well as the control group were well matched for age and gender. The platelet membrane fluidity data for the two groups of relatives were similar. The combined group of first-degree relatives exhibited an increase in platelet membrane fluidity as reflected in a significant reduction in mean DPH anisotropy value as well as in the increased proportion of relatives who exhibited increased platelet membrane fluidity (DPH anisotropy < 0.1920). The prevalence of increased platelet membrane fluidity in the combined sample of asymptomatic first-degree relatives was 11.5 times higher than the respective value for the age- and sex-matched controls chosen without regard to family history and 3.2 times the respective value for the older control population (Fig. 1). This range reflected the estimates of the baseline rate of the platelet abnormality in the two control populations (2.9% or 1 of 34; 10.5% or 12 of 114), which did not significantly differ from one another. Furthermore, the variance in the anisotropy data from the combined group of relatives was significantly increased relative to the control value, but was similar to the respective variances for the demented probands and the larger cohort of demented patients from which they were chosen (Fig. 1). In summary, the increase in platelet membrane fluidity associated with Alzheimer's disease is a familial trait that aggregates in neurologically healthy, first-degree relatives of probands with Alzheimer's disease.

The implications of these results are manifold. Population and family studies conducted in the United States (26-30) and abroad (31) have uniformly found that first-degree relatives of patients with Alzheimer's disease are at a significantly higher lifetime risk of developing dementia, especially if the affected family member is a parent and the age of onset is before age 70. The observed 3.2-11.5-fold increase in the prevalence of the platelet membrane abnormality among first-degree relatives (primarily offspring) of probands with Alzheimer's disease strongly suggests that this cellular change is related to, but antedates, the onset of symptoms of dementia. Furthermore, this finding excludes nonspecific concomitants of chronic illness or medication history as the cause of the increased platelet membrane fluidity observed in patients with Alzheimer's disease.

Population and family studies have suggested that a significant fraction, even a majority, of the cases of Alzheimer's disease may result from a familial disorder that places first-degree relatives at a lifetime risk approaching 50% (26-30,32). Based on these reports, we have analyzed our family data for evidence that the increased platelet membrane fluidity associated with Alzheimer's disease might potentially provide a useful genetic marker for familial Alzheimer's disease. The observed 3.2-11.5-fold increase in the frequency of cases with increased platelet membrane fluidity among the first-degree relatives of probands with Alzheimer's disease is similar to the reported 3.6-6.9-fold increase in the 85-90-year lifetime risk of developing Alzheimer's disease in this high-risk group (26-32). Moreover, the mean of the 2.9-10.5% range of cases with increased platelet membrane fluidity in the control group is approximately half of the respective value for the 8-18% estimates of 85-90-year lifetime risk of Alzheimer's disease in the general population (26-32). This finding is consistent with the approximate 50% prevalence of the platelet membrane abnormality in our patients with Alzheimer's disease. As predicted for an inherited trait, relatives with increased platelet membrane fluidity were almost exclusively related to probands who exhibited this phenotype (Table 2). Moreover, the proportion of individuals exhibiting increased platelet membrane fluidity among the first-degree relatives of probands of the same phenotype, 57% (13 of 23), did not significantly differ from the 50% expected for

TABLE 2 Relationship of Platelet Membrane Fluidity in Probands with "Probable" Alzheimer's Disease to Platelet Membrane Fluidity in Asymptomatic First-Degree Relatives

Probands	First-Degree Relatives	
	Increased Fluidity	Normal Fluidity
Increased fluidity	13 (8M/5F)	10 (4M/6F)
Normal fluidity	2 (1M/1F)	18 (6M/12F)

Relatives with increased platelet membrane fluidity (DPH anisotropy <0.1920) were significantly more likely to be related to probands with increased platelet membrane fluidity than probands with normal platelet membrane fluidity (DPH anisotropy $\geqslant 0.1920$); $p = 0.0015$, one-tailed Fisher's exact test (19).

an uncommon but fully penetrant autosomal dominant trait. Males and females in this group of relatives were affected at approximately equal frequencies, consistent with this pattern of inheritance.

While our family data were consistent with the hypothesis that increased platelet membrane fluidity may result from the inheritance of an uncommon but highly penetrant autosomal dominant gene(s), as suggested by others for at least some cases of Alzheimer's disease (26,30-33), the data presented above do not exclude other genetic and nongenetic causes for this cell membrane alteration associated with Alzheimer's disease. To resolve this ambiguity, we conducted a complex segregation analysis of continuous DPH anisotropy values obtained from 14 pedigrees containing 26 nuclear families (A. Chakravarti, S. Slaughenhaupt, G.S. Zubenko, unpublished results). The probands were 4 sequential cases of autopsy-confirmed Alzheimer's disease and 10 sequential cases of probable Alzheimer's disease diagnosed by currently accepted clinical criteria (22), and were chosen without knowledge of their platelet membrane fluidity values. These families included a total of 95 relatives between the ages of 16 and 85 years.

The segregation analysis was performed using the quantitative DPH anisotropy data under a defined model of inheritance termed the mixed model, as proposed by Morton and MacLean (34) and extended by Lalouel and Morton (35). This model assumes that a continuous variable (x) results from the independent contributions of a major locus, a multifactorial transmissible component, and random environmental effects. The object of the analysis was to assess the evidence for the segregation of a major locus affecting platelet membrane fluidity in the presence of other causes of familial aggregation. In order to satisfy the distributional assumptions of the mixed model, the family data were first adjusted against a normalized control sample. The resulting normalized data were subjected to complex segregation analysis using the computer program POINTER (35), with which the $\log_e$ likelihood and maximum likelihood parameter estimates were calculated.

The general model obtained was that of a single major locus, with additive allelic effects and a gene frequency of 0.56 for the allele causing increased platelet membrane fluidity. Furthermore, there was no residual polygenic variation once the major locus was included. In comparison, a sporadic model with no inheritance could be clearly rejected (χ^2=27.46, 4 df, $p < 2 \times 10^{-5}$). The most general transmission model, the multifactorial model, gave an estimated heritability of 79% and could also be rejected against the general mixed model (χ^2=14.24, 3 df, p=0.0026). Next, major locus models were evaluated, but both the single-locus dominant (χ^2=12.84, 2 df, p=0.0016) and the recessive (χ^2=12.15, 2 df, p=0.0024) models were rejected. A single-locus additive model fit the family data as well as the mixed model (χ^2=0.16, 2 df, p=0.69), providing no evidence for the inclusion of other genetic or nongenetic determinants of the platelet membrane alteration associated with Alzheimer's disease. Therefore, the segregation analysis suggested that platelet membrane fluidity, as reflected by a continuum of DPH anisotropy values, is controlled by the inheritance of a single locus with two alleles with additive effects: one causing increased fluidity (*a*) and one causing normal fluidity (*A*). The allele *a* causing increased fluidity had an estimated frequency of q=0.56 ± SE 0.06.

In our previous studies, a cutoff value of <0.1920 was chosen for DPH anisotropy at 37°C to define increased platelet membrane fluidity. The genetic model was useful for calculating penetrances of the various genotypes using this threshold. Based on the assumption that q=0.56, the penetrance of homozygotes *aa* was 76% and of heterozygotes *Aa* was 1%. The penetrance of *aa* could be increased to 90% by defining the cutoff value at 0.1940. However, this was accompanied by a higher frequency (4%) of heterozygotes being affected. Resetting the cutoff of 0.1920-0.1940 resulted in the reclassification of only one individual into the affected group. Therefore, the genetic model supports the validity of the 0.1920 threshold for increased platelet membrane fluidity.

When q=0.56 and DPH anisotropy <0.1920, approximately 98% (P [aa/affected] = P [affected/aa] P[aa] /P[affected] = 0.9797) are *aa* and 2% are *Aa*. Thus in matings between affected and normal subjects, the common mating types are *aa* X *AA* and *aa* X *Aa*, and their relative frequencies are approximately 0.28 and 0.72. Based on these estimates, the average segregation probability for affection in such families is approximately 0..36±SE 0.04 (0.5X0.72; 36), a value not significantly different from the previous empirical value 0.57 ± SE 0.10 (19; χ^2=0.39, 1 df, p=0.53). Therefore, while the inheritance of the fluorescence anisotropy of DPH-labeled membranes on a continuous scale is best represented by a single-locus model with two condominant alleles, the inheritance of increased platelet membrane fluidity, as defined by DPH anisotropy values <0.1920, more closely resembles a trait produced by the inheritance of a highly penetrant, recessive allele that is quite common in the population. Indeed, family data and segregation patterns of familial Alzheimer's disease merit reconsideration in light of the possibility that the relevant gene(s) may be more common than previously proposed (26, 30-33).

Our segregation data indicate that the alteration of platelet membrane fluidity associated with a subtype of Alzheimer's disease is determined by the inheritance of a single major locus. They do not allow us to deduce whether this locus represents an Alzheimer's gene or a gene that modifies the expression of Alzheimer's disease. However, these results now justify linkage studies of platelet membrane fluidity with Alzheimer's disease, which may settle this issue. Under either outcome, our findings make mapping and cloning strategies of the *PMF* locus a reasonable goal.

Finally, it should be noted that the genetic model does not exclude the possibility of an essential interaction with one or more pandemic environmental factors. Under this circumstance, the genetic model is not fatalistic. For example, the altered expression of a viral receptor, gut transport system, or metabolic pathway may lead to the development of Alzheimer's disease only in the presence of the relevant infectious agent or toxin. Successful therapeutic strategies could include interventions that are as simple, in principle, as the development of a vaccine or the elimination of an environmental toxin. Furthermore, therapeutic strategies that delay the age of symptomatic onset in those individuals who show the diathesis could have a significant effect on the public health problem posed by this late-onset, neurodegenerative disorder.

REFERENCES

1. Blass, J.P., and Zemcov, A. (1984). Alzheimer's disease: A metabolic systems degeneration? *Neurochem. Pathol.* 2: 103-114.
2. Hollander, E., Mohs, R.C., and Davis, K.L. (1986). Antemortem marker for Alzheimer's disease. *Neurobiol. Aging* 7: 367-387.
3. Zubenko, G.S., Cohen, B.M., Growdon, J., and Corkin, S. (1984). Cell membrane abnormality in Alzheimer's disease. *Lancet* 2: 235.
4. Zubenko, G.S., and Cohen, B.M. (1985). Biophysical alterations in cell membranes associated with psychotherapeutic drug exposure, psychopathology, and aging. *Psychopharm. Bull.* 21: 631-640.
5. Zubenko, G.S., and Malinakova, I. (1987). Temperature dependence of the molecular dynamics of platelet membranes in Alzheimer's disease. *Biol. Psychiatry* 22: 987-994.
6. Zubenko, G.S., Cohen, B.M., Boller, F., Reynolds, C.F., et al. (1987). Platelet membrane abnormality in Alzheimer's disease. *Ann. Neurol.* 22: 237-244.
7. Zubenko, G.S., Cohen, B.M., Reynolds, C.F., Boller, F., et al. (1987). Platelet membrane fluidity in Alzheimer's disease and major depression. *Am. J. Psychiatry* 144: 860-868.
8. Hicks, N., Brammer, M.J., Hymas, N., and Levy, R. (1987). Platelet membrane properties in Alzheimer and multi-infarct dementias. *J. Alzheimer's Dis. Assoc. Disord.* 1: 90.
9. Zubenko, G.S., Malinakova, I., and Chojnacki, B. (1987). Proliferation of internal membranes in platelets from patients with Alzheimer's disease. *J. Neuropathol. Exp. Neurol.* 46: 407-418.
10. Pettegrew, J.W., Minshew, N.J., Cohen, M.M., Kopp, S.J., et al. (1984). P-31 NMR changes in Alzheimer's and Huntington's disease brain (abstract). *Neurology* 34: 281.
11. Barany, M., Chang, Y., Arus, C., Rustan, T., et al. (1985). Increased glycerol-3-phosphorylcholine in post-mortem Alzheimer's brain (letter). *Lancet* 1: 517.
12. Chia, L.S., Thompson, J.E., and Moscarello, M.A. (1984). X-ray diffraction evidence for myelin disorder in brain from humans with Alzheimer's disease. *Biochim. Biophys. Acta* 775: 308-312.
13. Zubenko, G.S. (1986). Hippocampal membrane alteration in Alzheimer's disease. *Brain Res.* 385: 115-121.

14. Zubenko, G.S., and Teply, I. (1988). Longitudinal study of platelet membrane fluidity in Alzheimer's disease. *Biol. Psychiatry* 24: 918-924.
15. Zubenko, G.S., and Cohen, B.M. (1985). Effects of phenothiazine treatment on the biophysical properties of platelet membranes for psychiatric patients. *Biol. Psychiatry* 20: 384-396.
16. Zubenko, G.S., Huff, F.J., Becker, J., Beyer, J., et al. (1988). Cognitive function and platelet membrane fluidity in Alzheimer's disease. *Biol. Psychiatry* 24: 925-936.
17. Zubenko, G.S., Brenner, R.P., and Teply, I. (1988). EEG correlates of increased platelet membrane fluidity in Alzheimer's disease. *Arch. Neurol.* 45: 1009-1013.
18. Zubenko, G.S., Huff, F.J., Beyer, J., Auerbach, J., et al. (1988). Familial risk of dementia associated with abnormal platelet membrane fluidity in Alzheimer's disease. *Arch. Gen. Psychiatry* 45: 889-893.
19. Zubenko, G.S., Wusylko, M., Cohen, B.M., Boller, F., et al. (1987). Family study of platelet membrane fluidity in Alzheimer's disease. *Science* 238: 539-542.
20. McKhann, G., Drachman, D., Folstein, M.F., Katzman, R., et al. (1984). Clinical diagnosis of Alzheimer's disease: Report of the NINCDS-ADRDA work group under the auspices of the Department of Health and Human Services Task Force on Alzheimer's disease. *Neurology* 34: 939-944.
21. Khachaturian, Z.S. (1985). Diagnosis of Alzheimer's disease. *Arch. Neurol.* 42: 1097-1105.
22. Folstein, M.F., Folstein, S.F., and McHugh, P.R. (1975). "Mini-mental state": A practical method for grading the cognitive state of patients for the clinician. *J. Psychiatry Res.* 12: 189-198.
23. Blessed, G., Tomlinson, B.E., and Roth, M. (1968). The association between quantitative measures of dementia and senile change in the cerebral grey matter of elderly subjects. *Br. J. Psychiatry* 114: 797-811.
24. Zubenko, G.S., and Cohen, B.M. (1985). Effects of psychotropic agents on the physical properties of platelet membranes in vitro. *Psychopharmacology* 86: 369-373.
25. Corash, L., Tan, H., and Gralnick, H.R. (1977). Heterogeneity of human whole blood platelet subpopulations, I: Relationship between buoyant density, cell volume, and ultrastructure. *Blood* 49: 71-87.
26. Heston, L.L., Mastri, A.R., Anderson, V.E., and White, J. (1981). Dementia of the Alzheimer type: Clinical genetics, natural history and associated conditions. *Arch. Gen. Psychiatry* 38: 1085-1090.
27. Heyman, A., Wilkinson, W.E., Hurwitz, B.J., Schmechel, D., et al. (1983). Alzheimer's disease: Genetic aspects and associated clinical disorders. *Ann. Neurol.* 14: 507-515.
28. Breitner, J.C.S., and Folstein, M.F. (1984). Familial Alzheimer's dementia: A prevalent disorder with specific clinical features. *Psychol. Med.* 14: 63-80.
29. Silverman, J.M., Breitner, J.C.S., Mohs, R.C., and Davis, K.L. (1986). The reliability of the family history method in Alzheimer's disease and related dementias. *Am. J. Psychiatry* 143: 1279-1282.

30. Mohs, R.C., Breitner, J.C.S., Silverman, J.M., and Davis, K.L. (1987). Alzheimer's disease: Morbid risk among first-degree relatives approximates 50% by 90 years of age. *Arch. Gen. Psychiatry* 44: 405-408.
31. Larsson, T., Sjogren, H., and Jacobson, G. (1963). A clinical, sociomedical and genetic study. *Acta Psychiatr. Scand.* 39: 1-259.
32. Breitner, J.C.S., Folstein, M.F., and Murphy, E.A. (1986). Familial aggregation in Alzheimer dementia: I. A model for age-dependent autosomal dominant inheritance. *J. Psychiatr. Res.* 20: 31-43.
33. St. George-Hyslop, P.H., Tanzi, R.E., Polinaky, R.J., Haines, J.L., et al. (1987). The genetic defect causing familial Alzheimer's disease maps on chromosome 21. *Science* 235: 885-890.
34. Morton, N.E., and MacLean, C.J. (1974). Analysis of family resemblance. 3. Complex segregation of quantitative traits. *Am. J. Hum. Genet.* 26: 489-503.
35. Lalouel, J.-M., and Morton, N.E. (1981). Resolution of linkage for irregular phenotype systems. *Hum. Hered.* 31: 312-321.

15

The Search for Possible Neuropsychological Associations and Other Early Markers in Familial Alzheimer's Disease

LINDA A. WINTERS-MINER / *Familial Alzheimer's Disease Research Foundation, Tulsa, Oklahoma*

DAVID STRYKER / *Eastern Nazarene College, Quincy, Massachusetts, and Metropolitan State Hospital, Belmont, Massachusetts*

ROGER C. BURGUS / *City of Faith Medical and Research Center, Tulsa, Oklahoma*

GARY D. MINER / *Familial Alzheimer's Disease Research Foundation, Tulsa, Oklahoma, and City of Faith Medical and Research Center, Tulsa, Oklahoma*

INTRODUCTION

In 1980, we started planning a long-term prospective study on possible neuropsychological associations with familial Alzheimer's disease (FAD). The actual study started in 1982 as we began assessing members of families appearing to have a genetic predisposition for Alzheimer's disease. The purpose was to find associations, biomarkers, or "risk factors" that could predict those destined to get FAD prior to actual diagnosis. The assessment battery consisted of neuropsychological tests, interviews, and interviewer observations, the sum of which required about 2 hr to administer. Over the next 4 years we traveled across the United States to locations of subjects to conduct the testing. The information derived will allow us to build a discriminate function model testing risk factor hypotheses.

Differences were found between the at-risk and the not-at-risk groups. We studied a "homogeneous" group of people having a higher probability of similar causes for their disease than a group chosen randomly from the population. The group studied was homogeneous in that it:

1. was familial, rather than sporadic, in cases of AD.
2. appeared to originate from the same geographic area.
3. had a specified age of onset that appeared to be more or less consistent within families.
4. had families with a large number of cases compared to other families in which only a small number of family members were, or had been, affected.
5. appeared to fit an autosomal dominant mode of genetic inheritance.

Study of such a homogeneous group had the potential advantage of providing cleaner data due to the natural control existing in the families themselves: a number of subjects tested had nonaffected parents, thus these can be considered as internal controls.

Family pedigrees were studied in a genetic-epidemiological fashion similar to that suggested by Schull and Weiss (1) and Mary-Claire King (2). The psychometric tests were given to members of familial Alzheimer's disease families, under the age of onset, to look for premorbid putative risk factors. Of particular interest were the possibilities of bimodality of the at-risk vs. not-at-risk groups (defined by having or not having an affected parent). A large part of this chapter will deal with the preliminary data from our neuropsychological marker study, with suggestions for further studies of this type. In addition, other biomarker studies that are currently being conducted or need to be done in the future will be reviewed briefly.

SEARCH FOR NEUROPSYCHOLOGICAL ASSOCIATIONS

Due to the insidious nature of the disease, early symptoms of Alzheimer's disease such as memory deficits may be masked by compensatory mechanisms that are difficult to spot even by affected persons themselves. Therefore, traditional tests of intelligence and vocabulary may not pick up very early differences. This is especially true for an intelligent individual: when one word will not come to mind, synonyms abound so that compensatory mechanisms may be present for a long time before their effectiveness is exhausted. Furthermore, a major problem facing researchers using neuropsychological instruments is the differentiation of psychiatric diagnoses from other degenerative brain disorders (3,4). Thus many tests, involving different brain areas and functions, were used. Also included were traditional tests of intelligence.

Review of Background Work

Of great interest was the fact that Goudsmit et al. (5) reported that two FAD families originated from the same area in Russia, the "Pale settlement" of Ashkenazi Jews. A good history of the development of this settlement is provided by Goodman (6). Certain inherited disorders occur with increased frequency in

Jews of this eastern European origin (6-8). Although some of these diseases were described in the 1880s, most have been recognized during the past three decades. Goodman (6) made two interesting observations concerning these disorders: most involve the central nervous system and, three of them (Tay-Sachs, Gaucher's, and Niemann-Pick disease) share a common metabolic pathway. It is not known if this is a random finding or if it indicates a particular genetic relationship.

One early report (9) provided strong evidence for a biological distinction between FAD and sporadic dementia of the Alzheimer's type (DAT). This work showed that brain suspensions caused in vitro cell fusing in 10 of 17 FAD cases (59%) but in only 3 of 17 sporadic DAT cases (17%); the percentage of sporadic cases was not statistically different from the nonneurological control patients. Since one-third of patients with various other chronic neurological disorders exhibit cell fusion activity, this may be related to secondary neurological changes rather than being directly connected to the causes of these diseases.

Low performance IQ prior to onset has been reported in two patients with Alzheimer's disease (10) and also in one of two currently unaffected family members of a FAD family; these two show increased aneuploidy, which was hypothesized to be a predictor of disease in FAD families. Whether or not low performance relative to verbal is a possible predictor was one of the goals of this study. Later work by Coolidge et al. (11) found a discriminant function algorithm to differentiate dementia from depression. Again, the relative strength of the verbal scores generated the predictive relationship; the vocabulary scaled score was greater than or equal to twice the Block Design scaled score with a 74% correct prediction rate for dementia. Whether or not such scores would predict prior to diagnosis had yet to be demonstrated.

Duara et al. (12) compared neuropsychological measures with positron emission tomographic (PET) scans that included three patients who had first-degree family members also affected by Alzheimer's. Their 21 demented patients showed consistent patterns in the neuropsychological measures and in metabolic abnormalities, even among the "mildly" impaired subjects. The study also showed a progression of hemispheric metabolic asymmetry, according to level of impairment, with the frontal right hemispheric area appearing normal. (It is interesting that in our interviewing of FAD family members, they often reported that their affected relative responded to music, generally a right hemisphere activity, even in severe stages of the disease when there was no response to verbal cues.) In the Duara study, the FAD subjects were pooled for analysis according to severity of symptoms: mild, moderate, or severe. The neuropsychological tests showed declines across levels, and also in retests over time. Furthermore, the PET scanning showed abnormalities earlier than was possible with computed tomographic (CT) scans, according to the authors.

Neary et al. (13) also used neurological testing in attempting to distinguish Alzheimer's dementia from non-Alzheimer's dementia. Prospective data were collected from 24 patients with a diagnosis of primary cerebral atrophy. Eighteen of these were classified as having Alzheimer's and classified into four subgroups according to pathological-chemical-CT activity (from cerebral biopsies). The six non-Alzheimer's subjects did not show changes in these variables. Three of the Alzheimer's patients had family histories of AD. Among the Alzheimer's subjects (including the familial ones) abnormalities occurred in perceptuospatial, executive, and memory functions but social conduct and personality measures remained the same. For the non-Alzheimer's groups there were fewer abnormalities, except for memory, and social conduct and personality changes did occur. Progressive cognitive deterioration with stable personalities characterized the AD patients. However, Rubin and Morris (14) have shown that personality changes are common in mild AD and increase as the illness progresses.

RATIONALE FOR THE STUDY

Early prediction is important to allow a better understanding of the natural history and for the identification of early lesions or defects; genetic counseling; and early prescription of medication, if treatment is available. Early treatment of most diseases leads to better prognosis, and the same might be expected for Alzheimer's disease. Therefore, early identification of individuals at risk will be important as treatment modalities become available. Also, identification of those family members at low or no risk for the disease may aid in alleviating their fears of developing the disease and in genetic counseling.

This study attempted to identify early risk factors by doing the following.

1. Giving neuropsychological tests to members of FAD families (members both at risk and not at risk), thus using natural controls within the families.
2. Prospectively studying such family members to observe any predictive patterns of change and/or disease state.
3. Developing a discriminate function capable of predicting AD as early as possible; it was hoped that AD might be reliably predicted before the onset of any debilitating symptoms.

METHODS

Subjects

Familial

The 49 subjects in these analyses all came from families that appear to have a genetic form of AD. Autopsy confirmations on several family members from each of the families lent credence to what the families had known for years: senility was being passed down through the generations.

The subjects were classified into two groups: those who had a confirmed (by autopsy) or suspected parent with Alzheimer's disease, and those whose parents did not develop the disease and had passed the age of onset.

Age

The subjects ranged in age from 17 to 49 years. The risk group averaged age 35.9, while the not-at-risk group averaged 32.3. This difference did not achieve significance (t=1.37, df=3, n=43) (see Fig. 1).

Sex

In the at-risk group, there were 17 men and 18 women; in the not-at-risk group, there were 5 men and 5 women.

Socioeconomic Status

The subjects lived in Ohio, Kansas, Missouri, Indiana, California, and Oklahoma, with the majority living in California and Oklahoma. Using the Hollingshead (15) Yale Station, Two-Factor Index, the 49 subjects averaged 39.7, SD=14.9, range 11-65. This puts them in the middle of the third class, which was the middle class as well. These Hollingshead scores were normal across all the subjects and risk vs. not-at-risk groups means were essentially the same: 99 for the at-risk group and 101 for the not-at-risk group.

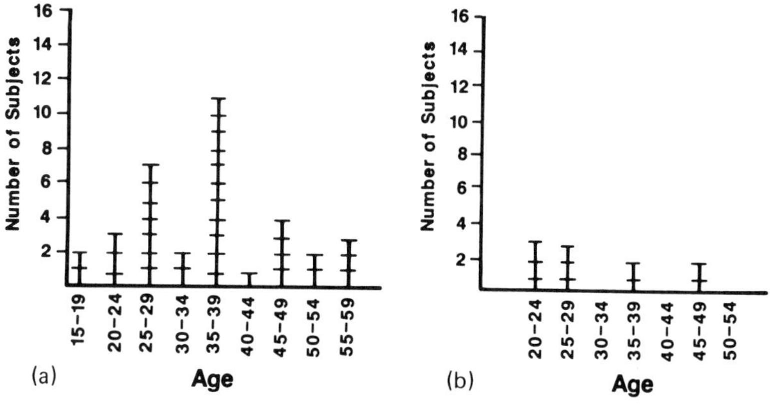

FIGURE 1 Comparison of age range in: (a) the at-risk group versus (b) controls.

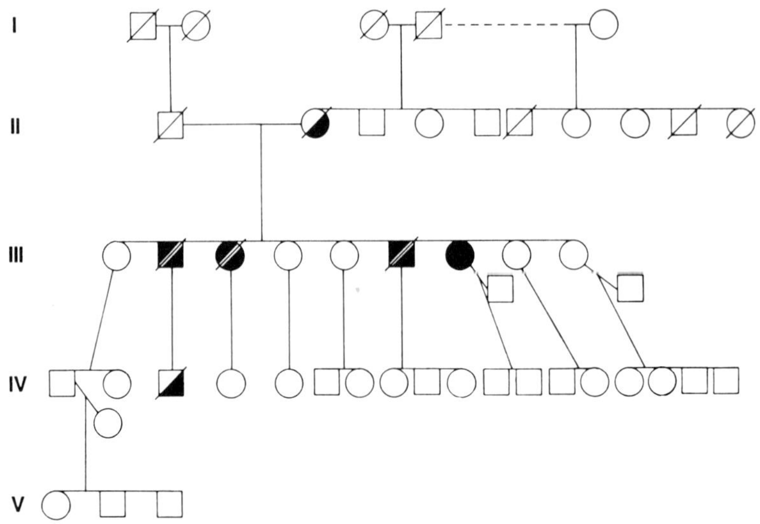

FIGURE 2 Pedigree chart of the K family. Darkened circles (females) and squares (males) represent cases of AD.

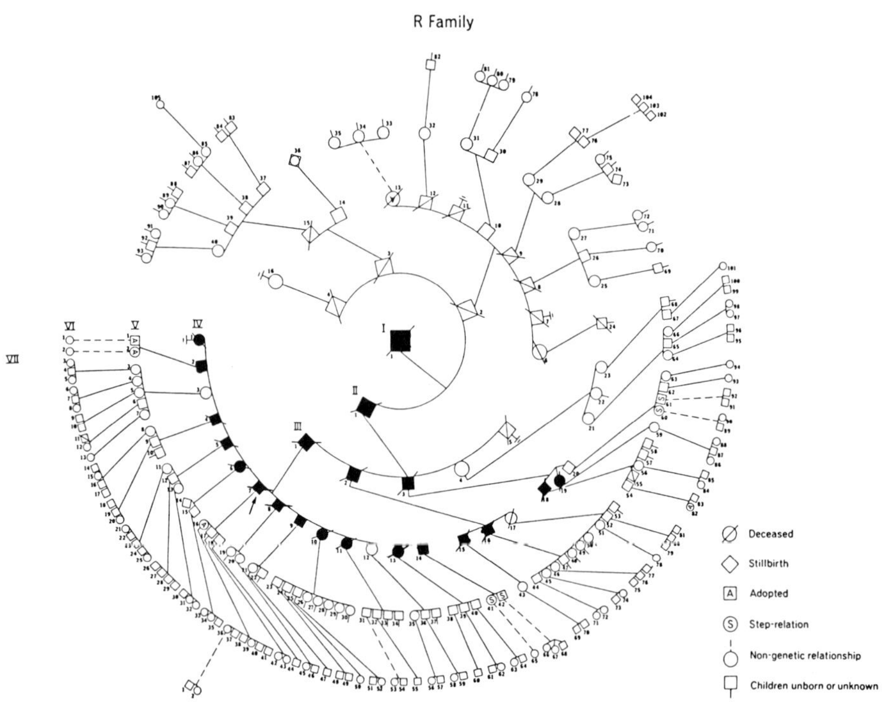

FIGURE 3 Pedigree chart of the R family.

Family Pedigrees

The 49 subjects of this study came from two large FAD families. These two pedigrees are shown in Figures 2 and 3. Many of the members in the younger generations that were tested are not shown in Figure 2, but Figure 3 shows most of the members of its family. In the family in Figure 2, 4 of 9 sibs of generation III have been affected; in the family in Figure 3, 12 of 14 sibs have been affected in generation IV.

Assessment Devices

The 2 hr battery consisted of the elements listed in Table 1.

The Wechsler Adult Intelligence Score's (WAIS) subtests of arithmetic reasoning, digit span, and similarities, measured verbal IQ. Block design, picture arrangement, and digit symbols measured performance IQ. The following tests were used for measuring "left hemisphere" functions: Shipley abstractions (a test for mild intellectual impairment, especially abstract thinking) (16), and the controlled word association test (17,18). For nonverbal "right hemisphere" functions, the following were used: judgment of line direction test (19), facial recognition (20, 21), and the visual recognition test (22,23).

The tests described above took about 60 min to administer and sampled various aspects of mental functioning. If mild deficits were to exist, one of these tests should have detected them. The testing booklets and materials are available

TABLE 1 Battery of Tests

Structured interview and Eysenck personality test
Wechsler Adult Intelligence Scale
Arithmetic reasoning
Digit span
Similarities
Block designs
Picture arrangement
Digit symbols
Six neuropsychological tests (NEURO)
Shipley abstractions (verbal)
Controlled word association (verbal)
Judgment of line direction (nonverbal)
Facial recognition (nonverbal)
Tinker-Toy test (executive ability)
Visual retention test (Benton's)
Torque test

from Psychological Corporation or from the University of Iowa Benton Laboratory of Neurology, Division of Behavioral Neurology, Department of Neurology, Iowa City, Iowa.

The Tinkertoy test (3,24) measured executive functioning, and measures of laterality were obtained by use of a finger-tapping test (25). Other tests included a "torque" test (26,27), described later in this chapter, the Boston naming test (28), and the Moss recognition span test (29).

A short structured interview (developed by the authors for this study) gained pertinent information about the family and elicited possible premorbid symptoms not identified by the test battery listed above. Questions involved family history, childhood and adolescent development, personal goals and decision making processes, marital and family history, education, social history, job history, and questions relating to any unusual behaviors. The Eysench personality inventory (30) concluded the assessment.

The subjects were tested by "blind" interviewers; the interviewer did not know the "risk" status of the subject. Likewise, all scoring of the tests was also blind. Normed data from the WAIS test and six of the neuropsychological tests, hereinafter referred to as NEURO (see Table 1) were entered onto subject-coded protocol sheets before undergoing statistical analysis. Since one of the purposes of this study was to seek a hypothesis, high-powered statistical packages were not used. Rather, prior to use of the usual statistical tests, the protocol sheets (Fig. 4) were

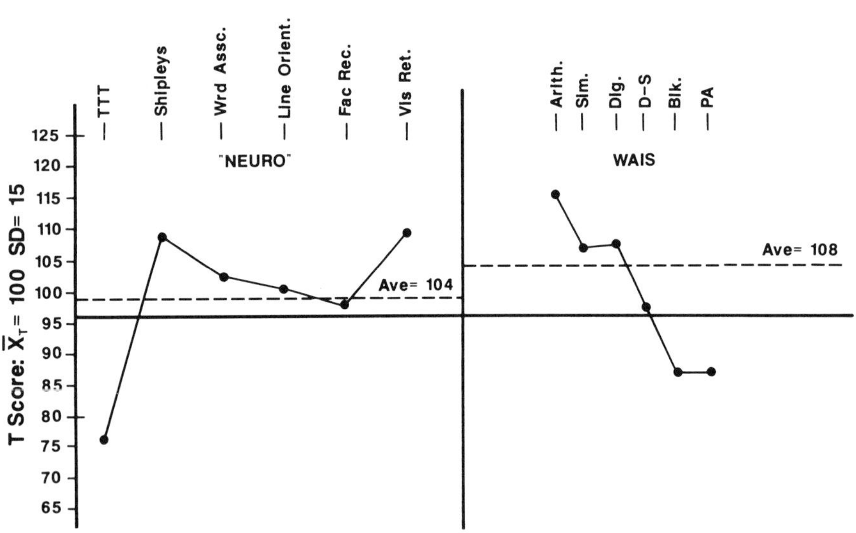

FIGURE 4 Sample protocol sheet on which each subject's scores for the NEURO and WAIS tests were plotted.

examined by looking at groups spread across a display board (this may be an unorthodox procedure, but some hunches emerged).

RESULTS

NEURO Variables

Scores from the six WAIS tests and the six NEURO tests (Table 2) were normed over the entire group (mean=100, SD=15) and two averages for each subject were found: a WAIS average and a NEURO average. Table 2 shows the correlations of these scores and with age.

Figure 5 shows the scatter plot of the average (NEURO) scores by age for the at-risk subjects and the not-at-risk subjects. Four of the subjects had a parent who died before the age of onset; these subjects were placed in a ? category since there was no way we would be able to establish their risk.

A chi-square compared those who scored at or below T=96 vs. those who scored above 96 by risk or not risk. This chi-square approached significance ($p < 0.1$; see Fig. 6).

The at-risk group appeared to exhibit an age-related curve, while the not-at-risk group did not. Significant correlations in Table 2 include a negative correlation between age and average NEURO score for the at-risk group. As the age of the subject increased, the average NEURO score decreased. There was not a significant correlation between the age and normed, averaged WAIS scores for this group. By contrast, the not-at-risk group did not show a correlation between age and either the NEURO or the WAIS measures.

Comparisons of Low NEURO, at-Risk, and Not-at-Risk Groups

Verbal Versus Performance

Given the algorithm used by Coolidge et al. (11), this study looked at subtests within the WAIS. The test most "verbal" was the similarities subtest; the most

TABLE 2 Correlations of Age, WAIS Average, and NEURO Tests Average

	NEURO	WAIS	Overall (n)	At risk (n)	Not at risk (n)
Age	-0.379*	0.117	49		
	-0.457**	0.015		35	
	-0.273	0.221			10

$H_0 : r = 0$
*$p < 0.05$
**$p < 0.01$

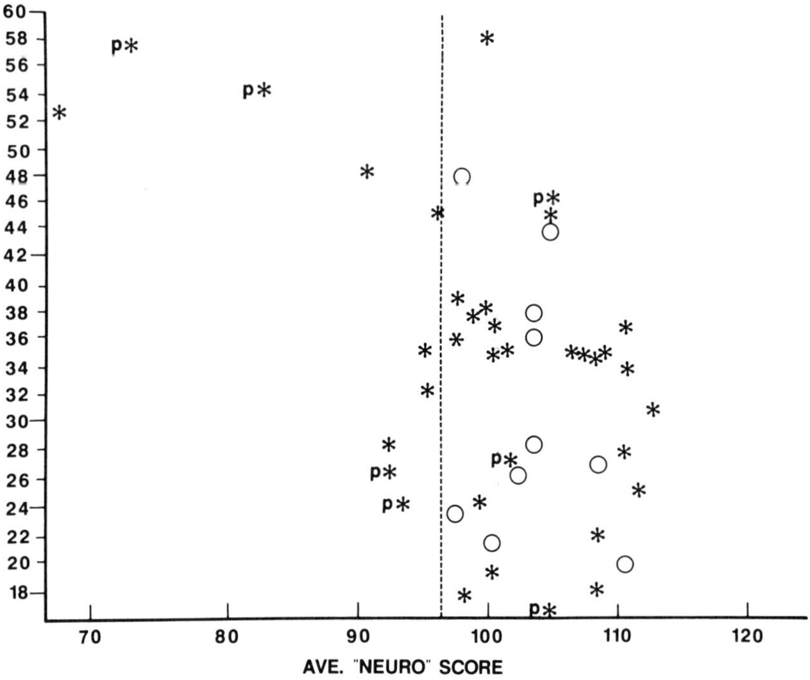

FIGURE 5 A scatter plot of the NEURO scores for each of 45 subjects. * = At risk: those with a parent with AD; p* = probable risk: those subjects whose parents are under the age of onset for FAD, and who therefore have a 50% risk or a 0% risk; O = control (not at risk).

Ave T		Risk	Not Risk
	≤96	10	0
	>96	25	10

$\chi^2 = 3.28$ df= 1

$.05 < p < .1$

FIGURE 6 Chi-square comparison of those who scored at or below T = 96 versus those above T = 96 by risk versus control.

TABLE 3 WAIS Similarities-Block Design Score

	$\overline{X}$	n
All subjects	2.6	45
At risk	6.5	35
Not at risk	-9.6	10

"nonverbal" was the block design test. These scores were not available on one of the not-at-risk subjects and on seven of the at-risk subjects. Comparing available data gave some interesting results. The block design normed score was subtracted from the similarities normed score. For all subjects (n=37), the average difference was +2.6 (see Table 3). However, the at-risk group (n=28), averaged +6.5 whereas the not-at-risk group (n=9) averaged -9.6.

When we looked at the low-scorer at-risk group (n=8) compared with the not-at-risk group (n=9) across ages (see Fig. 7), there appeared to be an age-related function for the at-risk group.

These trends are consistent with Cook's (10) and Coolidge's (11) findings of relative low performance scores noted in patients with early Alzheimer's disease.

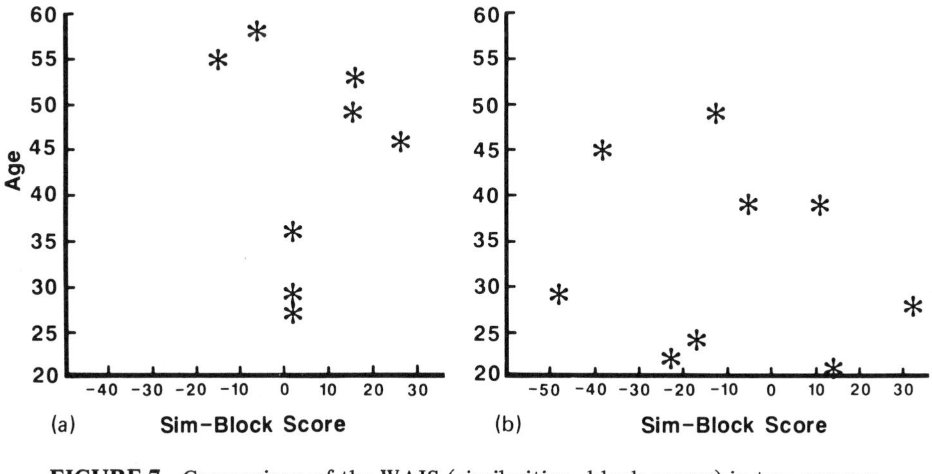

FIGURE 7 Comparison of the WAIS (similarities - block scores) in two groups: (a) low NEURO, at-risk (n=8) versus (b) control (not-at-risk) subjects (n=9).

	TORQUE	NO-TORQUE
AT-RISK	5	5
NOT-AT-RISK	1	9

$X^2 = 7.67$, df=1, $p < 0.01$

FIGURE 8 A chi-square comparison of torque/no-torque versus at risk (low score NEURO)/controls.

Torque

Torque, as defined by Blau (26), is the developmental persistence of atypical circle-making with either hand. Very young children typically draw circles in either direction. Instructed in school to make counterclockwise movements, most children, by the time the corpus collusum is fully myelinated (at about age 11), always make counterclockwise circles with the dominant hand and most of the time with the nondominant hand. The persistence of clockwise circles into adulthood, particularly with the dominant hand, is associated with schizophrenia (26,27) and also with creativity (31). Because drawing circles is a quick device, this test was added to the battery on the premise that it might yield something of interest. In the chi-square examination (Fig. 8), "torque" was counted present if it occurred in either hand over six trials. "No torque" meant that all six circles were drawn counterclockwise.

With one degree of freedom, the chi-square of 7.67 was significant. The variable, torque, occurred more frequently in the low-scoring at-risk group than in the not-at-risk group. Among the total at-risk group (n=35) torque appeared in 46% of the subjects, as opposed to 10% in the not-at-risk group.

TABLE 4 Similarities Minus Block Designs: Torque vs. No Torque

	All At Risk (n = 28)	Not At Risk (n = 9)
$\bar{X}_{\text{s-b (no-torque)}}$	6.3	32 (only one)
$\bar{X}_{\text{s-b (torque)}}$	6.8	-14.8

TABLE 5 At-Risk: Similarities Minus Block Designs: Torque vs. No Torque

Low Scores on NEURO At Risk, <=96, n=8		High Scores on NEURO At Risk, >96, n=20	
$\bar{X}$	1.8	$\bar{X}$	7.7
s-b (no-torque) n=4		s-b (no-torque) n=13	
$\bar{X}$	8.8	$\bar{X}$	5.7
s-b (torque) n=4		s-b (torque) n=7	

Torque and Similarities-Block Design

Table 4 shows that the presence of torque appeared to produce a positive similarities/minus block design score, whereas the no torque condition appeared to produce a lower score or a negative score. However, when the at-risk group was classified according to low (<96) NEURO score vs. high (>96) NEURO score, there appeared to be some kind of interaction (see Table 5).

DISCUSSION

If genetics plays a part in AD, these gene(s) probably have pleiotropic effects that present as chemical and neuropsychological markers that appear sometime during the lifespan, with some probably present prior to clinical onset. These early markers should be detected in approximately one-half of family members.

This neuropsychological marker study has really only begun. From the information presented here, some directions are emerging that may prove useful in building an algorithm to be tested out (a) over time, as family members are diagnosed; and (b) as additional members are tested and new families are located. Therefore, the following discussion must be considered tentative in nature but hopeful as a beginning.

Neuropsychological tests have differentiated early AD from other dementing conditions. With the natural controls that exist in FAD, there is the hope that neuropsychological tests might usefully determine some measure of risk for the disease and also help to determine very early pathogeneses.

The battery of tests did seem to differentiate groups: at-risk vs. not-at-risk. This was particularly true for the six NEURO tests, by which a subgroup of the larger at-risk group was differentiated. For this group, an age function seemed to be operating.

Of particular interest is the fact that the subject with the lowest score was diagnosed 2 years later as having AD. We suspect that these tests are sensitive to very early disease states. However, the sensitivity may drop off the farther away one gets from the disease.

The variable of "torque" deserves some additional study. A recent study correlated positron emission tomography (PET) (12) scans with severity of disease. It is interesting that in the "mild" cases the brain area delineated as initially implicated was area 14, the right superior parietal. Lesions in this area might produce problems with sensorimotor or kinesthetic tasks such as using scissors, or with handwriting or visuospatial disturbances that could interfere with such tasks as the block constructions (32). The fact that counterclockwise circles (torque) were drawn more often by the at-risk group than the not-at-risk group may not be of any particular consequence, or it may prove to be some sort of marker. Perhaps for those at-risk subjects who also score low on the neurological tests, the presence of torque may indicate initial pathological changes. For those who score high, the presence of torque may indicate some bent toward creativity rather than pathological change. This is consistent with other studies in which torque has been associated with pathological change and creativity (26,27,31).

Koss et al. (33) observed lateral asymmetries in glucose metabolism for patients with early-onset AD that were not seen in the late-onset subjects. They found more visuospatial impairment in the presenile patients, which correlated with the right hemisphere hypometabolism as measured by PET scans. Since age of onset for our subjects tends to be in the 40s, it is conceivable that torque might serve as a marker. Other putative markers are being discovered. Weinreb et al. (31) reported enhanced sensitivity to the antiproliferative effect of interferon (IFN) in early-onset AD. It is interesting that the IFN receptor has been mapped to the distal arm of chromosome 21, trisomy 21 cells are abnormally sensitive to IFN, and there are neuropathological and pedigree associations between AD and trisomy 21 (Down's syndrome).

The new neuropsychological marker data presented in this chapter are promising and more data are forthcoming. Certainly there is a need for longitudinal studies such as this one (4). The FAD families play a crucial role in expediting the research. Coordination of research among researchers and institutions lessens possible "harassment" of families. We have experienced excellent cooperation from family members, and are continuing this study by retesting subjects at intervals and adding new subjects. Tests are added or deleted as the premorbid model is built.

Early and accurate diagnosis of AD was identified as a crucial research issue by the National Institute on Aging, the American Association of Retired Persons, the National Institute of Neurological and Communicative Disorders and Stroke, and the National Institute of Mental Health during a joint meeting held in 1985 (35). The usefulness of early markers can only be reiterated, and will be maximally useful only when we know who and when to test. Areas that need to be further developed to find early markers and establish more accurate diagnostic

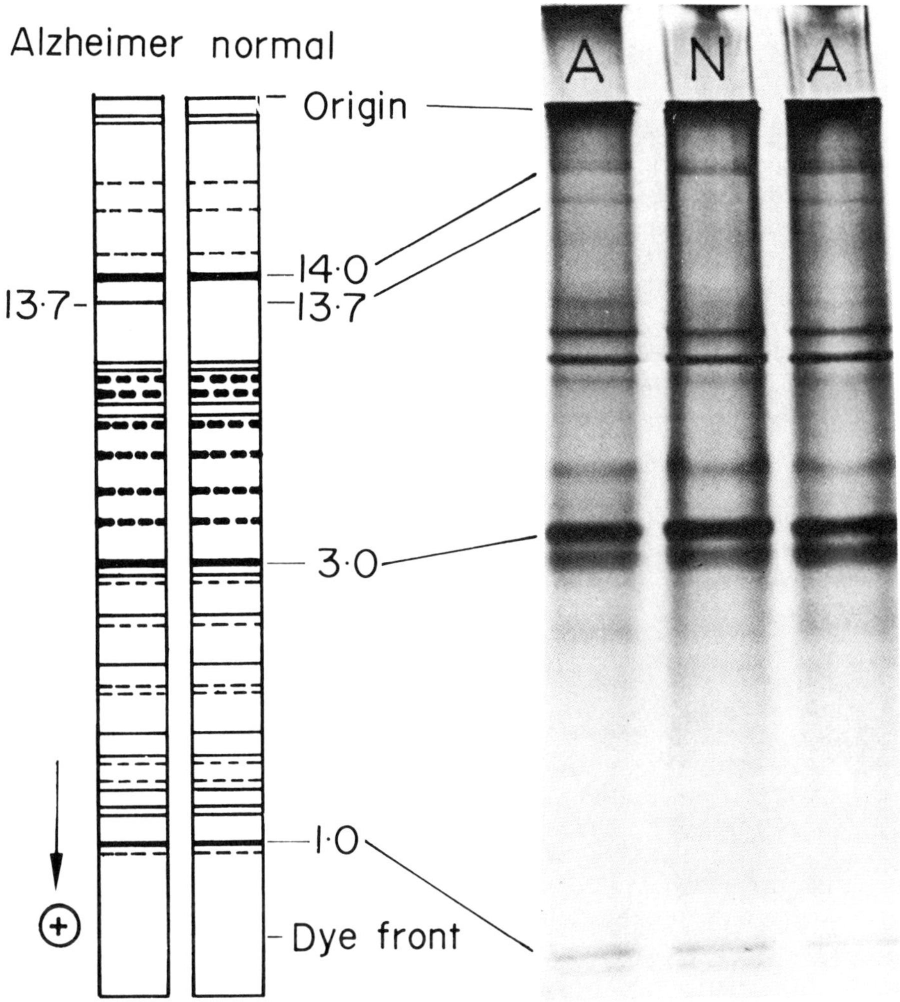

FIGURE 9 This figure illustrates a slab acrylamide gel electrophoretic separation of human brain proteins in Alzheimer's disease and controls. The diagram represents a composite of all human brain protein polymorphisms found in our normal population and is not drawn precisely to scale. In addition, not all bands are clearly reproduced in the photograph, accounting for the discrepancy between the diagram and the photo. Protein 13.7 has been detected in all 5 Alzheimer brains examined. The acrylamide system is as follows: 5 mM-Tris-phosphage pH 7.1 brain extract; Tris-chloride-glycine pH 8.4 continuous pH, discontinuous ionic strength; high voltage pulsed power; 20-4.5% step acrylamide gel gradient (from the bottom to the top of the gel: 2 cm 20%, 1 cm 16%, 1 cm 12%, 1 cm 8%, 1 cm 6%, 0.5 cm 4.5% acrylamide). The direction of protein migration is toward the anode. (From ref. 36.)

methods include neuropsychological and other behavioral measures, biological and chemical markers, neuroimaging strategies, and neuropathological indexes.

Miner et al. (36) in 1976 reported a unique brain protein in Alzheimer tissue, called protein 13.7 (see Fig. 9 and Table 6). Further work (unpublished) indicated that this protein was of high molecular weight (around 250,000) and did not break into subunits under the standard SDS-electrophoretic separating systems. Table 6 provides data on this protein from 5 AD brain samples and 36 controls. Protein 13.7 was found in one Pick's disease brain (the only one sampled), but was not found in a Down's syndrome and several Huntington's disease samples among the 36 controls. Therefore, despite the lack of exclusive specificity for one dementing process, the statistical significance of the association of AD with protein 13.7 is high. Protein 13.7 has not been studied since 1976, as far as we know. Its potential as a biological marker for AD underscores the need for further research in this area.

TABLE 6 Summary of Occurrence of Protein 13.7 in Alzheimer and Control Brains

Alzheimer brains exhibiting protein 13.7
  No.'s 55 (56), 57 (61), 58 (62), 75 (63), and 82 (59) = total of 5 brains (our total Alzheimer population size)

Control population
  Not exhibiting protein 13.7
    No.'s 3 (69), 4 (25), 5 (46), 7 (41), 8 (NA), 9 (54), 11 (71), 13 (72), 14 (44), 15 (72), 16 (57), 17 (37), 18 (66), 20 (80), 21 (56), 22 (72), 23 (NA), 24 (82), 25 (91), 26 (19), 27 (19), 28 (NA), 35 (70), 36 (73), 39 (62), 40 (80), 43 (NA), 52 (NA) = total of 29 brains
  Exhibiting protein 13.7 No.'s 6 (57) and 32 (61)
  Exhibiting protein 13.7 at low concentrations (appears to be approx. ½ concentration)
    No.'s 1 (57), 2 (74), 10 (54), 12 (60) and 19 (84)

Population frequency of 13.7 (at high concentration): 2/36 = 0.06

Population frequency of 13.7 (high + low concentration): 7/36 = 0.20

Probability of protein 13.7 occurring in all members of a sample size of 5 Alzheimer brains based on the null hypothesis that this protein should only occur at the (1) population frequency of 0.06: $x^2 = 39.24$, $p < 0.001$. Population frequency of 0.20 $x^2 = 27.24$, $p < 0.001$.

The number in parentheses following each brain code number is the age at death; NA = information not available.
From ref. 36.

Current studies involving potential identification of chemical and other markers are being conducted at many AD research centers around the world. These involve studies ranging from fingerprint pattern analysis in relatives of patients with AD to micromeasurements of aluminum in brain tissue. The following list provides a sampling of these current studies:

1. Met-enkephalin in blood plasma and CSF (37)
2. Red blood cell choline (38)
3. Fingerprint patterns (39,40)
4. Noncognitive psychiatric symptoms (41)
5. Ca^{2+} channel binding studies in AD brain (42)
6. Genetic linkage studies (43,44)
7. Chromosome 21 DNA amounts (45)
8. Antibody assay tests to proteins associated with paired helical filaments and other brain abnormalities in AD (46-48)

The long-term objectives of research of this nature is to identify some biological, neuropsychological, chemical, and/or neuropathological marker involved in AD. This can lead to development of diagnostic screening and, therefore, improved diagnosis. Today, incorrect diagnosis is thought to be common, perhaps ranging from 10 to 30% of cases (49,50). Needed is a continuing effort to define the disease precisely and to develop methods of definitively distinguishing AD from other nervous system diseases. The types of research discussed in this chapter are working toward these goals.

REFERENCES

1. Schull, W.J., and Weiss, K.M. (1980). Genetic epidemiology: Four strategies. *Epidemiol. Rev.* 2: 1-18.
2. King, M.C. (1981). Genetic epidemiology. Paper given at Symposium on Genetic Epidemiology at Annual Meeting of Society for Epidemiologic Research, Salt Lake City, June.
3. Lezak, M.D. (1983). *Neuropsychological Assessment.* New York, Oxford University Press, p. 579.
4. Khachaturian, Z.S. (1985). Progress of research on Alzheimer's disease: Research opportunities for behavioral scientists. *Am. Psychol.* 40(11): 1251-1255.
5. Goudsmit, J., White, B.J., Weitkamp, L.R., Keats, B.J.B., Morrow, C.H., and Gajdusek, D.C. (1981). Familial Alzheimer's disease in two kindreds of the same geographic and ethnic origin: A clinical and genetic study. *J. Neurol. Sci.* 49: 79-89.
6. Goodman, R.M. (1979). *Genetic Disorders Among the Jewish People.* Baltimore, The Johns Hopkins University Press, pp. 12-16.
7. Meals, R.A. (1971). Paradoxical frequencies of recessive disorders in Ashkenazic Jews. *J. Chron. Dis.* 23: 547-558.

8. Mourant, A.E., Kopec, A.C., and Domaniewska-Sobczak, K. (1978). *The Genetics of the Jews* (Research Monographs of Human Population Biology, general editor, G. Ainsworth Harrison) New York, Oxford Clarendon Press.
9. Moreau-Dubois, M.C., Brown, P., Goudsmit, J., Cathala, F., and Gajdusek, D.C. (1981). Biologic distinction between sporadic and familial Alzheimer's disease by an in vitro cell fusion test. *Neurology* 31: 323-325.
10. Cook, R.H., Ward, B.E., and Austin, J.H. (1979). Studies in aging of the brain: IV Familial Alzheimer disease relating to transmissible dementia, aneuploidy, and microtubular defects. *Neurology* 29: 1402-1412.
11. Coolidge, F.L., Peters, B.M., Brown, R.E., and Harsch, T.L. (1985). Validation of a WAIS algorithm for the early onset of dementia. *Psychol. Rep.* 57: 1299-1302.
12. Dura, R., Grady, C., Haxby, J., Sundaram, M., Cutler, N.R., Heston, L., Moore, A., Schlageter, N., Larson, S., and Rapoport, S.I. (1986). Positron emission tomography in Alzheimer's disease. *Neurology* 36: 879-887.
13. Neary, D., Snowden, J.S., Bowen, D.M., Sims, N.R., Mann, D.M.A., Benton, J.S., Northen, B., Yates, P.O., and Davison, A.N. (1986). Neuropsychological syndromes in presenile dementia due to cerebral atrophy. *J. Neurol. Neurosurg. Psychiatry* 49: 163-174.
14. Rubin, E.H., and Morris, J.C. (1987). Progression of personality changes in dementia. *J. Am. Geriatr. Soc.* 35: 89 (abstract).
15. Hollingshead, A.B. (1957). Two factor index of social position. 1965 Yale Station, New Haven, Connecticut.
16. Shipley, W.C. (1940). A self-administering scale for measuring intellectual impairment and deterioration. *J. Psychol.* 9: 371-377.
17. Benton, A.L. (1968). Differential behavioral effects in frontal lobe disease. *Neuropsychologia* 6: 53-60.
18. Benton, A.L., and Hamsher, K.deS. (1976, revised 1978). Multilingual Aphasia Examination, University of Iowa, Iowa City.
19. Benton, A.L., Varney, N.R., and Hamsher, K.deS. (1978). Visuospatial judgment: A clinical test. *Arch. Gen. Psychiatry* 35: 364-367.
20. Benton, A.L., and VanAllen, M.W. (1968). Impairment in facial recognition in patients with cerebral disease. *Cortex* 4: 344-358.
21. Benton, A.L. (1980). The neuropsychology of facial recognition. *Am. Psychologist* 35: 176-186.
22. Benton, A.L. (1962). The visual retention test as a constructional praxis task. *Confin. Neurol.* 22: 141-155.
23. Benton, A.L., Spreen, O., Fangman, M.W., and Carr, D.L. (1967). Visual retention test, administration C: Norms for children. *J. Special Ed.* 1(2): 151-156.
24. Lezak, M.D. (1982). The problem of assessing executive functions. *Int. J. Psychol.* 17: 281-297.
25. Reitan, R.M., and Davison, L.A. (1974). *Clinical Neuropsychology: Current Status and Applications.* New York, Hemisphere..
26. Blau, R.H. (1977). Torque and schizophrenic vulnerability: As the world turns. *Am. Psychologist* 31: 997-1005.

27. Kay, S.R. (1979). Significance of torque in retarded mental development and psychosis: Relationship to antecedent and current pathology. *Am. Psychologist* 34: 357-362.
28. Kaplan, E., Goodglass, H., and Weintraub, S. (1983). *Boston Naming Test.* Philadelphia, Lea and Feiger.
29. Moss, M.B., Albert, M.S., Butters, N., and Payne, M. (1986). Differential patterns of memory loss among patients with Alzheimer's disease, Huntington's disease, and alcoholic Korsakoff's syndrome. *Arch. Neurol.* 43: 239-246.
30. Eysenck, H.J., and Eysenck, S.B.G. (1963). *Eysenck Personality Inventory.* San Diego, California, Educational and Industrial Testing Service.
31. Miner, L.A., Lachenbruch, P.A., Nasrallah, H.A., Miner, G.D., and Lemke, J.H. (1981). Predicting children's nonverbal creativity from gender, torque and eye movements. Paper given to psychiatric epidemiology fellows at Annual Meeting of Society for Epidemiologic Research, Salt Lake City, June.
32. Walsh, K.W. (1981). *Neuropsychology: A Clinical Approach.* New York, Churchill Livingstone, pp. 188-223.
33. Koss, L., Friedland, P., Ober, A., and Jagust, J. (1985). Age at onset as an important determinant in Alzheimer-type dementia: Evidence from physiological imaging (abstract). *J. Clin. Exp. Neuropsychol.* 7 (2): 132-178.
34. Weinreb, H.J., Buskirk, D.R., Amador, R., Fillit, H.M., and Zabriskie, J.B. (1987). Enhanced lymphocyte interferon sensitivity in Alzheimer's disease (abstract). *J. Am. Geriatr. Soc.* 35: 85.
35. Khachaturian, Z.S. (1985). Diagnosis of Alzheimer's disease. *Arch. Neurol.* 42: 1097-1103.
36. Miner, G.D., Trapp, G.A., McSwigan, M., and Heston, L.L. (1976). Alzheimer's disease: human brain protein 13.7. *J. Neurochem.* 26: 605-607.
37. Valentine, J.L., Richter, R.W., Plotnikoff, N.P., and Patten, M.S. (1987). Blood and CSF determination of met-enkephalin in Alzheimer's disease. Paper presented at First International Symposium on Familial Alzheimer's Disease, October 22-23, Tulsa, Oklahoma.
38. Folstein, M.L., Tune, L.E., Miller, B.O., and Jenden, D. (1987). RBC choline as a potential peripheral marker. Paper presented at First International Symposium on Familial Alzheimer's Disease, October 22-23, Tulsa, Oklahoma.
39. Seltzer, B., and Sherwin, I. (1987). Fingerprint patterns in relatives of patients with Alzheimer's disease. Paper presented at First International Symposium on Familial Alzheimer's Disease, October 22-23, Tulsa, Oklahoma.
40. Nee, L.E., and Polinsky, R.J. (1987). Fingerprint patterns in subjects at risk for inherited Alzheimer's disease. Paper presented at First International Symposium on Familial Alzheimer's Disease, October 22-23, Tulsa, Oklahoma.
41. Ross, C.A., Zweig, R.M., Hedreen, J.C., Steele, C., Price, D.L., and Folstein, M.L. (1987). Non-cognitive psychiatric symptoms and brain stem pathology in AD. Paper presented at First International Symposium on Familial Alzheimer's Disease, October 22-23, Tulsa, Oklahoma.

42. Williams, R.G., Oibo, J.A., Ibok, I., Miner, G.D., and Colvin, R.A. (1988). Brain calcium channel binding sites are altered in Alzheimer's disease (abstract). Paper presented at 'PATHOBIOLOGY OF ALZHEIMER'S DISEASE', the Fifth Paulo Foundation International Symposium, June 17-19, 1988, Helsinki, Finland.
43. Brown, W.T., Robakis, N.K., Devine-Gage, E., Wu, Y., and Wisniewski, H.M. (1987). Linkage studies of familial Alzheimer's disease and other familial dementias. Paper presented at First International Symposium on Familial Alzheimer's Disease, October 22-23, Tulsa, Oklahoma.
44. St. George-Hyslop, P., Gusella, J., Nee, L., Polinsky, R., Tanze, R.E., Hobbs, W., Myers, R., Haines, J., and Conneally, P.M. (1987). Genetic linkage approaches to Alzheimer's Disease. Paper presented at First International Symposium on Familial Alzheimer's Disease, October 22-23, Tulsa, Oklahoma.
45. Schweber, M. (1987). Down's syndrome and the measurement of chromosome 21 DNA amounts in Alzheimer's disease. Paper presented at First International Symposium on Familial Alzheimer's Disease, October 22-23, Tulsa, Oklahoma.
46. Gaskin, F., Kingsley, B.S., and Fu, S.M. (1987). Auto- and allo-antibodies reactive with neurofibrillary tangles and astrocytes in Alzheimer's disease. Paper presented at First International Symposium on Familial Alzheimer's Disease, October 22-23, Tulsa, Oklahoma.
47. Iqbal, K., Iqbal, I.G., and Wisniewski, H.M. (1987). Role of neuronal cytoskeleton in the biology of Alzheimer's disease. Paper presented at First International Symposium on Familial Alzheimer's Disease, October 22-23, Tulsa, Oklahoma.
48. Sparkman, D.R., and White, C.L. (1987). Cell and molecular biology of Alzheimer's Disease. Paper presented at First International Symposium on Familial Alzheimer's Disease, October 22-23, Tulsa, Oklahoma.
49. National Institute on Aging Task Force (1980).
50. McKhann, G., Drachman, D., Folstein, M., Katzman, R., Price, D., Stadlan, E.M. (1984). Clinical diagnosis of Alzheimer's disease: report of the NINCDS-ADRDA work group under the auspices of Department of Health and Human Services Task Force on Alzheimer's disease. *Neurology* (NY) 34: 939-944.

16

Advances in the Therapy of Alzheimer's Disease

EZIO GIACOBINI and ROBERT BECKER / *Southern Illinois University School of Medicine, Springfield, Illinois*

Definitive treatment of Alzheimer's disease (AD) will depend upon an understanding of the causes and pathogenesis of this degenerative disease. Techniques derived from studies of molecular genetics will identify individuals at high risk (1). These studies may also characterize the molecular defect(s) derived from the genetic expression of the disease, but we view them as future developments that will not have clinical application for at least one to two decades. Shorter-term progress in the understanding of basic alterations of neurotransmitters, neuromodulators, and growth factors may lead to the development of ameliorative or palliative therapies that attenuate the expression of symptoms and possibly even slow the disease process.

Fundamental aspects of the basic pathological nature of Alzheimer's disease are not yet fully understood. There is still a basic lack of understanding of the relationships among clinical pathological changes such as plaques, tangles, and amyloid formation and the cause and course of the disease itself (2,3). The most widely held formulation of the disease's pathogenesis has associated plaques, tangles, and amyloid accumulation with the progression of the disease (4). This has recently been challenged, and the importance of neuronal loss has been stressed (5).

We believe that the accumulation of the pathological stigma (plaques and tangles) is not in synchrony with the disease progression and there is not sufficient accumulation of amyloid to produce the characteristic symptoms (2). Two points can be argued: dementia can occur without (e.g., Pick disease) or with a few plaques and tangles, and there is not a close enough relationship between pathological characteristics and dementia. There is a subgroup of AD patients with preserved mental status and numerous neocortical plaques (3). If there is no direct causal sequence between amyloid formation and dementia, the former could be

TABLE 1 Future Developments in Treatment of Alzheimer's Disease

Mechanism of action	Class of drug	Preferred route of administration
Classic neurotransmission	New cholinomimetics (inhibitors of agonists)	Oral or i.v.c.
Modulation of neuro-transmission	Neuropeptides (somatostatin, NPY)	i.v.c.
Trophic effects or neuronal rescue	NGF or other trophic factors	i.v.c.
Inactivation of protease inhibition (β-amyloid cleavage)	Specific enzyme inhibitors or reactivators	Oral or i.v.c.

only a secondary effect. Therefore, therapy directed towards preventing or decreasing the accumulation of amyloid may not alter the course of the dementia. A second possibility is that excessive amyloid formation or accumulation is a quantitative expression of aging that is present in the normal individual as well as in the AD patient.

Based on our present understanding of the process, there are at least three potentially therapeutic strategies for patients with Alzheimer's disease. First, the accumulation of amyloid could be arrested or reversed in the individuals at risk. To date, there is no means to identify these persons. Second, the rate of progression could be slowed in individuals already diagnosed with AD. Third, symptomatic expression could be suppressed or reduced without attentuation of the pathological characteristics. If neuronal death is the primary process and amyloid is a secondary event, the first task will be particularly difficult to accomplish. Thus, the second and the third approaches may be more feasible and realistic. This chapter will address these different approaches (Table 1).

THE MOLECULAR GENETIC APPROACH

Within the last 3 years, evidence has accumulated that a genetic abnormality is present in patients with some forms of AD. It has been suggested that the primary defect in the pathogenesis of one form of AD is a regulatory disturbance involving the amyloid gene represented on chromosome 21. Recent studies have shown that duplication of the amyloid gene in Down's syndrome (trisomy 21) can indeed be correlated with the excessive accumulation of amyloid in the brain. This has not been found in patients with AD (6). In the absence of a demonstration of gene duplication, several possibilities are still open to explain the excessive deposition: a defect in amyloid gene regulation, a defect in the β-amyloid protein cleavage, specific amyloid protein modifications, and changes in amyloid protein turnover regulation. Some of these mechanisms may be amenable to pharmacological intervention. Using hybridization techniques, Lewis et al. (7) found that mRNA encoding amyloid-β-protein precursor was present in neocortical neurons from the brain of both control subjects and patients with AD. This suggests that this protein precursor is a natural constituent of certain cortical cells. The same authors found that a subpopulation of neurons that show a decrease in precursor amyloid-β-protein mRNA in healthy brain developed neurofibrillary tangles (NFT) but not neuritic plaques. However, it appears that the expression of precursor amyloid-β-protein mRNA is necessary but not a sufficient prerequisite for NFT formation. Other factors such as long axonal projections, a distinctive pattern of corticocortical connections, and high levels of nonphosphorylated neurofilament protein may all contribute to making a neuron more vulnerable to the deposition of amyloid-β-protein (7). It is interesting to note that the amyloid protein precursor mRNA is specifically increased in nucleus basalis and locus ceruleus, which suggests that increased production of the precursor in these nuclei may play an important role in the deposition of cerebral amyloid in AD (8). Amyloid deposition represents a biochemical and pathological process that is not restricted to AD or Down's syndrome but is a common feature not only of the aging human brain but also of other mammalian species. Isolation and cloning of the amyloid gene will make it possible to transmit the defective gene to laboratory animals to produce models of excessive amyloid expression. This step will certainly help in the search for drugs that alter the production and accumulation of the amyloid protein, which could be a feasible strategy at the molecular-genetic level.

The recent studies of the genetic aspects of AD have found that the gene coding and expressing for the β-amyloid precursor is not increased in AD patients; only the accumulation of amyloid in the CNS is increased. The studies by Tanzi et al. (9) and Kitaguchi et al. (10) suggest that the presence of a proteoglycan receptor-type site related to chromosome 21 with a possible function being the activation of a protease inhibitor specific for the β-amyloid molecule cleavage. Several cellular roles for the glycosylation of the amyloid peptide precursor have been discussed, including cell adhesion, ion transport, and regulation of an endogenous protease inhibitor. This protease inhibitor, which is encoded by a DNA sequence designated HL124i, may influence the metabolism of the amyloid protein precursor (APP), protecting the molecule from degradation by certain proteases that have not been well identified (9,10). Inhibition of this protease could prevent amyloidogenesis by blocking up-regulation of the gene. Therapy could be developed to alter the function of the protease inhibitor. On the other hand, the protease inhibitor may be beneficial in decreasing amyloidosis because it prevents the cleavage of the β-protein from the membrane. Therefore, inactivation of this inhibitor could achieve the opposite effect and actually increase amyloidosis instead of decreasing it. With regard to the type of proteases involved in this process, it has been demonstrated that the APP molecule blocks trypsin activity in vitro and could therefore be similar to a chimotrypsin-G (10). Additional proteases of the α-chimotrypsin type have been postulated for the amyloidotic process. Any therapy directed towards influencing such a protease inhibitor needs to be targeted specifically to brain cells at concentrations high enough to act selectively on the specific cells carrying abnormally high levels of the inhibitor. Besides its expression in nerve cells, cerebral vessels, and meninges, the amyloid gene is also expressed in cells of the kidney, heart, and other organs. It can be assumed that adverse effects may follow complete suppression of amyloid formation or excessive breakdown. Because amyloid is expressed ubiquitously in cell tissues of the body as a universal protein, high regional selectivity might be required for therapeutic effect. Fetal brain shows a uniform high expression of the amyloid gene (9). In the adult brain cortex, particularly in the temporal cortex, it seems to be more clearly represented (9). Recent findings by Tanzi et al. (9, 11) indicate the presence of the two amyloid messages (APP_1 and APP_2), the levels of which are affected differently by AD. APP_2 mRNA increases specifically in the basal forebrain and in the entorinal cortex. If this finding is confirmed, it may allow higher specificity for potential drugs, inhibiting selectively the protease inhibitor (APP_1) expressed by the AD brain. The final question is: If it is available, how would such an inhibitor be administered? It seems that the intraventricular (i.v.c.) route would be particularly suitable to concentrate and amplify the effect of the drug in brain. The delivery of other macromolecules (peptides, proteins) that might also be considered in future therapy (such as neuropeptides or growth factors) may also be more effective if administered i.c.v. They may also require administration by this route because of the blood-brain barrier or other similar factors. Before we can use this route of administration effectively, we need to obtain detailed information about ventricular penetration, intracerebral diffusion, and transport of these potential drugs and macromolecules (Table 1).

THE SEARCH FOR A THERAPEUTIC NEUROPEPTIDE

Brain neuropeptides are synthesized and released by many types of nerve cells. In the hypothalamus, various peptidergic neurons synthesize and release macromolecules that stimulate or inhibit the release of hormones. In addition, neuropeptides are believed to function either as neurotransmitters or modulators of neurotransmitters. Neuropeptide-containing neurons form a class of cortical interneurons that make up approximately 5-10% of the total neuronal cell population of the brain (12). Of the neuropeptides identified in the human cortex, cholecystokinin (CCK), neuropeptide Y (NPY), and somatostatin (SS) are found in the highest concentrations and in most cell bodies while vasoactive intestinal peptide (VIP), substance P, corticotropin-releasing factor (CRF), and dynorphin are found in a smaller number of neurons (13).

Of all the neuropeptides studied in the aged or demented patient, only SS and, to a lesser degree, substance P and NPY seem to be decreased in a manner that systematically correlates with the stage of cognitive deterioration. Levels of VIP and CCK are not modified. Somatostatin regulates the release of growth hormone from the anterior pituitary gland. Immunocytochemical and electrophysiological evidence suggests that SS may also be a transmitter in the hippocampus (14). Somatostatin and NPY have been found to be reduced in postmortem samples of cerebral cortex hippocampus (15,16) and the cerebrospinal fluid (CSF) of AD patients (17-20). It is interesting that SS and NPY have been colocalized in abnormal neurites, which suggests a common origin from local intrinsic neurons (21). Somatostatin coexists also with acetylcholine (ACh) in cortical neurons (22) and SS receptors have been localized within the human cortex (23). Histochemical studies have shown an abundant innervation of the hippocampus by fibers containing markers for ACh that appear to project to the same dendritic areas of hippocampal nerves as SS-containing fibers (24). A possible coexistence of SS with ACh in other nerve cells, such as in cerebellum, has been suggested by Delfs et al. (22). It is noteworthy that i.v.c. administration of SS leads to an increase in ACh turnover and a decrease in ACh content in cortex (25); therefore, one could argue that SS administration may not be beneficial to neurons already depleted of this neurotransmitter. The association of choline acetyltransferase (ChAT), SS, and plaques in certain areas of the human cortex has also been discussed (24). In a double-blind placebo-controlled, crossover study, Cutler et al. (26,27) tested the effect of the SS analog L363.586 on AD patients. This molecule is 50 times more potent than the naturally occurring peptide. The peptide was given in intravenous (i.v.) infusion (40 μg four times each hour for 5.5 h). No effect on learning was found using neuropsychological evaluation. This is not entirely unexpected. Penetration of the brain by SS administered with the peripheral circulation has not been demonstrated. The peptide was not found in the CSF, which might indicate poor penetration in the CNS. Because of the widespread distribution of SS in CNS, it may be critical to achieve a high concentration of the peptide in CSF and CNS to achieve a facilitatory effect (Table 1).

Other peptides, in particular ACTH and its analog ACTH4-9 (ORG 2766), as well as vasopressin, have also been tested on AD patients with no evident benefit (28,29).

The involvement of the opioid system in AD has also been postulated. Naloxone has been shown to improve memory in animals and, therefore, blockade of opioid receptors has been attempted by using this substance in AD patients. The results obtained by Reisberg et al. (30), Tariot et al. (31), and Blass et al. (32) have not shown convincing evidence of changes in memory or cognitive function in these patients.

TABLE 2 Neuronotrophic and Neuritic Growth-Promoting Factors

Neuronotrophic factors		Neuritic growth-promoting factors
↓		↓
		Neuritic growth
Neuronal survival	→	
		Axonal guidance
↓		
Neuronal metabolism and neurotransmission	→	Axonal regeneration and sprouting

Source: Modified from Varon et al. (139).

The high polarity and low lipid solubility of many neuropeptides create major obstacles with these kinds of treatment. Except for the amounts entering the circumventricular organs, little of the substance enters the brain or the spinal cord with systemic administration. It is, therefore, highly unlikely that therapeutical levels can be achieved with parenteral administration, as has been tried with the SS experiments.

THE TROPHIC FACTOR APPROACH

Nerve growth factor (NGF) acts on the cholinergic neurons of the nucleus basalis that degenerate in AD. This has led to the suggestion that this growth factor may be involved in causing the disease (33). Basal forebrain neurons, immunoreactive to NGF receptors that colocalize with ChAT, are severely affected in AD and to some extent in demented patients with Parkinson's disease. It has been proposed that the death of specific cell populations in the CNS of AD patients may be due to loss, low delivery, or low utilization of neurotrophic factors derived from target neurons or supporting glial cells (33). These neurotrophic factors are acting on neuronal survival as well as on neuronal metabolism and neurotransmitter synthesis in specific cell populations (Table 2). The NGF is selectively taken up by ascending cholinergic nerve terminals and retrogradely transported to cell bodies located in basal forebrain nuclei (34,35). The NGF receptors have been localized in cholinergic neurons of the human basal forebrain (36). In the rat, it has been demonstrated that continuous infusion of NGF prevents basal forebrain neuronal death after fimbria fornix transection (37). The continuous infusion of exogenous 7S NGF (100 μg/week) intraventricularly spares 50% of the neurons in the medial septum and 100% in the diagonal band of Broca (37). Intraventricular injections or infusions of NGF in young adult rats reverse cholinergic cell body atrophy, promote behavioral recovery, and ameliorate spatial memory impairment in aged rats (38-40). These data provide evidence that NGF is able to promote survival and improve ability to perform in adult animals with cholinergic deficits similar to those seen in AD. Some NGF receptors have been demonstrated in the human brain. Decreased or equal levels of mRNA for NGF have been found in the CNS of AD patients (33,36,41,42). Goerdert et al. (42), however, did not find evidence for decreased NGF mRNA in the cerebral cortex of AD patients. Schweitzer (40) demonstrated that monoclonal antibodies to the NGF receptor can pass with its antigen-binding site intact from CSF into regions of the rat brain that contain NGF receptors. Therefore, it seems rational to use an intraventricular infusion of this molecule in the CSF to achieve maximally effective doses in the CNS. Thus, protease inhibitors, neuropeptides, and NGF are all examples of future applications or new approaches using an intracerebral route for the treatment of AD (Table 1).

For macromolecular treatment, an experimental therapy based on NGF administration poses several basic questions and requirements. Nerve growth factor is a protein with a sufficiently large molecular weight of high polarity and lipid insolubility not to permit systemic treatment. If high concentrations are required in strategic locations (e.g., nucleus basalis) of the CNS, systemic administration is not suitable. The first requirement for such therapy would be the availability of a highly pure human type of β-NGF protein with very high biological activity. Such a protein could be administered i.v.c. Presently available NGF proteins obtained by recombinant techniques or from purification from human organs (e.g., placenta) do not yet seem to meet the required standards. Most important is their lack of biological activity.

The quantitative requirements of such a therapy also need to be worked out in detail in experimental models. It is likely that milligram quantities of NGF protein will be necessary for a single treatment cycle. Such quantities are not yet available; however, they might be provided soon by recombinant techniques. The next questions center on when to start the treatment and how long to administer it. Beneficial effects are to be expected only at the initial phases of cell degeneration. This poses the problem of an early diagnosis. In our view, cortical biopsy combined with use of biochemical markers (43) might reveal early signs of degeneration of cholinergic neurons and, therefore, could be useful to determine the need for therapy with trophic factors. Nerve growth factors are likely to be ineffective in stages of advanced degeneration of the nerve cell. In general, animal models should be developed to determine the critical point for initiating therapy and the duration (weeks or months) of the treatment; the effect of drugs that potentiate or mimic NGF's action on its receptor; modalities of i.v.c. infusion of macromolecules; toxicology, severity, and frequency of side effects and complications; and any carcinogenic effect.

To address questions concerning drug delivery to brain, experiments are presently in progress in our laboratory as well as in our clinic with patients undergoing

TABLE 3 Trophic and Neurite Growth-Promoting Factors as Possible Candidates for AD Treatment

Neuronotrophic factors
Nerve growth factor (NGF)
Brain-derived neurotrophic factor (BDNF)
Ciliary neuronotrophic factors (CNTFS)
Neuritic growth-promoting factors
Polyornithine binding neurite-promoting factors (PNPFs)
Neurite extension factor (NEF)
Anchorage-dependent neurite-promoting factors

See Varon et al. (139) for a review.

i.v.c. treatment with cholinomimetic drugs (43). These experimental treatments attempt to optimize effects of prolonged intracerebral therapy and reduce the severity and frequency of complications.

The field of neuronotrophic and neuritic growth promoting factors has expanded to include several more or less well identified protein molecules (Table 3). New neuronotrophic factors are being identified. However, their purification and characterization are still far from the level reached for NGF. It is also possible that what we now believe to be a single growth factor may in fact include several components of a larger family. The molecular mechanisms of action of these factors is still largely unknown, which may prevent the selective use of these proteins in therapeutical approaches. Particularly deficient is our knowledge of possible involvement of growth factors in the regeneration of adult and aging neurons. The main question remaining is whether adult and/or aging nerve cells have preserved their capacity to react to the same factor that is present and active during the developmental phase.

THE ACETYLCHOLINE APPROACH: CHOLINOMIMETIC DRUGS

Of all the approaches in experimental AD treatment, the cholinergic one is by far the most developed. Multiple cholinergic deficits seen in AD have been well documented (Table 4). Choline acetyltransferase, the synthetic enzyme for acetylcholine (ACh), is consistently reduced by 60-95% in the cortex and hippocampus of AD patients compared to age-matched controls (44-47). Significant reductions are also observed in the high-affinity choline uptake (HACU) (48,49), in vitro synthesis of ACh, and release during depolarization (50,51). Presynaptic muscarinic (not postsynaptic) and nicotinic receptor binding (43,52,53), ACh

TABLE 4 Six Brain Systems Most Often Affected by Alzheimer's Disease

	Representation of Cholinergic Systems	
	Neurons	Projections
Neocortex (Frontal parietotemporal)	+	++
Hippocampus	–	+++
Amygdala	–	++
Basal forebrain	+++	–
Locus ceruleus	–	+
Raphe	–	+

TABLE 5 Biochemical Changes in Cholinergic Markers That Correlate with a Positive Diagnosis of Alzheimer

	Neural		Extraneural		
Marker	Cortical biopsy or autopsy	CSF	Lymphocytes	Erythrocytes	Plasma
Nicotinic receptor binding	Decrease (presynaptic)		Decrease		
Muscarinic receptor binding	No difference (postsynaptic)		Decrease		
ChAt activity	Decrease	Not measured			
AChE activity	Decrease	Decrease		No difference	BuChe No difference
Release of ACh	Decrease				
ACh synthesis	Decrease				
HACU	Decrease	Increased Ch levels			
Altered Ch metabolism	Decrease	Increased Ch levels		Increased Ch levels	Ch nc difference

content and acetylcholinesterase (AChE) activity of cortex (54), and AChE activity in cerebrospinal fluid (CSF) (55,56) are also reduced (Table 5). The reduction of these presynaptic cholinergic markers is closely associated with a marked loss of cells in the nucleus basalis of Meynert that project to cortex (57). By contrast, postsynaptic muscarinic receptor mechanisms appear to be relatively spared in AD patients (43,45,47,58). The reductions in cortical and CSF cholinergic markers are closely correlated with the extent of neuropathological change (senile plaques) and with the severity of cognitive impairment (43,44,46,51,55,56, 59-62).

When corrections are made for tissue losses, the decrease in ChAT activity closely reflects that reported for morphological degeneration (63). Reduced activity of ChAT is correlated with the degree of cognitive impairment (63). Deficits of cholinergic markers seen in cortical biopsies are not as widespread as non-cholinergic deficits detected postmortem (autopsies) (43,63). The involvement of the cholinergic system in dementias and the hypothesis that correction of its deficits may produce significant clinical improvement are further supported by the fact that several degenerative disorders of CNS are associated with severe cholinergic cell degeneration (Table 6), and three major demential syndromes (Alzheimer's, Parkinson's and Korsakoff's) show a significant involvement of cholinergic neurons (Table 7).

TABLE 6 Disorders Associated with Cholinergic Cell Degeneration

Alzheimer's disease
Parkinson's disease
Korsakoff's psychosis
Down's syndrome
Gerstmann Straussler syndrome
Parkinson dementia complex of Guam
Dementia pugilistica

TABLE 7 Major Dementias with Involvement of CNS Cholinergic Neurons

Alzheimer's disease
Parkinson's disease
Korsakoff's psychosis

The effectiveness of cholinomimetic drugs for AD treatment will probably be limited by the progression of the disease, side effects, and possible development of tolerance. However, the major question is whether or not the substantial cholinergic deficit measurable in AD patients is of functional significance. We will not be able to answer this question until we are able to produce a significant, sustained long-term enhancement of cholinergic function and measure its effect on memory and cognitive function. Such a result has not yet been feasible with the cholinergic agents tested and the type of administration used so far (64-66) (Table 8).

Table 8 summarizes the drug trials in progress using cholinergic drugs. Two major groups of drugs are represented: ChE inhibitors and cholinergic agonists mainly of the muscarinic type. Table 9 documents therapeutic attempts based on the use of drugs or compounds, the action of which is not directly attributed to the cholinergic system. This group includes a broad spectrum of drugs from potassium-channel blockers (aminopyridines) to nootropic drugs and gangliosides. A critical analysis of the available data reveals that ChE inhibitors are the only drugs tested so far that produce significant, reproducible, short-lasting therapeutic effects in double-blind, randomized, crossover clinical trials of at least 12 weeks total duration. Many studies reported in Table 9 are flawed due to poor documentation, short duration of the trial, small number of patients, and non-double-blind, placebo-containing trials. In this review, we will, therefore, concentrate mainly on attempts using ChE inhibitors, particularly the most recent attempts in our laboratory, and on the use of the second and third generations of these compounds.

Oral Physostigmine Studies

Results From Other Laboratories

Several studies found consistent, albeit quite modest, improvement in the neuropsychological test performance of AD patients after i.v. infusion of physostigmine (Phy) (55,65,67,68) or tacrine (THA) (69). However, in dose-response studies, the maximum improvement varied considerably across patients, and only about 20-25% of patients showed pronounced and reproducible improvement at their optimum doses of Phy (55,65,69). Other studies have confirmed a beneficial effect of i.v. administration of these reversible ChE inhibitors in some patients with dementia of the Alzheimer's type (70-72). Discrepant results after a single fixed dose (0.5 mg) of Phy (73) may reflect a relatively narrow therapeutic window for the drug with i.v. administration (55,65). Mixed results were also obtained after intramuscular (i.m.) or subcutaneous (s.c.) Phy, but a number of patients did improve when the drug was given alone (74) or with a low dose of lecithin (75). Case studies (70,76) found no change in recall, but reductions in frequency of intrusions and constructional praxis were found in Alzheimer's disease patients

TABLE 8 Cholinergic Drugs Undergoing Testing for Treatment of Alzheimer's Disease

Category	Drug	Administration	Country	Side effects	No. of patients	Memory effect	Cognitive effect
I	Physostigmine	Oral	USA	Nausea, anticholinergic effects	Several hundred	+	(+)
		i.v.				+	?
		i.v.c.				+	–
I	THA	Oral	USA	Hepatoxicity	300	++	+
			Sweden	Nausea	10	++	+
			Canada	Anticholinergic effects	22	++	+
I	Metrifonate	Oral	USA	Anticholinergic effects	10	–	–
I	Huperzine A	Oral	China	–	Several hundred	+	–
I	Heptylphysostigmine	Oral	Italy	–	10	–	–
II	Bethanechol	i.v.c.	USA	Nausea and vomiting at beginning	8	+/?	+/?
II	R-86	Oral	USA-Europe	Nausea, vomiting, salivation, sweating	500	(+)/?	0
II	Oxotremorine	Oral	USA	Strongly toxic	10	0	0

I, Chel: cholinesterase inhibitors; II, ACh Ag: cholinergic agonists; +, mild, transient effect; ++, moderate effect, long-lasting; 0, no effect; ?, uncertain effect; –, study in progress.

TABLE 9 Noncholinergic Drugs Undergoing Testing for Treatment of Alzheimer's Disease

Category	Drug	Administration	Country	Side effects	No. of patients	Memory effect	Cognitive effect
I	4-Aminopyridine	Oral	Holland	Agitation	14	(+)	?
I	3-4-Diphosphopyridine	Oral	USA	None	–	–	–
0	Phophatidylserine	Oral	Italy, Germany	None	142	(+)	–
II	Piracetam	Oral	Europe, USA	None	Several hundred	+/0	?/0
II	Oxiracetam	Oral	Italy USA	None	20 + 10 12	+/0 –	+/0 –
0	L-Acetylcarnitine	Oral	Italy	–	100	(+)	–
0	Gangliosides (GM_1)	Oral	Italy USA	–	20	–	–
III	THIP	Oral	USA	–	10	0	0
0	Captopril	Oral	USA (2 multi-center)	–	100	–	–
N	Somatostatin (SMS 2%-995)	i.v.c.	Sweden	None	8	(+)	0

I, amino pyridines, (K^+ channel blockers); II, Nootropic drugs; III, GABA agonist (tetraisoazololopyridine); 0, other; N, neuropeptide; +, mild, transient effect; ++, moderate effect, long-lasting; 0, no effect; ?, uncertain effect; –, study in progress.

after parenteral administration of Phy. However, no significant effect was found in two other studies with six to seven patients each after 1 mg Phy i.m. (77) or 10 and 20 μg/kg Phy s.c. with lecithin pretreatment (78).

Encouraging results have been reported when Phy or THA was administered orally to AD patients (67,68,74,75,79, 87). In these studies, ChE inhibitors were given in combination with lecithin (74,75,79-82,86,87) and/or repeatedly up to seven times a day for several days prior to neuropsychological testing. Peters and Levin (75) reported sustained improvement for up to 3-10 months in patients treated with oral Phy/lecithin combination. However, other studies that tested only after 1 or more months of repeated oral Phy alone (88,89) or with lecithin (78) were negative. Experiments in mice show a sustained beneficial effect on learning and memory following long-term (4-6 months) oral administration of THA (90). The diminishing efficacy of Phy (75,86,87) or THA (86) after prolonged administration in "responders" may be due to the progression of the degenerative effects of the disease. This may also indicate tolerance to the therapeutic effect of ChE inhibitors (66).

Results From Our Laboratory

In our studies (91), we sought to determine whether measurable inhibition of plasma and red blood cell (RBC) ChE activity could be used to define the kinetics of brain ChE inhibition and to estimate changes in brain ACh. Our findings suggest an interpatient variability of response on neuropsychological testing to the administration of ChE inhibitors based on the state of the individual's cholinergic system.

Neuropsychological test performance has been variable in virtually all positive studies of Phy in AD patients. Interindividual pharmacokinetic differences may account in part for interindividual differences. Inhibition of plasma and RBC ChE activity is readily quantified after administration of both reversible and irreversible ChE inhibitors, and RBC enzyme inhibition has been correlated with behavioral manifestations (92,93). Plasma prolactin, cortisol, and adrenocorticotrophic hormone (ACTH) levels were also examined in the Alzheimer's patients after oral Phy as putative markers of central cholinergic stimulation. Elevation of these neuroendocrine levels has been reported after Phy administered in relatively high i.v. doses (94-96), and the magnitude of the response was highly correlated with the effect of drug on mood (97). Kumar et al. (98) showed a significant positive correlation between the effect of Phy (i.v.), an increase of cortisol, and the decrease of ChE activity in plasma. Physostigmine increased plasma cortisol with greatest difference at time points after 90 min following drug administration. Development of neuroendocrine markers of the efficacy of Phy may help to establish the optimal regimen for consistent cognitive improvement in Alzheimer's dementia.

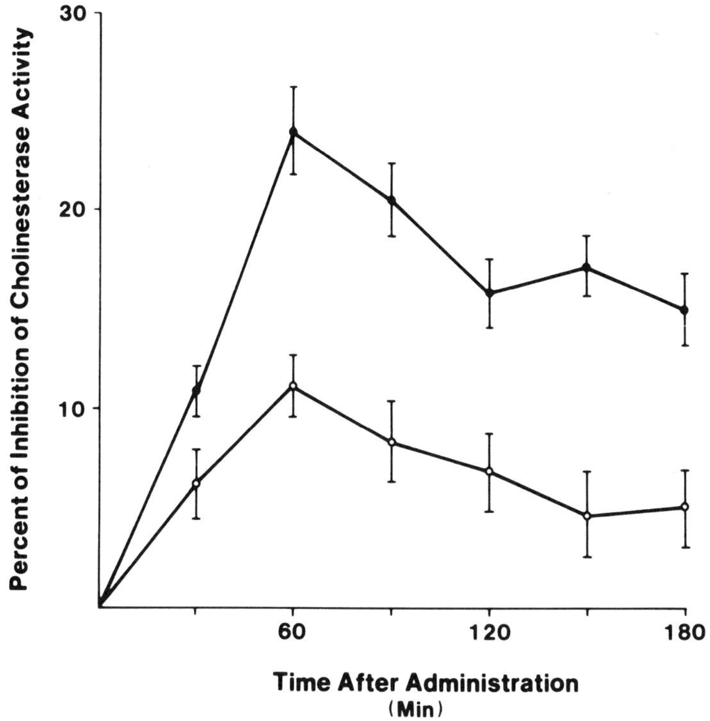

FIGURE 1 Inhibition of ChE in plasma (0) and red blood cells (0) is expressed as a percentage of the mean of the two predrug values as baseline. Results are mean ± S.E. as percentage for 10 patients. ChE activity was determined in triplicate for all plasma samples and for RBC baseline and 60 min points. The RBC activity was expressed per mg hemoglobin in each sample (modified from ref. 91).

Cholinesterase Inhibition

Inhibition of plasma ChE increased to a maximum at 60 min after oral administration of 60 μg/kg Phy (Fig. 1). Plasma ChE activity was inhibited compared to predrug baseline in all patients, but varied quantitatively from 12% to 33% maximum inhibition. Mean inhibition at 60 min was 23.9% ± 2.2%, and mean peak inhibition was 25.1 ± 2.0% (n=10). Inhibition of plasma ChE activity then declined from 60 to 120 min, but plateaued at 15-17% inhibition from 120 to 180 min. Sixty percent of the maximal effect on plasma ChE persisted for up to 3 hr after oral Phy.

Red blood cell (RBC) ChE activity was also inhibited maximally at 60 min. However, the magnitude of inhibition of RBC AChE activity (11.1 ± 1.5% at 60 min) is less than the inhibition of plasma ChE activity (Fig. 1).

Neuropsychological Test Performance

Analysis of variance of the neuropsychological test scores showed no significant difference between performance after Phy and neostigmine as active placebo. In both drug conditions, performance tended to deteriorate by 3 hr.

Conclusion

Oral Phy administration shows considerable variation in the pharmacokinetics of absorption and metabolism. The low efficacy of the doses that can be tolerated by most patients may account for the modest and inconsistent clinical effect after acute oral administration. However, our studies suggest that blood measures of ChE inhibition and neuroendocrine response may be useful for monitoring the biological efficacy of other inhibitors such as THA or other regimens, including the multiple-dose daily administration of Phy,which may be more effective therapeutically than acute Phy administration in reversing the memory deficit.

Physostigmine and Scopolamine i.v. Trials

Plasma Butyrylcholinesterase Inhibition

Physostigmine (Phy) was administered to 12 patients with mild to moderate AD (NINCDS criteria) as i.v. infusion according to the diagram shown in Figure 2. After a "best dosage"-finding phase (300, 600, 900, 1200 $\mu g/m^2$ during 3 weeks), the "best dosage" of Phy, saline (placebo), and a dose of scopolamine (0.161 $\mu g/kg$) were administered i.v. over a 2.5-hr period in counterbalanced order in a double-blind design. During a second phase (replication phase) of three weeks duration the "best dosage" producing highest total number of correct word or picture identifications was tested against saline placebo and 0.161 mg/m^2 i.v. scopolamine in a randomized double-blind study. Prior to receiving Phy, all patients received 0.1 mg glycopyrolate i.v. All patients received 12.4 g lecithin per day. Figure 2 shows the pattern of inhibition of butyrylcholinesterase (BuChE) in plasma of three patients and three normal controls during a 6 hr period. Maximum BuChE inhibition is 28% at approximately 2.5 hr after the infusion is started. The appearance and duration of side effects, mainly nausea, and the period of neuropsychological testing are also reported (Fig. 2). A steady state of BuChE inhibition is reached after 1 hr, lasting approximately 1.5 hr. In this time period a steady-state concentration of approximately 4 ng/ml Phy is reached during the last 30 min of infusion, with a linear relationship between BuChE inhibition and Phy dosage. Individual variations are seen in both patients and controls. Figure 3 shows the dose-response relationship for the percentage BuChE inhibition in plasma in 12 AD patients following i.v. infusion of Phy. The percentage inhibition at steady-state inhibition (105-135 min) increases linearly from approximately 15% at the 300 $\mu g/m2$ dosage to 35% at the 1200 $\mu g/m2$ dosage (Fig. 3). These data allow us to estimate the ChE inhibition in brain at various

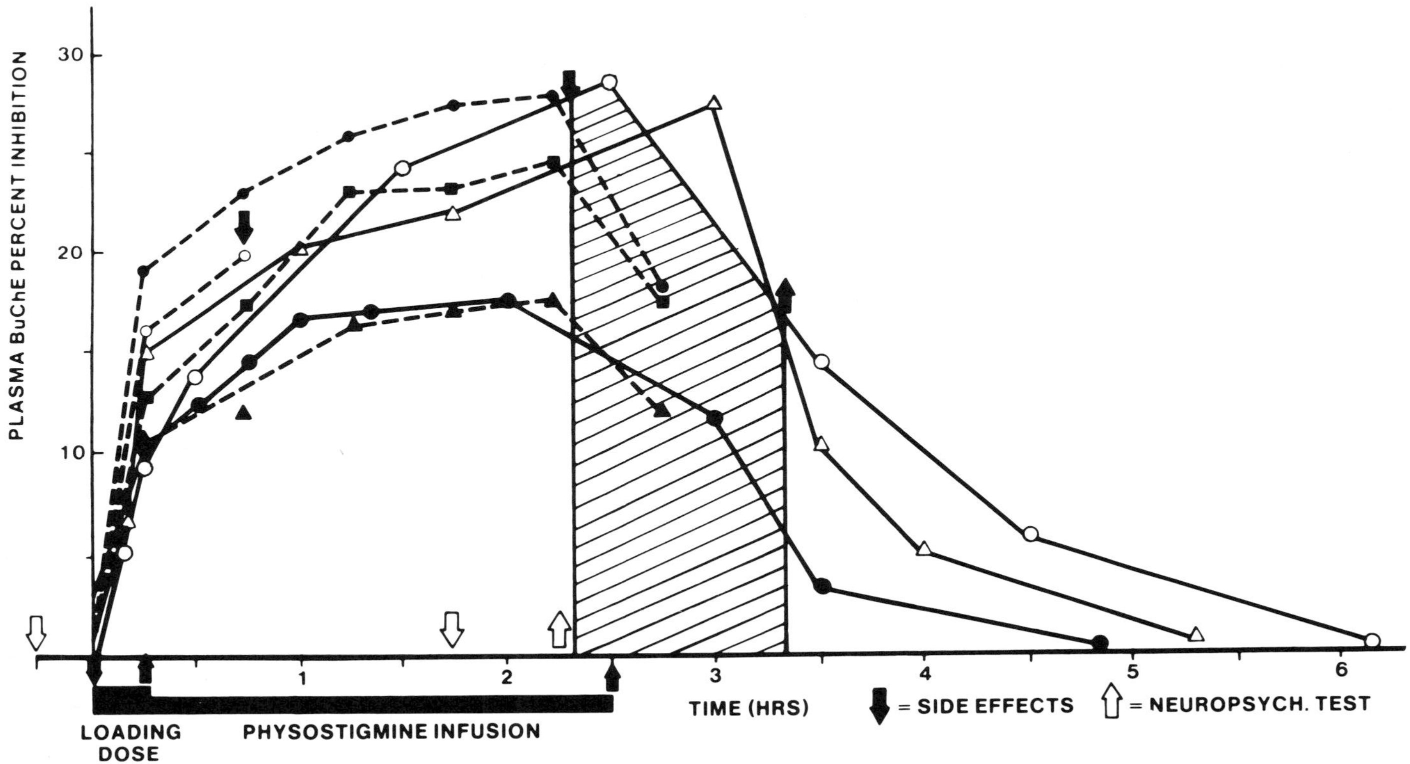

FIGURE 2 Percentage BuChE inhibition in plasma in three normal subjects (---) and three AD patients (——) following i.v. infusion of Phy. Start and end of injection as well as side effects and neuropsychological testing is reported. The shadowed area represents the period of maximal intensity of side effects.

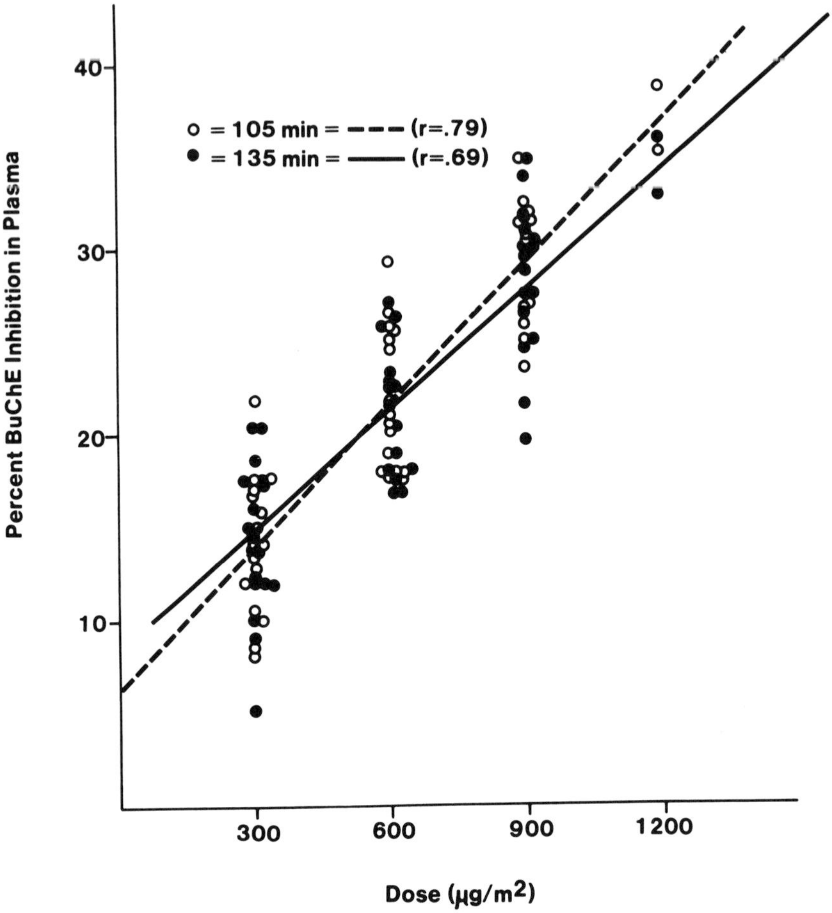

FIGURE 3 Dose-response relationship of Phy i.v. infusion in 12 AD patients. Data are presented at 105 and 135 min after starting of the infusion. Linear regression analysis shows r' = 0.88 p<.001 (105 min) and r'' = 0.83 p<0.001.

levels of plasma ChE inhibition by using the model we have developed in the rat (99). This model estimates brain ChE inhibition following Phy i.v. and i.m. at 100% of the steady state (99).

Memory Effect

In the word recognition task, the patient reads or identifies aloud 12 high-imagery words or pictures that are then randomly mixed with 12 words or pictures (dis-picture whether it was a "new" or "old" word or picture (trial 1). This procedure is then repeated for two more trials with the same target words or pictures but with a new set of distractor items for each trial.

The data were analyzed using a signal detection analysis. Using paired-t comparisons it was found that the patients scored significantly better with Phy than with scopolamine ($p=0.019$) on trial 1, and that there was a trend toward better memory performance with Phy versus placebo ($p=0.061$) for trial 1. Scopolamine impaired memory by an average of 9% compared to saline.

There was a significant learning effect across the three trials for the two memory measures (d': $p=0.02$; SI: $p=0.03$), which appears to be due to improved performance on trial 2 versus trial 1. There was no significant difference on the responsivity measures across the three trials.

In conclusion, only in trial 1 of the three learning trials did we find a statistically significant effect on memory when we compared the three drug conditions (Phy, placebo, and scopolamine). Both the magnitude and duration of the effect are small. The best-dosage Phy-induced memory improvement (dosage-finding phase) correlated with best-dosage improvement during replication phase. This finding supports the concept that "cholinergic responders" (i.e., patients who show memory improvement with Phy) tend to do so consistently, which suggests that this drug improves memory in a subpopulation of AD patients. This is consistent with other published studies demonstrating a modest but unequivocal effect of cholinergic enhancement using Phy on memory in Alzheimer's patients (100). We replicated the finding of Mohs and Davis (101) that the major effect of Phy on recognition memory was to decrease incorrect "yes" responses (false alarms) rather than increasing correct "yes" responses (hits). Mohs and Davis (101) concluded that Phy selectively decreases the number of false alarms, suggesting that the cholinergic system is important for the inhibition of inappropriate responses and that one effect of decreasing cholinergic activity may be to lower the threshold for initiating certain kinds of responses. Our study extends the finding of Mohs and Davis (101) by showing that while Phy decreased "false alarms" compared to the placebo trial, scopolamine increased "false alarms," while neither drug changed the number of "hits." Thus, our study demonstrated opposite effects on "false alarm" responses as a result of increasing cholinergic activity with Phy and decreasing cholinergic activity with scopolamine. These findings add further support to the hypothesis of Mohs and Davis (101) that cholinergic manipulation affects response inhibition. Our data also supports the concept that "cholinergic responders" do exist in a population of AD patients.

Physostigmine i.v.c. Study

Results From Other Laboratories

Intraventricular medication has been used when the administration of systemic agents has failed to influence the disease process. The rationale for i.v.c. drug administration is that there is better penetration of the drug in the brain than with systemic administration; higher doses can be delivered directly to the brain; and systemic toxic effects are reduced because the total dose is lower.

A first preliminary report on intracranial cholinergic drug infusion in patients with AD has been published by Harbaugh et al. (102). The clinical trial involved the use of an implantable infusion system connected to a Silastic intracranial catheter. Four patients were infused during 3 week intervals with the cholinergic agonist bethanecol chloride (0.05-0.7 mg/da6). The results are encouraging, with reported decreased confusion, increased initiative, and improved memory. A second study of cholinomimetic i.v.c. therapy on 12 patients was published by Fox et al.)103), who also used bethanechol chloride. During insertion of the i.v.c. catheter for long-term infusion, these authors performed a left frontal cortical biopsy, which confirmed the clinical diagnosis of AD in all cases. A third study with bethanechol is being published by Penn et al. (104). At this point it is important to compare the clinical effects of two different strategies, such as direct receptor stimulation (bethanechol studies) and ACh enhancement through AChE inhibition (this study). Both studies suggest that i.v.c. drug infusion is feasible in AD patients, and more extensive studies on local delivery of drugs are now being funded (105).

Results From Our Laboratory

Experiments on Animals We have demonstrated that i.v.c. administration of very small doses (10-20 μg/kg) of Phy in dogs produces significant (50%) and long-lasting inhibition (up to 3 hr) of AChE activity in cerebrospinal fluid (CSF), with few side effects (106). These dosages inhibit AChE in selective brain regions including striatum, hippocampus, and cortex. These areas contain cholinergic cells and terminals that are affected by AD. The medulla oblongata and pons are much less seriously affected.

Additional evidence for the effectiveness of the i.v.c. route is provided by our recent study in the rat (99). The administration of 4 =g Phy i.v.c. produced a 45% and 73% inhibition of AChE activity in cortex and hippocampus, respectively. At 30 min, ACh was increased by 18% and 22% in striatum and hippocampus, respectively. No increase was seen at this time point in the medulla oblongata. At this dosage, the rat showed, however, a higher frequency of side effects than the dog. Rats are known to be more sensitive to the effects of ChE inhibitors than most mammalian species.

FIGURE 4 Effect of various dosages of Phy administered i.v.c. to an AD patient on AChE activity in CSF (upper curves) and plasma (lower curves). The pattern of Phy concentrations in CSF is also shown following an 8 μg single dose i.v.c.

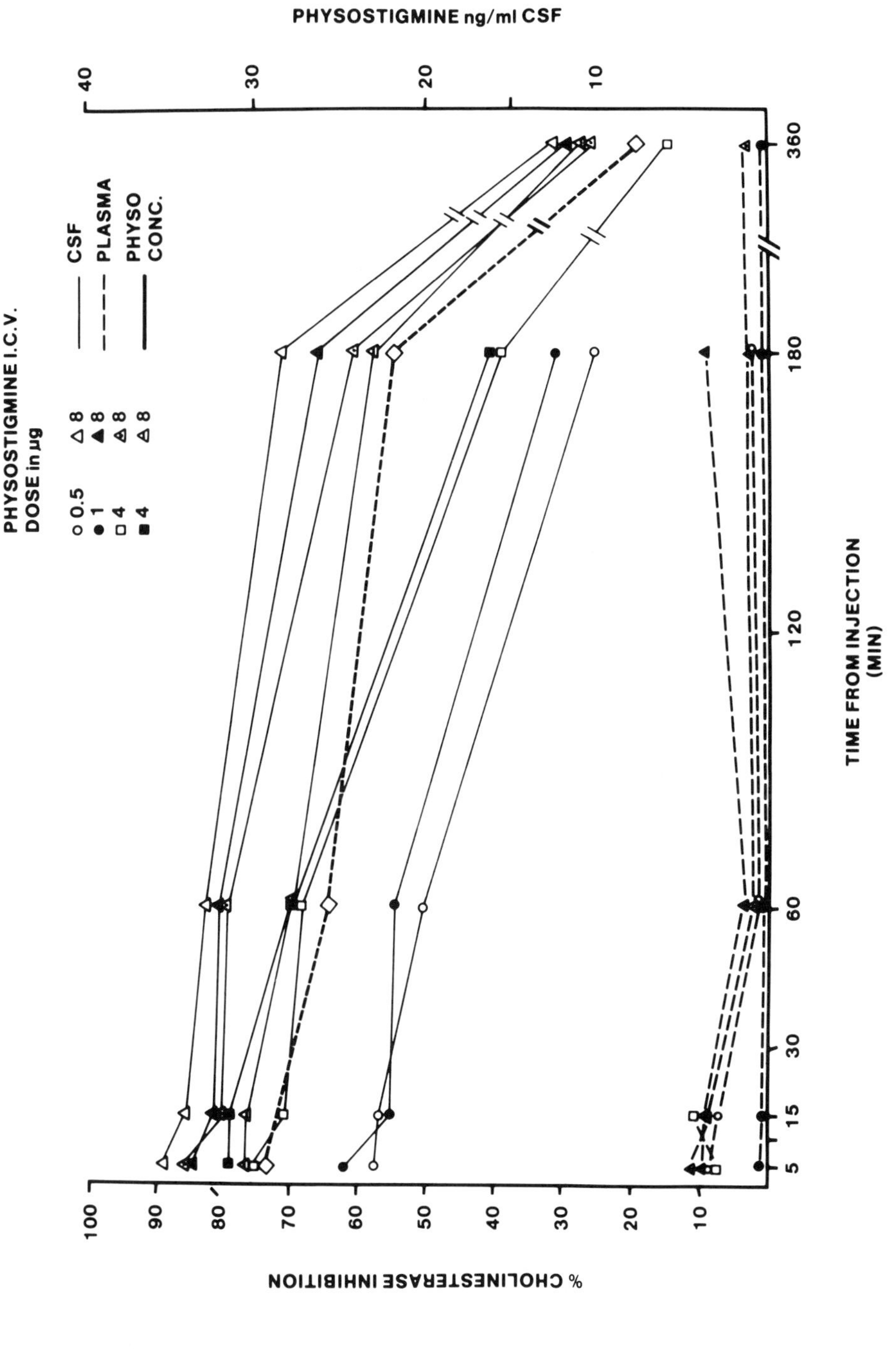
PHYSOSTIGMINE ng/ml CSF
40
30
20
10
PHYSOSTIGMINE I.C.V.
DOSE in µg
○ 0.5
● 1
□ 4
■ 4
△ 8
▲ 8
CSF
PLASMA
PHYSO CONC.
% CHOLINESTERASE INHIBITION
100
90
80
70
60
50
40
30
20
10
TIME FROM INJECTION (MIN)
5
15
30
60
120
180
360

DeSarno and Giacobini (107) have shown that chronic administrations of Phy i.v.c. (4 µg, twice daily during 14 days) produce a desensitization of cholinergic nicotinic receptors, which leads to an increase in binding sites (up-regulation) for [^{3}H] nicotine in hippocampus and cortex. The same treatment increases significantly the release of [^{3}H] ACh from the hippocampal slices. These experimental data correlate with the effects of Phy seen on cortical slices from biopsies of AD patients (43) and on the effect of the same drug on ACh release in the CSF of treated patients reported in the next section.

Clinical i.v.c. Trials Our preliminary results are from a continuing pilot study in which we will treat six severely demented (CDR 2.5-3) patients with i.v.c. Phy infusion. Figure 4 summarizes the results obtained in the treatment of a 75-year-old patient with a 5 year history of the disease and a CDR score of 2.5. Several

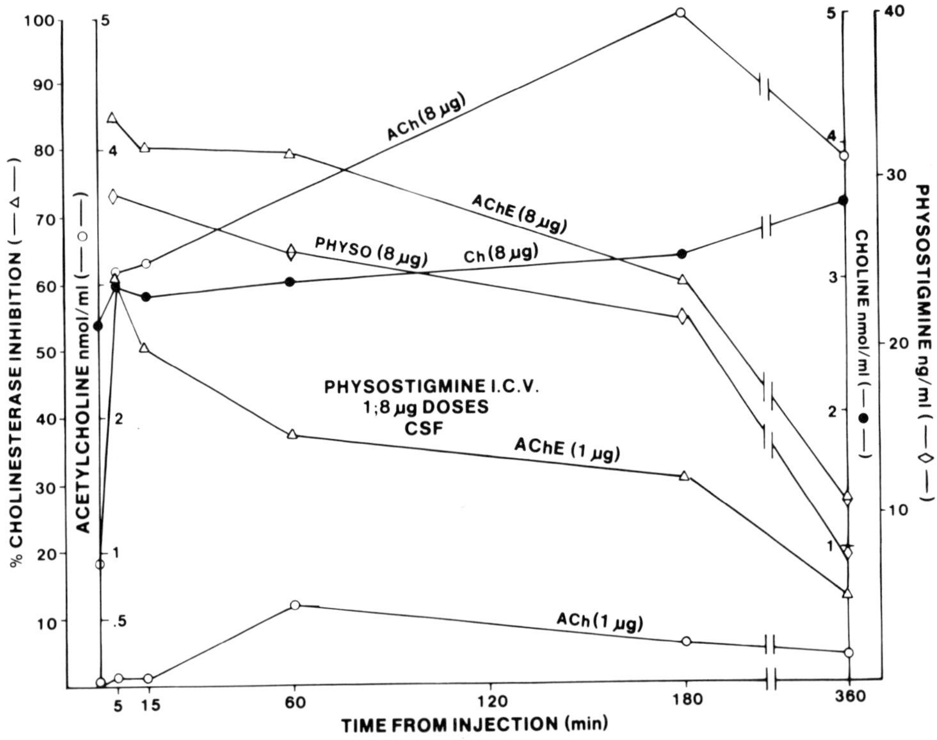

FIGURE 5 The effect of a single dose of 8 µg Phy on ChE activity, ACh, and Ch concentrations and Phy concentrations in CSF of an AD patient. In the ACh control, AChE was not inactivated immediately following collection of CSF.

dosages of Phy ranging from 0.5-8 μg were administered i.v.c. through the reservoirs in single administrations at different sessions. Figure 4 shows the results of nine consecutive experimental trials on the percentage inhibition of CSF (upper curves) and plasma (lower curves) ChE activity. At 5 min from starting the injection, the lowest dosage range (0.5-1 μg) inhibited CSF AChE by 60%; at 180 min AChE activity was still 30% inhibited. The middle dosage (4 μg) caused 75% and 45% AChE inhibition at 5 min and 180 min, respectively; however, at 360 min AChE activity was inhibited by only 20%. The highest dosage (8 μg), administered in four trials, resulted in 85% inhibition at 5 min and 70% inhibition at 180 min. At 360 min, AChE activity was still 30% inhibited. Contrary to the high degree of CSF ChE inhibition, plasma BuChE was maximally inhibited only 10% at the highest dosage and 3% after 60 min. For comparison, in the same figure, the CSF concentration of Phy is reported following the 8 μg dosage. The concentration curve of Phy follows closely ChE inhibition, decreasing from the 5 min value of 20 ng/ml to 7 ng/ml at 360 min. Figure 5 shows the effect of administration of an 8 μg i.v.c. dosage of Phy on the same patient on several cholinergic parameters as well as on Phy concentration in the CSF. For comparison, in the same figure, the CSF ACh levels are reported following a lower (1 μg) dosage administration. The most significant effect of the higher dose is a fivefold increase of ACh in CSF; from 0.9 nmol/ml to a peak value of 5 nmol/ml at 180 min. It is interesting to note that at 360 min, ACh levels are still elevated (4 nmol/ml) in spite of the low level of ChE inhibition in CSF (30%). Contrary to the rapid and sustained increase in ACh, choline (Ch) levels are fairly constant throughout the trial. This would suggest that the CSF pool of Ch was not utilized to synthesize the ACh recovered in CSF. Inhibition of AChE activity and levels of Phy follow a parallel trend throughout the experiment.

These results suggest that following a single dosage i.v.c. injection of Phy, causing 85% inhibition of AChE in CSF, ACh is released from the CNS into the CSF and is maintained at high steady state levels during a period of at least 6 hr. If CSF ACh and Ch levels reflect closely extracellular fluid concentrations in the brain, as suggested by animal experiments (108), high and sustained cerebral ACh in CSF would be a direct result of Phy i.v.c. administration. This represents one of the major goals established for our therapy (64,66). This result has not been achieved by any other route of administration, either in experimental animals or in humans (66,109).

As predicted by our dog model (106), i.v.c. Phy produces few peripheral side effects. Our patient, who was evaluated closely for cardiovascular, respiratory, and gastrointestinal symptoms, did not show side effects. No side effects could be recorded throughout the duration of the trial, not even at the highest Phy dosage (8 μg). In particular, no peripheral side effects were present and the patient appeared to be little bothered by the Phy injection. This demonstrates that Phy can be safely injected i.v.c. in an elderly AD patient, producing high levels of CNS inhibition of ChE with little peripheral effect. Most significant is the long-lasting fivefold increase in ACh. The patient was tested with our memory battery prior to the trial, the day of the trial before the injection, and at 1, 3, and 6 hr following Phy injection. The scores on the cognitive portion of the Alzheimer Disease and Associated Disorders Association (ADADA) scale improved on the trial with respect to placebo on double-blind trial. There was an indication of a positive drug effect on the word recognition subtest. However, at times, the patient seemed to be more irritable or sleepy. Due to the slow mixing and low turnover rate of CSF ($t_{1/2}$ = 3.5 hr), the amount of Phy taken up by the brain from the CSF can be more easily estimated at late (≥180 min) times than at early ones. At 180 min, if one assumes uniform distribution, approximately 50% of the injected Phy is still present in CSF. Therefore, the CSF is acting as a slow release system for Phy, causing prolonged AChE inhibition in brain and preservation of high extracellular ACh levels, as reflected in CSF concentrations. Another interesting observation is the 44% increase in baseline CSF AChE activity from 5.38 ± 0.84 to 9.48 ± 0.67 nmol/ml/min at the higher dosages (8 μg). The same effect has been observed in the dog with i.v. injections. This is related to a stimulation of AChE release into the CSF (106,110).

Conclusions We report here a summary of three clinical studies (Table 10) performed on AD patients with Phy administered by three different routes (oral, i.v., and i.v.c.). Of these three approaches, the i.v.c. seems to be the most promising. Oral and single dose i.v. administrations show only modest and short-lasting improvement in neuropsychological test performance (Table 8). In addition, side effects such as nausea and dizziness, which limit these agents' use, are reltively

TABLE 10 Short-, Intermediate-, and Long-Acting Cholinesterase Inhibitors: Experimental 3-Drug Trial in Alzheimer Patients

Drug	Single dose (mg/kg)	Route	Half-life (min)	% Plasma BuChE inhib	No. of patients	Schedule
Physostigmine	0.06	Oral	22	24 (60 min)	12	Completed
Salicylate	0.01-0.02	i.v.		12-25 (120 min)	20	In progress
	0.001	i.v.c.		90 (5 min)	6	In progress
Tetrahydro-aminoacridine	150-200	Oral	80	60	18	In progress
Metrifonate	10	Oral	180	80-90	10	In progress

TABLE 11 Comparison of Pharmacological Properties of Three Reversible ChE Inhibitors: Experimental and Clinical Data

	Phy	THA	MTF
Acute LD_{50}[a] (mg/kg)	1.3 (rat)	25 (rat)	395 (rat) (DDVP=15)
Half-life (min)	15 (rat); 31 (dog); 22 (man)	80 (man)	180 (humans)
Peak time for maximal ChE inhibition[a] (min)	15	60	30
% Inhibition ChE at peak time[a]	60	40	75
Duration of inhibition[a] (min)	120	240	540
Recovery of 50% ChE activity[a] (min)	30	120	180
Recovery of 100% ChE activity[a] (min)	120	500	540
Side effects[b]	Mild-moderate	Moderate-strong	Mild or absent
% maximum increase of ACh in CNS[a] (1st administration)	70	70	45
% maximum increase of ACh in CNS[a] (2nd administration)	75	0 (no effect	30
Uptake of Ch[c]	Decreased	Decreased	No effect
Synthesis of ^{3}H-ACh[c] (dpm/mg prot)	372	113	338
Evoked release of ACh[c] (% of total dpm)	12	0 (Block)	5

DDVP, dichlorvos
[a]i.m. administration in the rat, Phy = 600 μg/kg; THA = 20 mg/kg; MTF = 80 mg/kg (111); [b]humans, therapeutic doses (86,91,112); rat (138); [c]caudate slices, rat (111).

common. The low efficacy of the oral and i.v. route is probably related to the short-lasting effect of the drug in the brain and the appearance of toxic effects at dosages that result in low BuChE inhibition in plasma. The i.v.c. route produces practically no BuChE inhibition in plasma and no peripheral side effects. On the other hand, the i.v.c. route does produce a high percentage inhibition of AChE in CSF and a demonstrable increase of ACh in the CSF. This effect lasts for at least 3 hr with single doses and does not produce side effects. Among the several noncholinergic drugs tested so far (Table 9), none has shown clear effects of memory improvement or cognitive enhancement. Some of them are still being tested and more results will be available shortly.

Table 10 reports the three major clinical trials in progress in our Alzheimer Center. Encouraged by the results of Summers et al. (86) and by the results obtained in animal trials with metrifonate (MTF) (99,111), we are now comparing the clinical effects of three cholinesterase inhibitors in AD patients.

The pharmacological properties of these three compounds are distinctly different (Table 11). Our preclinical trials emphasize these differences.

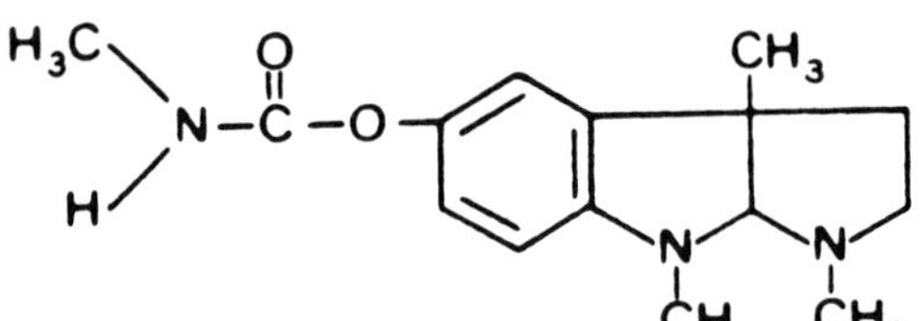

Physostigmine
(eserine)

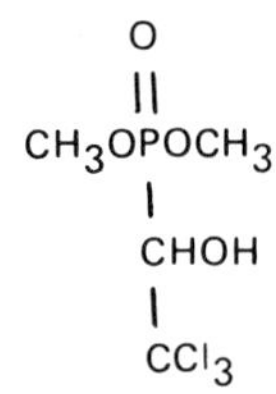

METRIFONATE

O,O - dimethyl - (1 - hydroxy - 2, 2, 2 - trichloroethyl) - phosponate

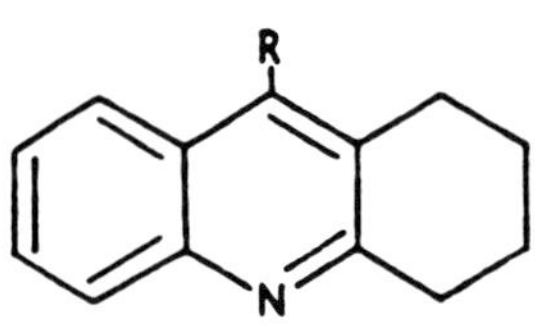

I

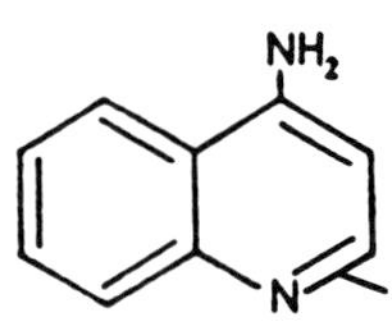

II

I, R = NH_2 = Tetrahydroaminoacridine

I, R = NHC_4H_9 = N - Butylaminotetrahydroacridine

I, R = H = Tetrahydroacridine

II = 4 - Aminoquinoline

FIGURE 6 General structure of physostigmine, metrifonate, and tetrahydroaminoacridine.

Although all three of these drugs—Phy, MTF and THA—are potent ChE inhibitors presently used in experimental treatment of AD (Fig. 6, Table 10) (66), they differ markedly with respect to several effects on ACh metabolism, increases in ACh levels, $[^3H]$ ACh release, $[^3H]$ Ch accumulation, and ChE inhibition. The mechanism for these differences is not yet fully understood.

Based on pharmacological results obtained in the rat (99), we have suggested that MTF, an organophosphorus ChE inhibitor acting as a slow-release agent with a longer action than both Phy and THA, is more likely to produce therapeutic effects in AD patients than the other inhibitors. There are significant differences between the effect of Phy and MTF given i.m. The ACh levels reach peak values in brain faster and are higher with Phy (500 μg/kg) than with MTF (80 mg/kg); however, duration of inhibition of ChE is four times longer after administration of MTF than after Phy (Table 11) (99). In humans, a dose of 10 mg/kg of MTF given orally produces an 80% inhibition of plasma ChE, which persists for 2-3 days without inducing significant side effects (112).

With regard to other specific differences between Phy and MTF, since the effect of the latter on the activity of ChE on brain is slower, it may allow for a more gradual build-up of the neurotransmitter and a more efficient nonenzymatic elimination. The rate of increase of ACh levels in brain may also be important in determining the severity of cholinergic side effects.

Independently of the drug, there seems to be a limit in the maximal level of ACh that will be reached in brain and, more important, in the length of the period during which increases in levels of ACh will be maintained (66). These factors are important in determining the therapeutic effect of the drug (66).

Our observations in an animal model can be relevant to the selection of a ChE inhibitor that is suitable for the treatment of cholinergic deficits in Alzheimer's patients. Our experimental results indicate that THA may not present any distinct advantage over either Phy or MTF in maintaining steady-state ACh levels in brain. On the contrary, our data show that THA's effect on brain ACh may not be as sustained as that of MTF (Table 11) (111). The selective downregulation of M_1 (muscarinic) subtype of receptors seen after chronic THA administration in the rat (113) may also lead to diminished efficacy of long-term THA treatment in AD.

THA and Metrifonate: First Clinical Results

Three studies of THA have been published to date (69,74,86). Very positive results have been reported in 17 patients by Summers et al. (86). A multicenter trial of THA is presently being conducted in the United States. Results from four unpublished studies recently added some additional support to the possible efficacy of THA in the treatment of Alzheimer's disease. There appears to be a high incidence of possible hepatotoxicity with the use of THA that may be dosage related (114). Because of these side effects and questions raised about the reliability of data reported by Summers et al. (86), the results of the multicenter trial must be available before a reasonable appraisal of the role of THA in Alzheimer's disease can be reached.

Only 17 patients treated by Summers et al. (86) have received THA for more than 1 week. All of the patients in this report improved drastically on a number of measures of memory and behavior. As might be expected, the amount of improvement was greater in the less severely affected patients. A number of problems have been considered to be unsatisfactorily addressed by the initial report and subsequent responses of the investigators to questions. This includes the use of unvalidated scales, lack of reported reliability, suspicion that behaviors in patients were evaluated not face-to-face but by telephone, and others. In addition, the revelation that patients who participated in the research were charged for the costs of the research, including the investigators' time, led to suspicions of the motives of the investigators that have furthered skepticism about the conduct of this study. The two earlier published studies both reported improvement

(a)

(b)

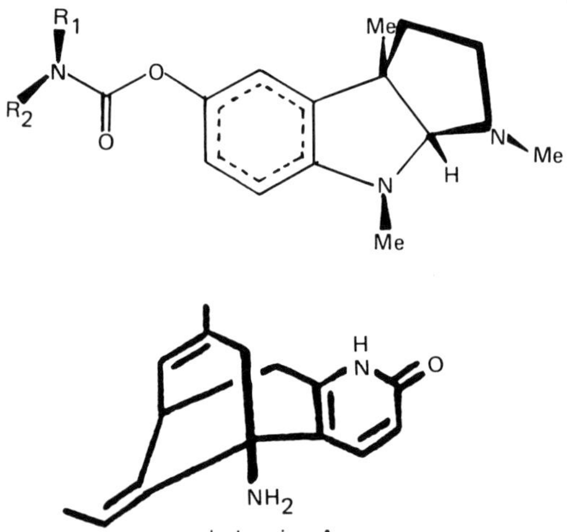

huberzine A

(5R, 9R, 11E) - 5 amino - 11 - ethylidinene 5, 6, 9,
10 - tetrahydro - 7 - methyl - 5, 9 - methanocycloocteno
[b]pyridin - 2 (1H) - one

FIGURE 7 (a). General structure of new physostigmine derivatives (from ref. 120). (b). Chemical structure of Huperzine A (from ref. 124).

in memory with THA. Summers et al. (69) found that less cognitively impaired patients improved with THA treatment if they were pretreated with lecithin.

In a recent report, Fitten et al. (115) found no improvement with THA in 10 patients treated for 1 week. Fauthier et al. (116) reported improvement on a THA-lecithin combination in an 8-week study, with a return to baseline neuropsychological test performance within 2 weeks of cessation of administration of THA. THA has also been administered to patients by Levy (114) and Nyback et al. (117). Both investigators found about 50% of patients improved. None of these more recent reports was fully double-blind.

Reports of side effects are variable, with up to 80% of patients being adversely affected in the study by Gauthier et al. (116). It has been suggested that dosages above 200 mg daily are associated with the appearance of side effects. Muscle stiffness, nausea, and vomiting have not been major problems that would limit the clinical use of THA.

Elevated liver enzyme levels in plasma have been observed in a number of studies (98,114,116-118). The multicenter trial of THA in the United States was interrupted because of elevation of liver enzymes. That trial has been restarted using lower dosages of THA. At present, there are questions about the results from the Summers et al. study (86), the small numbers of patients treated in other trials, the brief duration of treatment in these trials, and the frequent appearance of elevated liver enzyme levels in plasma of patients receiving THA. Thus, a final evaluation of the clinical utility of THA is not available.

CHOLINESTERASE INHIBITORS: THE THIRD GENERATION, HEPTYL-PHYSOSTIGMINE, AND THE HUPERZINES

The therapeutic application of Phy is reduced by its toxicity, adverse side effects, short half-life, narrow effective dosage range, and low bioavailability (91,119). This has stimulated pharmacologists to produce new ChE inhibitors with improved effects and lower toxicity.

New Physostigmine Analogs

In order to bypass these problems, a group of chemists at the Department of Pharmaceutical Chemistry of the University of Rome (120) have synthesized a new series of Phy analogs in which the methylcarbamic group has been substituted with 1-16 carbon atoms, long alkylcarbamic groups, and dialkylcarbamic groups (Fig. 7A). These have a higher lipophilicity and consequently a different body distribution and pharmacokinetics than Phy.

The anticholinesterase (antiChE) activity in vitro and in vivo, the acute toxicity, and some behavioral effects of a selected derivative, heptyl, have already been investigated (120,121).

This preliminary work indicates that heptyl-physostigmine (heptyl-Phy) is a more suitable inhibitor of ChE than Phy due to its greater lipophilicity and its longer inhibitory activity (Fig. 7A; heptyl, R_1 = C7H15, R_2 = H).

The main result emerging from the work of Brufani et al. (120) and Pomponi and Giacobini (121) is that the new compound heptyl-Phy exerts its antiChE activity at dosages significantly less toxic than Phy: the LD_{50} of heptyl-Phy is 35 mg/kg, while the same lethal effect is evident with a dosage of 0.6 mg/kg of Phy. Moreover, a powerful long-lasting inhibition of both brain and serum ChE activity is evident in rats and mice following heptyl-Phy administration (121).

At the behavioral level, the action of heptyl-Phy results in an antagonism of the stimulating effects of scopolamine, a well-known anticholinergic agent, on the locomotor activity of mice. The modifications of the electrocorticogram (ECoG) activity following administration of 10 mg/kg of heptyl demonstrate a typical increase in cholinergic functions. However, the most interesting result in terms of behavioral modifications is probably the effect of heptyl-Phy on passive avoidance learning, which may be interpreted in terms of enhanced consolidation processes (122).

The Huperzines

One of the characteristic features of substances modulating the effect of ACh in brain is that they occur as alkaloids or neurotoxins in nature (e.g., atropine and alpha-bungarotoxin). The division of the two major receptor categories of the cholinergic system is based on two groups of naturally occurring substances: nicotine and muscarine. Classic examples of anticholinergic drugs are atropine, scopolamine, and other related belladonna alkaloids that are widely distributed in nature, especially in the Solanaceae plants (*Atropa belladonna, Datura stramonium, Hyoscyamus niger,* and *Scopola carniolica*). Drugs inhibiting or inactivating AChE activity are no exception. Physostigmine (Phy), a ChE inhibitor, is an alkaloid obtained from the calabar bean, the dried seed of *Physostigma venenosum* used for treatment of glaucoma since 1877 and now for experimental treatment of Alzheimer's disease (119). Galanthamine is another example of a ChE inhibitor occurring in nature. In 1982, pharmacologists at the Chinese Academy of Science and the Shanghai School of Medicine isolated a new series of alkaloids from the plant *Huperzia serrata*, which they called huperzine A and B (123-125) (Fig. 7B). These alkaloids seem to possess remarkable antiChE activity (Fig. 8). They are powerful and reversible ChE inhibitors that produce an improvement in short-term as well as long-term memory in experimental animals (124) and in aged humans (126). Because of their potent pharmacological action and the low frequency of side effects, huperzine A and B might represent a valid alternative to both Phy (119) and THA (86) experimental treatment of Alzheimer's patients. Preliminary studies (125) suggest that huperzine A may be a more potent and selective inhibitor of AChE, with a lower toxicity and a higher therapeutic index

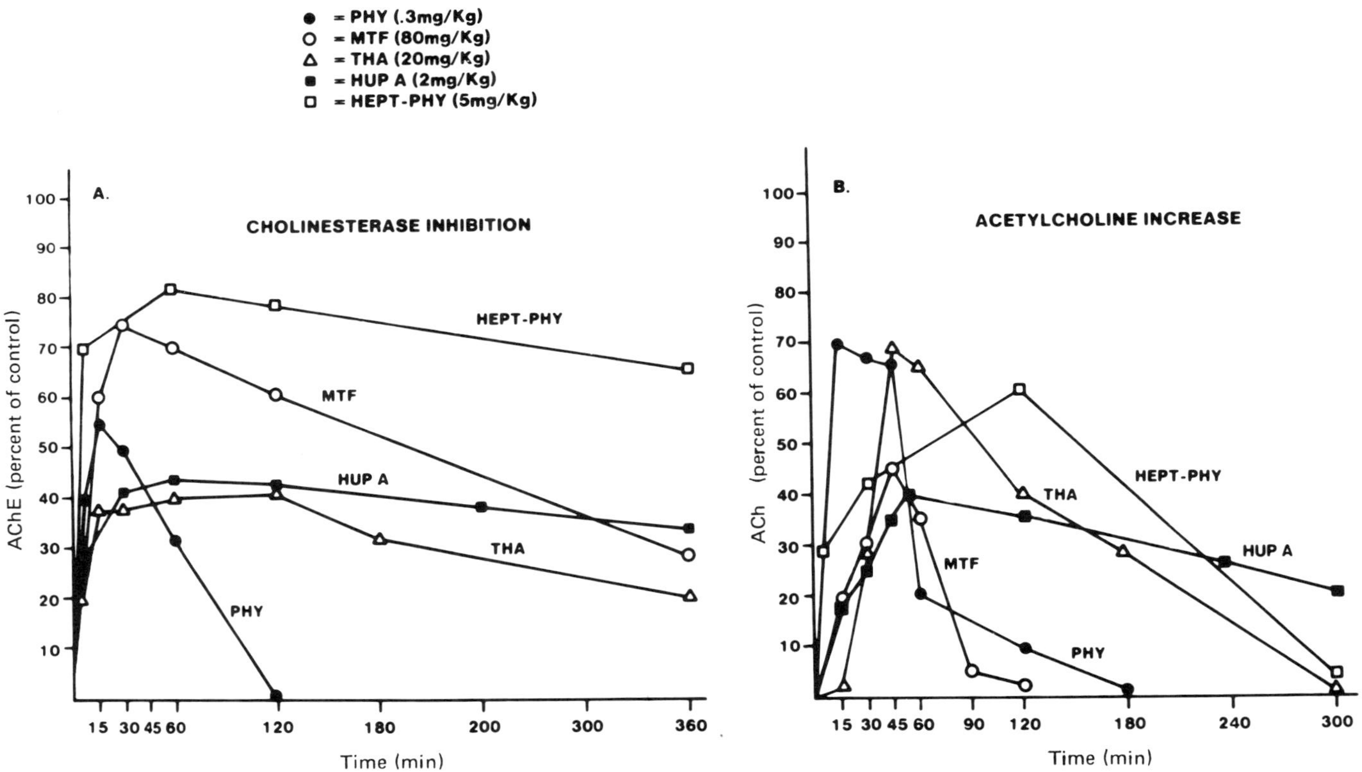

FIGURE 8 Comparison of the effect of five cholinesterase inhibitors on AChE inhibition and ACh levels in rat brain following a single dose of the drug administered i.m.

TABLE 12 Comparison of Therapeutic Indices of Five Cholinesterase Inhibitors

	Mice (i.p., μmole/kg)		LD_{50}	Rats (i.v., μmole/kg)		LD_{50}
Drug	Acute LD_{50}	ED_{50}	ED_{50}	Acute LD_{50}	ED_{50}	ED_{50}
Huperzine A	7.44	0.32	23.2	10.33	0.14	73.8
Huperzine B	97.65	3.75	26.0	171.02	0.58	294.9
Neostigmine	2.31	0.27	8.6	0.89	0.02	44.5
Physostigmine	1.94	0.50	3.9	1.23	0.17	7.2
Galanthamine	–	–		33.46	0.93	36.0

Source: Tang et al. (124).

than Phy (Table 12). Facilitation of retrieval (Y maze, discrimination performance) was produced by huperzine A in a dosage-dependent fashion (36-167 μg/kg) (124). Scopolamine (0.2 mg/kg s.c.), atropine (5 mg/kg s.c.), or hemicholinium (20 μg i.v.c.) antagonized the positive effect of huperzine A (0.1 mg/kg) on retrieval, but methyl atropine (2 mg/kg s.c.) did not. These results suggest that huperzine A may act on the central cholinergic system. Muscarinic receptors may be affected since muscarinic receptor blockers reversed the action of huperzine A, but their quaternary nitrogen derivatives such as methyl-atropine, which does not pass the blood-brain barrier, do not. These pharmacological effects obtained in animals support the effect observed in humans by Zhang (126).

Vincent et al. (127) from Roche Lab (Basel, Switzerland) have reported that different tests for cognitive performance show that huperzine A (μg/kg doses i.p.) is acting as a cognitive enhancing agent on rats, mice, and monkeys. Only at high dosages does huperzine A cause side effects that are antagonized by methscopolamine.

During the last year new data have been published with regard to the effect of huperzines A and B in the CNS. The latest results are those published by Yan et al. (128). They present evidence that both huperzine A and B potentiate muscle contraction in the rat's isolated phrenic nerve-diaphragm preparation and cause electroencephalographic (EEG) activation. Huperzine A was found to be more potent on the isolated phrenic nerve-diaphragm preparation than huperzine B, but less potent than Phy and neostigmine. Both huperzine A and B exert an anticurare effect on the sciatic-tibialis preparation. The activation effect on the rabbit EEG was also more pronounced for huperzine A (0.05 mg/kg i.v.) than for huperzine B. These results show that both drugs act on peripheral as well as central cholinergic mechanisms. Peripheral effects after use of the huperzines are less pronounced than after Phy, while the opposite is true for central effects.

Behavioral studies have been performed by the Chinese authors (124) on the effect of huperzine A on learning and retrieval with discrimination performance in rats using a Y maze. Huperzine A (36-167 μg i.p.) produced a dosage-dependency facilitation of retrieval that was antagonized by scopolamine and atropine (0.2 mg/kg s.c., 0.1 mg/kg s.c., respectively).

Evidence that huperzine A is effective, nontoxic, and/or useful in the treatment of AD in humans is derived from the study by Zhang (126). This author compared huperzine A with Hydergine in a double study of 100 aged patients with memory impairment (54 men, 46 women aged 46-82). According to Zhang, memory improved 1-4 hr after an injection of 30 μg huperzine A. The improvement was sustained for a period of 8 hr and was superior to that of 600 μg Hydergine. According to new results (Tang, personal communications), huperzine A has now been tested in over 200 patients with memory impairment including Alzheimer disease. To our knowledge, no other drug trials in patients have been done in patients outside China. The recent data obtained by Tang and Giacobini (129) on AChE inhibition and ACh metabolism in rat brain also support the hypothesis of a strong and sustained cholinomimetic effect in the CNS produced by the huperzines (Fig. 8).

THE CHOLINERGIC-ADRENERGIC APPROACH

Recent studies by Whitehouse and Unnerstall (130), Kalaria et al. (131), and Zweig et al. (132) emphasize losses of adrenergic neurons in the locus ceruleus (LC), as well as an increase in cortical beta-adrenergic receptors (Table 13) in patients with AD. This deficit may be a consequence of denervation supersensitivity due to loss of presynaptic input from LC. Such changes combined with severe cholinergic losses in the nucleus basalis (NB) and the decrease in nicotinic receptors seen by us (43) suggest that a combination of cholinomimetic drugs (AChE inhibitors, ACh agonists) and β-receptor agonists (Table 13) could be beneficial in slowing down the effect of denervation.

In addition, Davis et al. (133) have reported that the addition of an LC deficit produced by a lesion to animals with an NB lesion profoundly affects their response to cholinomimetic drugs. Physostigmine and oxotremorine, which are effective in reversing performance deficits in passive avoidance learning following an NB lesion, are without effect in animals with both LC and NB lesions. The addition of clonidine (an α-blocking agent) to Phy or oxotremorine restores the animal's performance to control levels. These experimental data also argue for a combined cholinergic/adrenergic type of therapy. The ideal drug would be a combination of a selective ChE inhibitor and a β-agonist or a specific nicotinic agonist and β-agonist that would maintain high levels of ACh, increase release, and slow down development of denervation hypersensitivity of adrenergic receptors.

TABLE 13 Two Major Neurotransmitter (NT) Systems Affected by Alzheimer's Disease

Localization	Percentage cell loss	NT	Presynaptic cortical receptors	Percentage loss	Postsynaptic cortical receptors	Percentage loss	Main symptoms	Potential treatment
Nucleus basalis	50-80[a]	ACh	Nicotinic[b]	60	Muscarinic[b]	0	Memory Cognitive	AChE inhibitors ACh agonists
Locus ceruleus	30-60[c]	NE	–	0	β_2[d]	40	Affective[e] Behavioral	β_2 agonists

[a]Ref. 140.
[b]Ref. 43.
[c]Refs. 132, 141.
[d]Refs. 130, 131.
[e]Hallucinations, depression, paranoid delusions, anxiety, aggressiveness.

GENERAL CONCLUSIONS ON COMPARATIVE STUDIES OF CHOLINESTERASE INHIBITORS FROM OUR LABORATORY

Figure 8 compares the effect of five ChE inhibitors on AChE inhibition and ACh levels in rat brain following i.m. administration of one single dose of the drug. The dosage has been selected based on the criterion ensuring a maximal increase in ACh levels in brain with high ChE activity inhibition at zero mortality level. Figure 8A shows that with MTF and heptyl-Phy it is possible to reach peak levels of 70-80% AChE inhibition within 30-60 min from administration. Huperzine A and THA produce lower peak levels of inhibition (40%); however, this is maintained for almost 6 hr with huperzine A and 3 hr with THA. Physostigmine produces a rapid (15 min) peak of 55% inhibition but this effect ends within 2 hr.

The effect on brain ACh levels is also markedly different for the different drugs. High ACh increases (70%) are obtained following both Phy and THA administration; however, particularly with Phy, this effect is short lasting (1 hr). Heptyl-Phy shows the most prolonged effect on brain ACh levels, with a peak at 2 hr. The effect of MTF instead is short lasting (1.5 hr).

It is important to note that Hallak and Giacobini (111) found major differences between the effects of three ChE inhibitors (Phy, THA, and MTF) in rat brain both with in vivo and in vitro experiments.

In particular, these inhibitors show varying effects after a second consecutive dose. After a second administration of Phy or MTF, an increase in brain ACh identical to that after the first administration is seen. However, with Phy both ChE activity and ACh level return to baseline while with MTF, ChE is still approximately 60% inhibited at the time that ACh has reached control values. A dissociation of these effects is even more pronounced with THA, since the second administration of this drug does not produce any increase in ACh despite persisting ChE inhibition (111). In fact, ACh levels continue to remain below control values, suggesting a decreased accumulation, perhaps due to reduced synthesis. However, a direct effect of THA, as well as of the other inhibitors, on ChAT activity can be ruled out by testing the effect of various concentrations of the drug on the purified enzyme.

The in vitro release of ACh from CNS slices also varies with the type of the drug and its concentration. it is known that ChE inhibitors decrease the electrically evoked release of ACh from striatum, hippocampal, and cortical slices (134, 135). In our experiments, release was suppressed by THA at a concentration of 1.4 mM, but not by Phy (0.1 mM) and MTF (1 mM). Indeed, Drukarch et al. (136) found that THA in a range of concentrations from 0.15 to 10 μM inhibits release of ACh from 5% to 47%, respectively, from neostriatal and neocortical rat brain slices. At a concentration of 3 μM, Phy produced a 66% decrease compared to a 44% decrease with THA used at the same concentration. This effect of THA is blocked by atropine. It is known that both THA and Phy interfere with nicotinic and muscarinic ligand binding, and that THA is more potent than

Phy at these receptors (137). Acute administration of THA (10 mg/kg s.c.) resulted in a 31% and 20% inhibition of HACU in P_2 fractions from rat hippocampus and cortex, respectively; however, Phy (0.88 mg/kg s.c.) also inhibited (by 44%) the HACU of the rat hippocampus (138).

These results reveal major differences in biochemical effects on rat brain including extent and duration of ChE inhibition, inhibition of ACh release, and increase in levels of ACh. Side effects are also markedly different in their time of appearance, duration, and severity. These findings suggest significant differences in mechanisms of action of various ChE inhibitors and, therefore, have potential clinical implications for a future symptomatic therapy of Alzheimer's disease patients.

The search for a pharmacological treatment of AD has started recently. The progress made in the last 2-3 years is remarkable, particularly since it has increased our knowledge on the effect of several types of drugs on the human brain. None of the drugs presently used experimentally is satisfactory, but important directions have been laid down by this initial work. We have discussed some of the most promising ones in this chapter.

ACKNOWLEDGMENTS

The work performed in the authors' laboratories was supported by National Institute of Aging grant AG05416-0161 to Ezio Giacobini, and National Institute of Mental Health grant MH41821-01 to Robert Becker, grants from the Southern Illinois University Foundation, the E.F. Pearson Foundation, and the State of Illinois, Department of Health.

REFERENCES

1. Rosenberg, R.N. (1986). *Neurogenetics, Principles, and Practice.* New York, Raven Press, pp. 95-99.
2. Terry, R.D., Hansen, L.A., DeTeresa, R., et al. (1987). Senile dementia of the Alzheimer type without neocortical neurofibrillary tangles. *J. Neuropathol. Exp. Neurol.* 46: 262-268.
3. Katzman, R., Terry, R., DeTeresa, R., Brown, T., Davies, P., Fuld, P., Renbing, X., and Peck, A. (1988). Clinical, pathological and neurochemical changes in dementia: A subgroup with preserved mental status and numerous neocortical plaques. *Ann. Neurol.* 23: 138-144.
4. Wisniewski, H.M., Merz, G.S., and Carp, R.I. (1985). Current hypothesis of the etiology and pathogenesis of senile dementia of the Alzheimer type. *Interdisc. Topics Gerontol.* 19: 45-53.
5. Terry, R.D. (1988). What, where and why are plaques. *Alzheimer Dis. Assoc. Disord.* 2: 223.

6. Rosenberg, R.N. (1988). Molecular genetics of Alzheimer's disease; recent advances (abst). Proceedings of the International Symposium on Alzheimer's disease, Kuopio, Finland.
7. Lewis, D.A., Higgins, G.A., Young, W.G., Goldgaber, D., Gajdusek, D.C., Wilson, M.C., and Morrison, J.H. (1988). Distribution of precursor amyloid-α-protein messenger RNA in human cerebral cortex: Relationship to neurofibrillary tangles and neuritic plaques. *Proc. Natl. Acad. Sci.* 85: 1691-1695.
8. Palmert, M.R., Golde, T.E., Cohen, M.L., Kovacs, D.M., Tanzi, R.E., Gusella, J.F., Usiak, M.F., Youngkin, L.H., and Youngkin, S.G. (1988). Amyloid protein precursor messenger RNAs; differential expression in Alzheimer's disease. *Science* 241: 1080-1084.
9. Tanzi, R.E., McClatchey, A.I., Lamperti, E.D., Villa-Komaroff, L., Gusella, J.F., and Neve, R.L. (1988). Protease inhibitor domain encoded by an amyloid protein precursor mRNA associated with Alzheimer's disease. *Nature* 528-530.
10. Kitaguchi, N., Takahashi, Y., Tokushima, Y., Shiojiri, S., and Ito, H. (1988). Novel precursor of Alzheimer's disease amyloid protein shows protease inhibitory activity. *Nature* 331: 530-532.
11. Tanzi, R.E., Gusella, J.F., Watkins, P.C., Bruns, G.A., St. George-Hyslop, P., VanKeuren, M.L., Patterson, D., Pagan, S., Kurnit, D.M., and Neve, R.L. (1987). Amyloid α protein gene: cDNA, mRNA distribution, and genetic linkage near the Alzheimer locus. *Science* 235: 880-884.
12. Beal, M.F., Kowall, N.W., and Mazurek, M.F. (1987). Neuropeptides in Alzheimer's disease. *J. Neural Transm.* 24: 163-174.
13. Jones, E.G., and Hendry, S.H.C. (1986). The peptide containing neurons of the primate cerebral cortex. In: *Implications of Neuropeptides in Neurological and Psychiatric Diseases*, J.B. Martin and J. Barchus (Eds.) New York, Raven Press, pp. 163-178.
14. Moore, S.D., Madamba, S., and Joels, M. (1988). Somatostatin augments the M-current in hippocampal neurons. *Science* 239: 278-280.
15. Davies, P., Katzman, R., and Terry, R.D. (1980). Reduced somatostatin-like immunoreactivity in cerebral cortex from cases of Alzheimer disease and Alzheimer senile dementia. *Nature* (London) 288: 279-280.
16. Rosson, M.N., Emson, P.C., Mountjoy, C.Q., Roth, M., and Iversen, L.L. (1980). Reduced amounts of immunoreactive somatostatin in temporal cortex in senile dementia of Alzheimer type. *Neurosci. Lett.* 20: 373-377.
17. Wood, P.L., Etienne, P., Lal, S., Gauthier, S., Cajal, S., and Nair, N.P.V. (1982). Reduced lumbar CSF somatostatin levels in Alzheimer's disease. *Life Sci.* 31: 2073-2079.
18. Francis, P.T., Bowen, D.M., Neary, D., Palo, J., Wikstrom, J., and Olney, J. (1984). Somatostatin-like immunoreactivity in lumbar cerebrospinal fluid from neurohistologically examined demented patients. *Neurobiol. Aging* 5: 183-186.
19. Serby, M., Richardson, S.B., Twente, S., Siekierski, J., Corwin, J., and Rotrosen, J. (1984). CSF somatostatin in Alzheimer's disease. *Neurobiol. Aging* 5: 187-189.

20. Atack, J.R., Beal, M.F., Mayu, C., Kaye, J.A., Mazurek, M.P., Kay, A.D., and Rapoport, S.I. (1988). Cerebrospinal fluid somatostatin and neuropeptide Y: Concentrations in aging and in dementia of the Alzheimer type with and without extrapyramidal signs. *Arch. Neurol.* 45: 269-274.
21. Kowall, N.W., and Beal, M.F. (1988). Cortical somatostatin, neuropeptide Y, and NADPH diaphorase neurons: Normal anatomy and alterations in Alzheimer's disease. *Ann. Neurol.* 23(2): 105-114.
22. Delfs, J.R., Zhu, C.-H., and Dichter, M.A. (1984). Coexistence of acetylcholinesterase and somatostatin-immunoreactivity in neurons cultured from rat cerebrum. *Science* 223: 61-63.
23. Uhl, G.R., Tran, V., and Snyder, S.H. (1985). Somatostatin receptors: Distribution in rat central nervous system and human frontal cortex. *J. Comp. Neurol.* 240: 288-304.
24. Morrison, J.M., Benoit, R., Magistretti, P.J., Ling, N., and Bloom, F.E. (1982). *Neurosci. Lett.* 34: 137.
25. Malthe-Sorenssen, D., Wood, P.L., Cheney, D.L., and Costa, E. (1978). Modulation of the turnover rate of acetylcholine in rat brain by intraventricular injections of tyrotropin-releasing hormone, somatostatin, neurotensin and angiotensin II. *J. Neurochem.* 31: 685-691.
26. Cutler, N.R., Haxby, J., Narang, P.K., May, C., Burg, C., and Reines, S.A. (1985). Evaluation of an analog of somatostatin (L363,586) in Alzheimer's disease. *N. Engl. J. Med.* 312: 725.
27. Cutler, N.R., Haxby, J., Kay, A.D., Narang, P.K., Lesko, L.J., Costa, J.L., Ninos, M., Linnoila, M., Potter, W.Z., Renfrew, J.W., and Moore, A.M. (1985). Evaluation of Zimelidine in Alzheimer's disease: Cognitive and biochemical measures. *Arch. Neurol.* 42: 744-748.
28. Soininen, H., Koskinen, T., Helkala, E.-L., Pigache, R., and Riekkinen, P.J. (1985). Treatment of Alzheimer's disease with a synthetic ACTH 4-9 analog. *Neurology* 35(9): 1348-1351.
29. Wilson, C.A. (1986). Society for Drug Research symposium: Senile dementia of the Alzheimer type. *Neurobiol. Aging* 7: 219-222.
30. Reisberg, B., Ferris, S.H., Anand, R., Mir, P., Geibel, V., and DeLeon, M.J. (1983). Effects of naloxone in senile dementia: A double-blind trial. *N. Engl. J. Med.* 308: 721-722.
31. Tariot, P.N., Sunderland, T., Weingartner, H., Murphy, D.L., Cohen, M.R., and Cohen, R.M. (1986). Naloxone and Alzheimer's disease. *Arch. Gen. Psychiatry* 43: 727-732.
32. Blass, J.B., Reding, M.J., Drachman, D., Mitchell, A., Glosser, G., Klatzman, R., Thal, L., Grenel, S., Spar, J.E., Larue, A., and Liston, E. (1983). Cholinesterase inhibitors and opiate antagonists in patients with Alzheimer's disease. *N. Engl. J. Med.* 309: 556.
33. Hefti, F., and Weiner, W.J. (1986). Nerve growth factor and Alzheimer's disease. *Ann. Neurol.* 20(3): 275-281.
34. Schwab, M.E., Otten, U., Agid, Y., and Thoenen, H. (1979). Nerve growth factor (NGF) of specific retrograde axonal transport and tyrosine hydroxylase induction in locus coeruleus and substantia nigra. *Brain Res.* 168: 473-483.

35. Seiler, M., and Schwab, M.E. (1984). Specific retrograde transport of NGF from neocortex to nucleus basalis in the rat. *Brain Res.* 300: 33-39.
36. Hefti, F., Hartikka, J., Salvatierra, A., Weiner, W.J., and Mash, D.C. (1986). Localization of nerve growth factor receptors in cholinergic neurons of the human basal forebrain. *Neurosci. Lett.* 69: 37-41.
37. Williams, L.R., Varon, S., Peterson, G.M., Wictorin, K., Fischer, W., Bjorklund, A., and Gage, F.H. (1986). Continuous infusion of nerve growth factor prevents basal forebrain neuronal death after fimbria fornix transection. *Proc. Natl. Acad. Sci.* 83: 9231-9235.
38. Will, B., and Hefti, F. (1985). Behavioral and neurochemical effects of chronic intraventricular-injections of nerve growth factor in adult rats with fimbria lesions. *Behav. Brain Sci.* 77: 17-24.
39. Fischer, W., Wictorin, K., Bjorklung, A., Williams, L.R., Varon, S., and Gage, F.H. (1987). Amelioration of cholinergic neuron atrophy and spatial memory impairment in aged rats by nerve growth factor. *Nature* 329: 65-68.
40. Schweitzer, J.B. (1987). Nerve growth factor receptor-mediated transport from cerebrospinal fluid to basal forebrain neurons. *Brain Res.* 423: 309-317.
41. Korsching, S. (1986). The role of nerve growth factor in the CNS. *Trends Neurosci.* 9: 570-573.
42. Goerdert, M., Fine, A., Hunt, S.P., and Ullrich, A. (1986). Nerve growth factor mRNA in peripheral and central nervous system: Lesion effects in the rat brain and levels in Alzheimer's disease. *Mol. Brain Res.* 1: 85-92.
43. Giacobini, E., DeSarno, P., Clark, B., and McIlhany, M. (1988). The cholinergic receptor system of the human brain. Neurochemical and pharmacological aspects in aging and Alzheimer. In: *Progress in Brain Research*, A. Nordberg (Ed.) Amsterdam, Elsevier.
44. Bowen, D.A., Smith, C.B., White, P., and Davison, A.M. (1976). Neurotransmitter related enzymes and indixes of hypoxia in senile dementia and other abiotrophies. *Brain* 99: 459-496.
45. Davies, P. (1979). Neurotransmitter-related enzymes in senile dementia of the Alzheimer type. *Brain Res.* 171: 319-327.
46. Perry, E.K., Tomlinson, B.E., Blessed, G., Bergmann, K., Gibson, P.H., and Perry, R.H. (1978). Correlation of cholinergic abnormalities with senile plaques and mental test scores in senile dementia. *Br. J. Med.* 42: 1457-1459.
47. Reisine, T., Yamamura, H.I., Bird, E.D., Spokes, E., and Enna, S.J. (1978). Pre- and postsynaptic neurochemical alterations in Alzheimer's disease. *Brain Res.* 159: 477-481.
48. Rylett, R.J., Ball, M.J., and Colhoun, E.H. (1983). Evidence for high affinity choline transport in synaptosomes prepared from hippocampus and neocortex of patients with Alzheimer's disease. *Brain Res.* 289: 69-175.
49. Sims, N.R., Bowen, D.M., Allen, S.J., Smith, C.C.T., Neary, D., Thomas, D.J., and Davison, A.N. (1983). Presynaptic cholinergic dysfunction in patients with dementia. *J. Neurochem.* 40: 503-509.

50. Blessed, G., Tomlinson, B.E., and Roth, M. (1968). The association between quantitative measures of dementia and of senile changes in the cerebral grey matter of elderly subjects. *Br. J. Psychiatry* 114: 797-811.
51. Neary, D., Snowden, J.S., Mann, D.M.A., Bowen, D.M., Sims, N.R., Northern, B., Yates, P.O., and Davison, A.N. (1986). Alzheimer's disease: A correlative study. *J. Neurol. Neurosurg. Psychiatry* 49: 229-237.
52. Mash, D.C., Flynn, D.D., and Potter, L.T. (1985). Loss of M2 muscarine re ceptors in the cerebral cortex in Alzheimer's disease and experimental cholinergic denervation. *Science* 228: 115-1117.
53. Whitehouse, P.J. (1987). Neurotransmitter receptor alterations in AD: A review. *Alzheimer Dis. Assoc. Disord.* 1: 9-18.
54. Richter, J.A., Perry, E.K., and Tomlinson, B.E. (1980). Acetylcholine and choline levels in post-mortem human brain tissue: Preliminary observations in Alzheimer's diseases. *Life Sci.* 26: 1683-1689.
55. Johns, C.A., Levy, M.I., Greenwald, B.S., Rosen, W.G., Horvath, T.B., Davis, B.M., Mohs, R.C., and Davis, K.L. (1983). In: *Banbury Report 15: Biological Aspects of Alzheimer's Disease*, Katzman (Ed.) Cold Spring Harbor NY, Cold Spring Harbor Laboratory, pp. 435-449.
56. Elble, R., Giacobini, E., and Scarsella, G.F. (1987). Cholinestereases in cerebrospinal fluid. *Arch. Neurol.* 44: 403-407.
57. Whitehouse, P.J., Price, D.L., Stuble, R.G., Clark, A.W., Coyle, J.T., and DeLong, M.R. (1982). Alzheimer's disease and senile dementia: Loss of neurons in the basal forebrain. *Science* 215: 1238-1239.
58. London, E., and Coyle, J.T. (1978). Pharmacological augmentation of acetylcholine levels in kainate-lesioned rat striatum. *Biochem. Pharmacol.* 27: 2962-2965.
59. Fuld, P.A., Katzman, R., and Davies, P. (1982). Instrusions as a sign of Alzheimer dementia: Chemical and pathological verification. *Ann. Neurol.* 11: 155-159.
60. Francis, P.T., Palmer, A.M., Sims, N.R., Bowen, D.M., Davison, A.N., Esiri, N.M., Neary, D., Snowden, J.S., and Wilcock, G.K. (1985). Neurochemical studies of early-onset Alzheimer's disease: Possible influence on treatment. *N. Engl. J. Med.* 313: 7-11.
61. Giacobini, E., Becker, R., Elble, R., Mattio, T., McIlhany, M., and Scarsella, G. (1987). Brain acetylcholine—a view from the cerebrospinal fluid. In: *Neurobiology of Acetylcholine Symposium*, Dun (Ed.) New York, Plenum Press, pp. 85-101.
62. Giacobini, E., Somani, S.M., McIlhany, M., Downen, M., and Hallak, M. (1987). Pharmacokinetics and pharmacodynamics of physostigmine after i.v. administration in beagle dogs. *Neuropharmacology* 26: 831-836.
63. Procter, A.W., Lowe, S.L., Palmer, A.M., Francis, P.T., Esiri, M.M., Stratmann, G.C., Najlerahim, A., Patel, A.J., Hunt, A., and Bowen, D.M. (1988). Topographical distribution of neurochemical changes in Alzheimer's disease. *J. Neurol. Sci.* 84: 125-140.
64. Giacobini, E. (1987). Models and strategies of cholinomimetic therapy of Alzheimer disease. In: *Cellular and Molecular Basis of Cholinergic Function*, Dowdall and Hawthorne (Eds.) England, Ellis Horwood, pp. 882-901.

65. Christie, J.E., Shering, A., Ferguson, J., and Glen, A.I.M. (1981). Physostigmine and arecoline: Effects of intravenous infusions in Alzheimer presenile dementia. *Br. J. Psychiatry* 138: 46-50.
66. Becker, R., and Giacobini, E. (1988). Mechanisms of cholinesterase inhibition in senile dementia of the Alzheimer type: Clinical, pharmacological and therapeutic aspects. *Drug Dev. Res.* 12: 163-195.
67. Mohs, R.C., Davis, B.M., Johns, C.A., Mathe, A.A., Greenwald, B.S., Horvath, T.B., and Davis, K.L. (1985). Oral physostigmine treatment in patients with Alzheimer's disease. *Am. J. Psychiatry* 142: 28-33.
68. Mohs, R.C., Davis, B.M., Greenwald, B.S., Mathe, A.A., Johns, C.A., Horvath, T.B., and Davis, K.L. (1985). Clinical studies of the cholinergic deficit in Alzheimer's disease. II. Psychopharmacologic studies. *J. Am. Geriatr. Soc.* 33: 749-575.
69. Summers, W.K., Viesselman, J.O., Marsh, G.M., and Candelora, K. (1981). Use of THA in treatment of Alzheimer-like dementia: Pilot study in twelve patients. *Biol. Psychiatry* 16(2): 145-153.
70. Muramoto, O., Sugishita, M., and Anda, K. (1984). Cholinergic system and constructional praxis: A further study of physostigmine in Alzheimer's disease. *J. Neurol. Neurosurg. Psychiatry* 47: 485-491.
71. Rose, R.P., and Moulthrop, M.A. (1986). Differential responsivity of verbal and visual recognition memory to physostigmine and ACTH. *Biol. Psychiatry* 21: 538-542.
72. Sullivan, E.V., Shedlock, K.J., Corkin, S., and Growdon, J.H. (1982). Physostigmine and lecithin in Alzheimer's disease. In: *Aging: Alzheimer's Disease–A Report of Progress*, Corkin et al. (Eds.) New York, Raven Press, pp. 361-367.
73. Ashford, J.W., Soldinger, S., Schaeffer, J., Cochran, L., and Jarvik, L.F. (1981). Physostigmine and its effects on 6 patients with dementia. *Am. J. Psychiatry* 138: 829-830.
74. Kaye, W.H., Sitaram, N., Weingartner, H., Ebert, M.H., Smallberg, S., and Gillin, J.C. (1982). Modest facilitation of memory in dementia with combined lecithin and anticholinesterease treatment. *Biol. Psychiatry* 17: 275-280.
75. Peters, B.H., and Levin, H.S. (1982). Chronic oral physostigmine and lecithin administration in memory disorders of aging. In: *Aging: Alzheimer's Disease–A Report of Progress*, Corkin et al. (Eds.) New York, Raven Press, pp. 421-426.
76. Smith, C.M., and Swash, M. (1979). Physostigmine in Alzheimer's disease. *Lancet* 1: 42.
77. Delwaide, P.J., Devoitille, J.M., and Ylieff, M. (1980). Acute effect of drugs upon memory of patients with senile dementia. *Acta Psychiatr. Belg.* 80: 748-754.
78. Wettstein, A. (1983). No effect from double-blind trial of physostigmine and lecithin in Alzheimer disease. *Ann. Neurol.* 13: 210-212.
79. Peters, B.H., and Levin, H.S. (1979). Effects of physostigmine and lecithin on memory in Alzheimer disease. *Ann. Neurol.* 6: 219-221.

80. Thal, L.J., and Fuld, P.A. (1983). Memory enhancement with oral physostigmine in Alzheimer's disease. *N. Engl. J. Med.* 308: 720.
81. Thal, L.J., Fuld, P.A., Masur, D.M., and Sharpless, N.S. (1983). Oral physostigmine and lecithin improve memory in Alzheimer's disease. *Ann. Neurol.* 13: 491-496.
82. Thal, L.J., Masur, D.M., Fuld, P.A., Sharpless, N.S., and Davies, P. (1983). Memory improvement with oral physostigmine and lecithin in Alzheimer's disease. In: *Banbury Report 15: Biological Aspects of Alzheimer's Disease*, Katzman (Ed.) Cold Spring Harbor, NY, Cold Spring Harbor Laboratory, pp. 461-469.
83. Davis, K.L., Mohs, R.C., Davis, B.M., Horvath, T.B., Greenwald, B.S. Rosen, W.G., Levy, M.I., and Johns, C.A. (1983). Oral physostigmine in Alzheimer disease. *Psychopharmacol. Bull.* 19: 451-453.
84. Davis, K.L., Mohs, R.C., Rosen, W.G., Greenwald, B.S., Levy, M.I., and Horvath, T.B. (1983). Memory enhancement with oral physostigmine in Alzheimer disease. *N. Engl. J. Med.* 308: 721.
85. Beller, S.A., Overall, J.E., and Swann, A.C. (1985). Efficacy of oral physostigmine in primary degenerative dementia. A double-blind study of response to different dose level. *Psychopharmacology* 87: 147-151.
86. Summers, W.K., Majorski, L.V., Marsh, G.M., Tachiki, K., and Kling, A. (1986). Oral tetrahydroaminoacridine in long-term treatment of senile dementia, Alzheimer type. *N. Engl. J. Med.* 315(20): 1241-1245.
87. Thal, L.J., Masur, D.M., Sharpless, N.S., Fuld, P.A., and Davies, P. (1986). Acute and chronic effects of oral physostigmine and lecithin in Alzheimer's disease. *Prog. Neuro-Psychopharmacol. Biol. Psychiatry* 10: 627-636.
88. Caltagirone, C., Gainotti, G., and Musullo, C. (1982). Oral administration of chronic physostigmine does not improve cognitive or amnesic performances in Alzheimer's presenile dementia. *Int. J. Neurosci.* 16: 247-249.
89. Jotkowitz, S. (1983). Lack of clinical efficacy of chronic oral physostigmine in Alzheimer's disease. *Ann. Neurol.* 14: 690-691.
90. Fitten, L.J., Flood, J.F., Baxter, C.F., Tachiki, K.H., and Perryman, K. (1987). Long-term oral administration of memory-enhancing doses of tacrine in mice: A study of potential toxicity and side effects. *J. Gerontol.* 42: 681-685.
91. Sherman, K.A., Kumar, V., Ashford, J.W., Murphy, J.W., Elble, R.J., and Giacobini, E. (1987). Effect of oral physostigmine in senile dementia patients: Utility of blood cholinesterase inhibition and neuroendocrine responses to define pharmacokinetics and pharmacodynamics. In: *CNS Disorders of Aging: Strategies for Intervention*, Strong et al. (Eds.) New York, Raven Press, pp. 71-90.
92. Grob, D., Harvey, A.M., Langworthy, O.R., and Lilienthal, J.L. Jr. (1947). The administration of di-isopropylfluorophosphate (DFP) in man. I. Effect on plasma and erythrocyte cholinesterease; general systemic effects; use in study of hepatic function and erythropoiesis; and some properties of plasma cholinesterase. *Bull. Johns. Hopkins Hosp.* 81: 217-244.
93. Bowers, M.B., Goodman, E., and Sim, V.M. (1964). Some behavioral changes in man following anticholinesterase administration. *J. Nerv. Ment. Dis.* 138: 383-389.

94. Risch, S.C., Cohen, R.M., Janowsky, D.S., Kalin, D.H., and Murphy, D.L. (1980). Mood and behavioral effects of physostigmine on humans are accompanied by elevations in plasma beta-endorphin and cortisol. *Science* 209: 1545-1546.
95. Davis, B.M., Brown, G.M., Miller, M., Friesen, H.G., Kastin, A.J., and Davis, K.L. (1982). Effects of cholinergic stimulation on pituitary hormone release. *Psychoneuroendocrinology* 7: 347-354.
96. Lewis, D.A., Sherman, B.M., and Kathol, R.G. (1984). Analysis of the specificity of physostigmine stimulation of adrenocorticotropin in man. *J. Clin. Endocrinol. Metab.* 58: 570-573.
97. Janowsky, D.S., Risch, C., Parker, D., Huey, L., and Judd, L. (1980). Increased vulnerability to cholinergic stimulation—affective disorder in patients. *Psychopharm. Bull.* 16: 29-33.
98. Kumar, V., Smith, R.C., Sherman, K.A., Ashford, W., Murphy, J., Giacobini, E., and Colliver, J. (1988). Cortisol responses to cholinergic drugs in Alzheimer's disease. *Intl. J. Clin. Pharmacol. Ther. Toxicol.*
99. Hallak, M.E., and Giacobini, E. (1987). A comparison of effects of two inhibitors on brain cholinesterase. *Neuropharmacology* 26(6): 521-530.
100. Brinkman, S.D., and Gershon, S. (1983). Measurement of cholinergic drug effects on memory in Alzheimer's disease. *Neurobiol. Aging* 4: 139-145.
101. Mohs, R.C., and Davis, K.L. (1982). A signal detectability analysis of the effect of physostigmine on memory in patients with Alzheimer's disease. *Neurobiol. Aging* 3: 105-110.
102. Harbaugh, R.E., Roberts, D.W., Coombs, D.W., Saunders, R.L., and Reeder, T.M. (1984). Preliminary report: Intracranial cholinergic drug infusion in patients with Alzheimer's disease. *Neurosurgery* 15(4): 514-518.
103. Fox, J.H., Penn, R., Clasen, R., Martin, E., Wilson, R., and Savoy, S. (1985). Pathological diagnosis in clinically typical Alzheimer's disease. *N. Engl. J. Med.* 313(22): 1419-1420.
104. Penn, R.D., Martin, E.M., Wilson, R.S., Fox, J.H., and Savoy, S.M. (1988). Intraventricular bethanechol infusion for Alzheimer's disease: Results of double-blind and escalating dose trials. *Neurology* 38: 219-222.
105. Cronin-Golomb, A. (1988). International study group on the pharmacology of memory disorders associated with aging. *Neurobiol. Aging* 8: 277-282.
106. Mattio, T., McIlhany, M., Giacobini, E., and Hallak, M. (1986). The effects of physostigmine on acetylcholinesterase activity of CSF, plasma and brain. A comparison of intravenous and intraventricular administration in beagle dogs. *Neuropharmacology* 25: 1167-1177.
107. DeSarno, P., and Giacobini, E. (1988). Modulation of acetylcholine release by nicotinic receptors in the rat brain. *J. Neurosci. Res.*
108. Tucek, S. (1984). Problems in the organization and control of acetylcholine synthesis in brain neurons. *Prog. Biophys. Mol. Biol.* 44: 1-46.
109. Hallak, M.E., and Giacobini, E. (1986). Relation of brain regional physostigmine concentration to cholinesterase activity, and acetylcholine and choline levels in rat. *Neurochem. Res.* 11(7): 1037-1048.
110. DeSarno, P., Giacobini, E., and Downen, M. (1987). Release of acetylcholinesterase from the caudate nucleus of the rat. *J. Neurosci. Res.* 18: 578-590.

111. Hallak, M., and Giacobini, E. (1988). Physostigmine, tacrine and metrifonate: The effect of multiple dosage on acetylcholine metabolism in rat brain. *Neuropharmacology*.
112. Nordgren, I., Holmstedt, B., Bengtsson, E., and Finkel, Y. (19??). Plasma levels of metrifonate and dichlorvos during treatment of schistosomiasis with Bilarcil. *Am. J. Trop. Med. Hyg.* 29(3): 426-430.
113. Flynn, D.D., Suarez, A., Cordoves, A., and Mash, D.C. (1987). Differential regulation of muscarinic receptor subtypes in the cerebral cortex by chronic tetrahydroaminoacridine administration. *Neurosci. Abst.* 13: 726.
114. Levy, R. (1987). Tetrahydroaminoacridine and Alzheimer's disease. *Lancet* 322.
115. Fitten, J., Perryman, K., and Gross, P. (1988). THA–memory and cognitive enhancement in mouse, monkey and man. In: *Current Research in Alzheimer Therapy*, E. Giacobini and R. Becker (Eds.) New York, Taylor and Francis, pp. 211-216.
116. Gauthier, S., Masson, H., Gauthier, L., Bouchard, R., Collier, R., Bacher, Y., Bailey, P., Becker, R., Gergman, H., Charbonneau, R., Dastoor, D., Gayton, D., Kennedy, J., Kissel, C., Krieger, M., Kushnir, S., Lamontagne, A., St-Martin, M., Morin, J., Nair, N.P.V., Neirinik, L., Ratner, J., Suissa, S., Tasfaye, Y., and Vida, S. (1988). Tetrahydroaminoacridine and lecithin in Alzheimer's disease. In: *Current Research in Alzheimer Therapy*, E. Giacobini and R. Becker (Eds.) New York, Taylor and Francis, pp. 237-246.
117. Nyback, H., Nyman, H., Ohman, G., Nordgren, I., and Lindstrom B. (1988). Preliminary experiences and results with THA for the amelioration of symptoms of Alzheimer's disease. In: *Current Research in Alzheimer Therapy*, E. Giacobini and R. Becker (Eds.) New York, Taylor and Francis, pp. 231-236.
118. Ames, D.J., Bhatal, P.S., Davies, B.M., and Fraser, J.R.E. (1988). Hepatotoxicity of tetrahydroaminoacridine. *Lancet* 887.
119. Giacobini, E., and Hallak, M.E. (1986). Anticholinesterase therapy of Alzheimer: From animal models to human applications. In: *Senile Dementias: Early Detection*, A. Bes et al. (Eds.) Paris, France, John Libbey Eurotext, pp. 337-341.
120. Brufani, M., Marta, M., and Pomponi, M. (1986). Anticholinesterase activity of a new carbamate, heptylphysositgmine, in view of its use in patients with Alzheimer-type dementia. *Eur. J. Biochem.* 157: 115-120.
121. Pomponi, M., and Giacobini, E. (1988). Neuropharmacological effects of heptyl-physostigmine.
122. Oliverio, A., Castellano, C., Iacopino, C., Pavone, F., Brufani, M., Marta, M., and Pomponi, M. (1986). Effects of physostigmine derivatives on cerebral cholinergic functions and their possible use in Alzheimer's disease. In: *Modulation of Central and Peripheral Transmitter Function*, G. Biggio, P.F. Spano, G. Toffano and G.L. Gessa (Eds.) Fidia Research Series, Symposia in Neuroscience III. Padova, Italy, Liviana Press, pp. 305-309.
123. Liu, J.S., Yu, C.M., and Zhou, Y.Z. (1986). The structures of Huperzine A and B, two new alkaloids exhibiting marked anticholinesterase activity. Can. J. Chem. 64: 827.

124. Tang, X.-C., Han, Y.-F., Chen, X.-P., and Zhu, X.-D. (1986). Effects of huperzine A on learning and retrieval process of discrimination performance in rats. *Acta Pharmacol. Sin.* 7(6): 507-511.
125. Wang, Y.-E., Yue, D.-X., and Tang, X.-C. (1986). Anti-cholinesterase activity of hyperzine A. *Acta Pharmacol. Sin.* 7(2): 110-113.
126. Zhang, S.-L. (1986). Therapeutic effects of hyperzine A on the aged with memory impairment. *New Drugs Clin. Rem.* 5(5): 260-262.
127. Vincent, G.P., Rumennik, L., Cumin, R., Martin, J., and Sepinwall, J. (1987). The effects of Huperzine A, an anticholinesterase inhibitor, on the enhancement of memory in mice, rats and monkey. *Soc. Neurosci. Abstr.* 237: 4.
128. Yan, X.-F., Lu, W.-H., Lou, W.-J., and Tang, X.-C. (1987). Effects of huperzine A and B on skeletal muscle and electroencephalogram. *Acta Pharmacol. Sin.* 8(2): 117-123.
129. Tang, X.-C., and Giacobini, E. (1988). Neuropharmacology of huperzine A in the rat.
130. Whitehouse, P.J., and Unnerstall, J.R. (1988). Neurochemistry of dementia. *Alzheimer Dis. Assoc. Disord.* 2: 159.
131. Kalaria, R.N., Andorn, A.C., and Harik, S.I. (1988). Alterations in adrenergic receptors in prefrontal cortex and in cerebral microvessels in Alzheimer's disease and normal aging. *Alzheimer's Dis. Assoc. Disord.* 2: 233.
132. Zweig, R.M., Ross, C.A., Hedreen, J.C., Steele, C., Cardillo, J.E., Whitehouse, P.J., Folstein, M.F., and Price, D.L. (1988). The neuropathology of aminergic nuclei in Alzheimer's disease. *Ann. Neurol.* 24: 233-242.
133. Davis, K.L., Haroutunian, V., and Kanof, P. (1988). Therapeutics of Alzheimer's disease for clinical and preclinical issues. *Alzheimer Dis. Assoc. Disord.* 2: 205.
134. Bourdois, P.S., Mitchell, J.F., Somogyl, G.T., and Szerb, J.C. (1974). The output per stimulus of acetylcholine from cerebral cortical slices in the presence or absence of cholinesterase inhibition. *Br. J. Pharmacol.* 52: 509-517.
135. Hadhazy, P., and Szerb, J.C. (1977). The effect of cholinergic drugs on [^{3}H-ACh release from slices of rat hippocampus, striatum and cortex. *Brain Res.* 123: 311-322.
136. Drukarch, B., Kits, K.S., Van der Meer, E.G., Lodder, J.C., and Stoof, J.C. (1987). 9-Amino-1,2,3,4-tetrahydroacridine (THA), an alleged drug for the treatment of Alzheimer's disease, inhibits acetylcholinesterase activity and slow outward K+ current. *Eur. J. Pharmacol.* 141: 153-157.
137. Nilsson, L., Hardy, J., Winblad, B., and Nordberg, A. (1987). Effect of Alzheimer cholinergic therapeutic agents in synaptic transmission in vitro. In: *Alzheimer's Disease–Dementia*, London, John Libbey, pp. 127-140.
138. Sherman, K.A., and Messamore, E. (1987). Comparison of tetrahydroaminoacridine and physostigmine after acute and chronic administration in rats. *Soc. Neurosci. Abstr.* 17: 77.1.
139. Varon, S., Manthorpe, M., Davis, G.E., Williams, L.R., and Skaper, S.D. Growth factors. *Adv. Neurol.* 4: 493-521.

140. Giacobini, E., Mussini, I., and Mattio, T. (1986). Aging of cholinergic synapses: Fiction or reality? In: *Dynamics of Cholinergic Function: Advances in Behavioral Biology*, Vol. 30, I. Hanin (Ed.) New York, Plenum Press, pp. 177-190.
141. Iversen, L.L., Rossor, M.N., Reynolds, G.P., Hills, R., Roth, M., Mountjoy, C.Q., Foote, S.L., Morrison, J.H., and Bloom, F.E. (1983). Loss of pigmented dopamine-α-hydroxylase positive cells from locus coeruleus in senile dementia of Alzheimer's type. *Neurosci. Lett.* 39: 95-100.

17

Clinical and Research Applications of Monspecific Antibodies to the Abnormal Proteins of Alzheimer's Disease

DENNIS R. SPARKMAN and CHARLES L. WHITE III / *University of Texas Southwestern Medical Center at Dallas, Dallas, Texas*

INTRODUCTION

Alzheimer's disease (AD) is a progressive degenerative dementia whose onset can be as early as the fourth and fifth decades of life (early onset), although in most cases it is first observed in the sixth and later decades (late onset). In many cases of early-onset AD, more than one family member will be affected, and it appears to be inherited through an autosomal dominant gene (1-4). The observed inheritance of AD in the early-onset families is thought to be due to the fact that most family members are still alive and the expression of the gene is observed more frequently. In the late-onset type, many potentially affected individuals do not survive to express the gene (3,4). Also, many individuals with Down's syndrome, which is due to a third chromosome 21, will develop AD neuropathological changes and dementia if they survive past age 35 (5,6). An increased incidence of Down's syndrome has been noted in AD families (3).

Since clinical diagnosis is at best only 80% accurate, specific diagnosis must rely on brain biopsy or a postmortem neuropathological examination of the brain. Gross examination of the brain reveals little, although atrophy has been noted in some cases (7). Microscopic examination reveals abundant neurofibrillary tangles (NFT) and neuritic plaques (NP), which are the histological hallmarks of AD. Also found are granulovacuolar degeneration, lipofuscin, and Hirano bodies (8).

The NFT and NP have been the two most studied lesions of AD. They are both abundant, composed of abnormal protein, and have been isolated. Here, we describe our work and that of others who have isolated these proteins and produced antibodies to them, and discuss how they are being used in research on AD and related dementias.

THE NEUROFIBRILLARY TANGLE

Cellular Pathological Findings

The NFT is a neuronal cytoplasmic inclusion that consists ultrastructurally of bundles and arrays of paired helical filaments (PHF). These neurons that are undergoing neurofibrillary changes will produce PHF in such amounts that most of the cytoplasmic space is occupied by the NFT, displacing cytoplasmic organelles and even the nucleus to the side (9). The NFT occur in specific brain regions such as the neocortex, hippocampus, nucleus basalis, and locus ceruleus. Since these regions are areas of the brain where cell loss occurs, it may be that the accumulation of PHF disrupts the cell's function and results in death (10).

Ultrastructurally, the PHF is composed of two 10 nm filaments that are wound around each other helically with a right-handed twist and a periodicity of 80 nm and are separated by a distance of 5 nm (11). These PHF do not resemble any normal cellular filament and their existence to date has been confined to human brain. The PHF have been shown by x-ray diffraction studies to have a beta-pleated sheet conformation, which accounts for their Congo red birefringence (12). They are also argentophilic and are routinely demonstrated by silver staining in formalin-fixed tissue sections (Fig. 1).

Isolation of Paired Helical Filaments

The PHF are a unique protein in that they are insoluble in sodium dodecyl sulfate (SDS) in the presence of a reducing agent at 100°C, as well as in most of the chaotropic salts that will solubilize most proteins (14). The insolubility of these proteins allowed for their purification. Ihara et al. (15) first isolated the NFT by homogenizing AD brain in SDS and 2-mercaptoethanol, followed by boiling and sucrose gradient centrifugation. Other procedures that do not use denaturing conditions have been reported (16), but we have found that these NFT still contain significant amounts of contaminating proteins. A procedure for isolating NFT by fluorescent-activated cell sorting (FACS) has been described using a fluorescent antibody (17) or dye (18).

We have used the SDS-extraction procedure (15) and added several modifications to break the NFT down to PHF, which are further purified (Sparkman and White, manuscripts submitted). The quality of the starting material will greatly determine the quality of the final PHF preparation. Tissue is chosen that is rich in NFT but relatively low in amounts of NP. In the initial extraction in SDS, 2 mM EDTA is added to help dissociate the tissue. The NFT isolated at the 1.4M-2.0M interface of the sucrose gradient are still large aggregates of PHF (Fig. 2a)

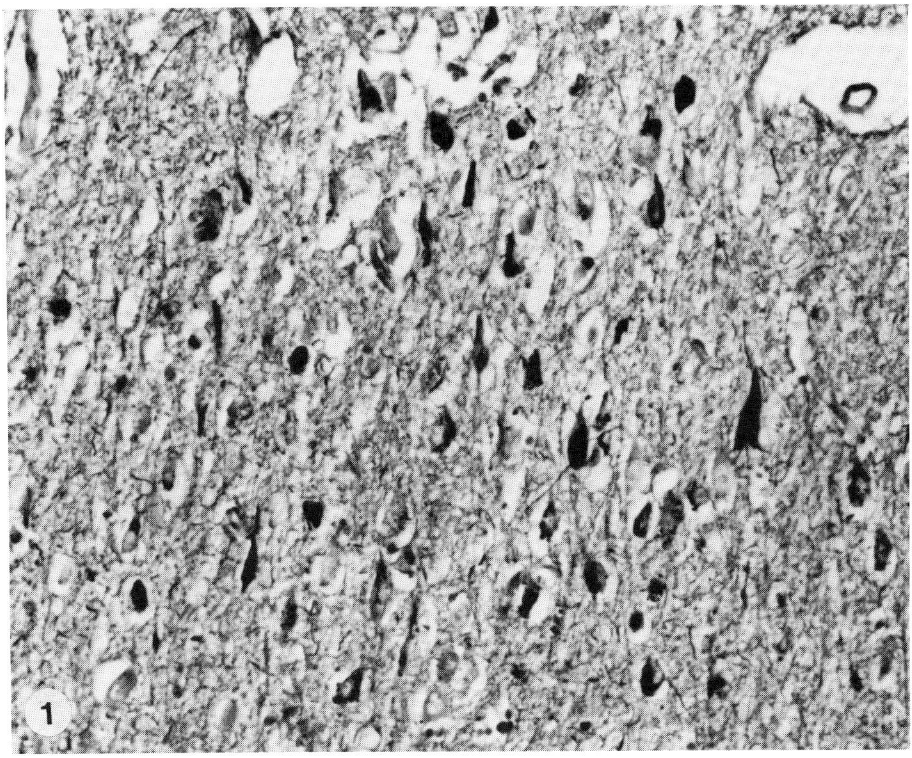

FIGURE 1 Formalin-fixed hippocampus from AD brain was parrafin sectioned and silver stained by the Sevier-Munger method (13).

and will still contain other SDS-insoluble proteins, especially lipofuscin. In order to purify the PHF further, the NFT are broken down by sonication and large aggregates removed by centrifugation at 10,000 g. The PHF are collected at 100,000 g and the procedure repeated several times to give a purified PHF preparation (Fig. 2b). The final preparation is a clear solution.

Antibodies to Paired Helical Filaments

Polyclonal antibodies have been produced to both the SDS-extracted NFT (10, 15,19,20) and the nondenatured NFT (21). The antibodies made from SDS-extracted PHF show good specificity toward NFT in tissue sections and PHF on Western blots (10,15,19,20). The antibodies made to the nondenatured PHF also react with NFT in tissue sections and PHF on Western blots, but they also

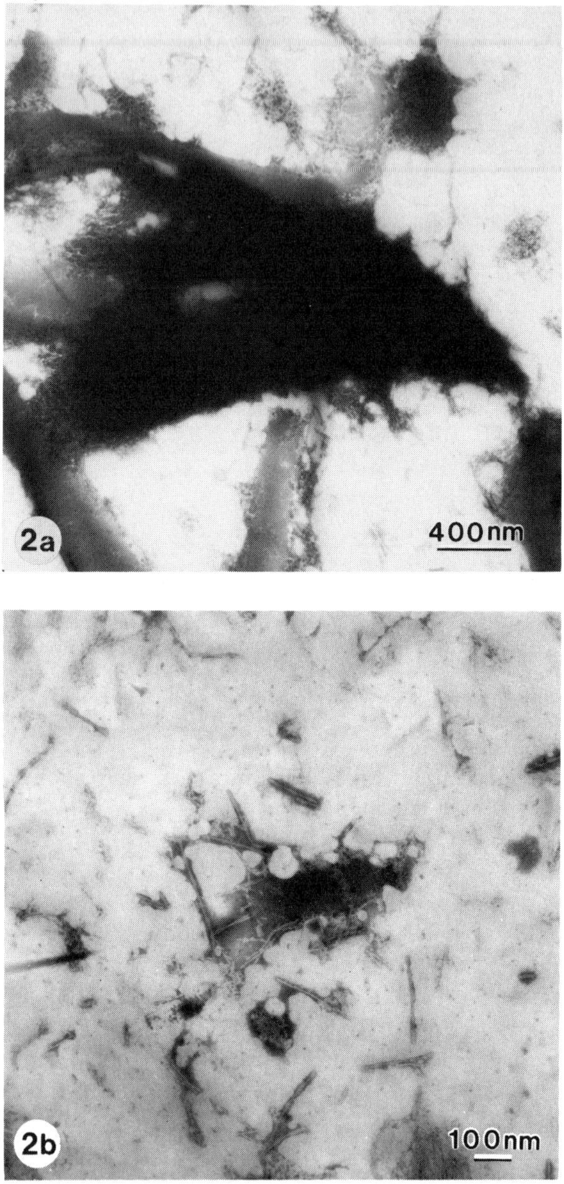

FIGURE 2 (a) An intact neurofibrillary tangle, negatively stained with 1% uranyl formate. (b) Individual PHF that were dispersed and further purified from the neurofibrillary tangle, negatively stained with 1% uranyl formate.

recognize additional proteins on the blots (21,22), which are probably contaminating proteins associated with the NFT.

Using our highly purified PHF preparation, we have developed a highly specific polyclonal antibody to PHF. The antibody was produced in a female New Zealand White rabbit by injecting 100 μg of a sonicated PHF preparation, emulsified in Freund's complete adjuvant, and injected intradermally at multiple sites along the back. Boosters were given at 3 and 6 weeks in complete and incomplete adjuvant, respectively. The rabbit is maintained by injecting 10 μg PHF in incomplete adjuvant every 6 weeks. This animal has produced antibodies to PHF for 2 years, has maintained a consistent titer, and has not produced any antibodies to any impurities that might still have been present in the antigen

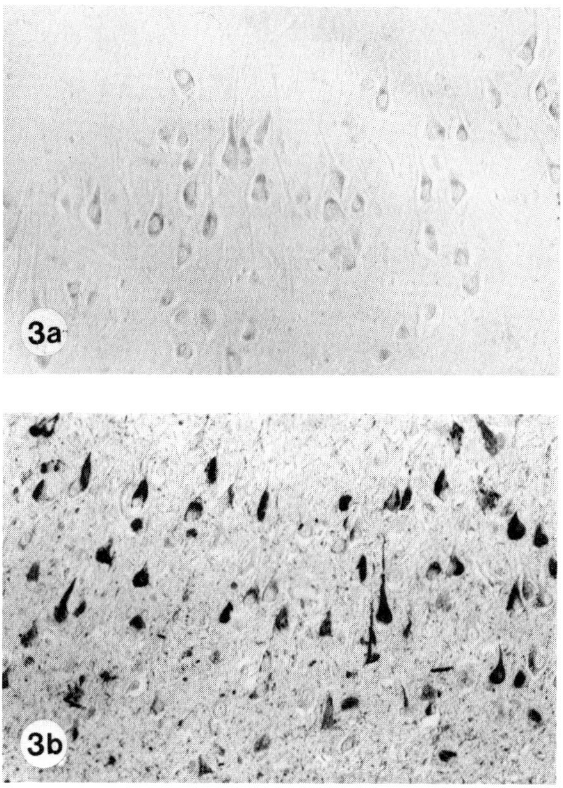

FIGURE 3 Immunohistochemistry of formalin-fixed, paraffin-sectioned (a) control and (b) AD brain after use of the anti-PHF serum.

preparation. By using one animal whose antiserum is well characterized, one eliminates the variability inherent in pooling many antisera from many less well characterized animals.

The antiserum was used to immunolabel the NFT in AD brains. Paraffin sections of 5 μm thickness from AD or normal controls were incubated with serial dilutions of either preimmune or immune serum. The sections were stained by the avidin-biotin immunoperoxidase method and photographed using Normarski optics. The anti-PHF serum labeled the NFT and degenerating neurites of the

FIGURE 4 Immunoblotting of proteins with the anti-PHF serum. Proteins were separated on a 5-15% polyacrylamide gradient gel, transferred to nitrocellulose, blocked with 5% nonfat dry milk, and incubated with 1:250 dilution of antibody. The antibody was visualized with [^{125}I] protein A and autoradiography. The anti-PHF antibody labeled only the excluded PHF in the AD lane and purified PHF.

NP, which contain PHF, but did not react with the control brain (Fig. 3). The preimmune serum did not react with either the normal or AD brain.

In order to show the specificity of the anti-PHF serum, the serum was absorbed with a normal control brain that did not contain any NFT or NP and with an NFT-rich region of AD brain. The antiserum absorbed with the control brain still stained the NFT and neurites of the NP with a reduction in background staining, while absorption with the AD brain eliminated all staining in the sections. By using the normal brain to absorb out any contaminating antibodies, the antiserum is made monospecific to the PHF. Western blotting of brain samples and purified PHF shows that the antibody specifically labels the PHF in the AD brain and the purified PHF, but does not label any soluble proteins in any of the brain fractions (Fig. 4).

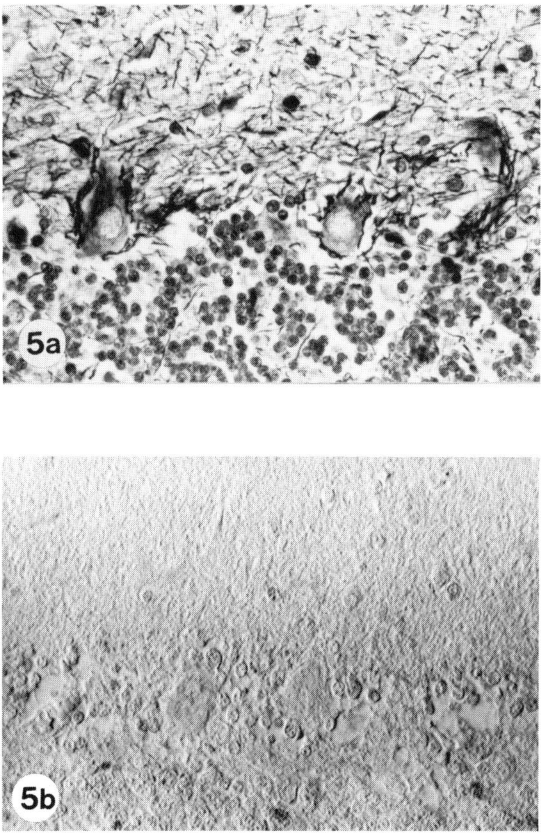

FIGURE 5 Formalin-fixed, paraffin-sectioned AD cerebellum was (a) silver stained or (b) reacted immunohistochemically with the anti-PHF antibody.

The anti-PHF serum was tested against AD tissue known not to contain NFT and NP, such as the cerebellum. Classic silver staining of fixed cerebellum shows intense staining of the neurofilaments in the basket fibers around Purkinje cells (Fig. 5a), while the anti-PHF serum does not react with any of the cells (Fig. 5b). Other cellular inclusions, such as the Lewy bodies, have also shown no immunoreactivity. The Pick bodies of Pick's disease have also reacted with this antiserum (23) and similar cross-reactivity has been reported independently (24).

The anti-PHF serum also stains the PHF in the degenerating neurities that surround the amyloid core of the NP (Fig. 6). The PHF of the neurities must share epitopes with the PHF of the cell body and may be the same. To date, no in-depth study of the neuritic PHF has been undertaken, but one study has shown that they have the same dimensions as those in the NFT (25).

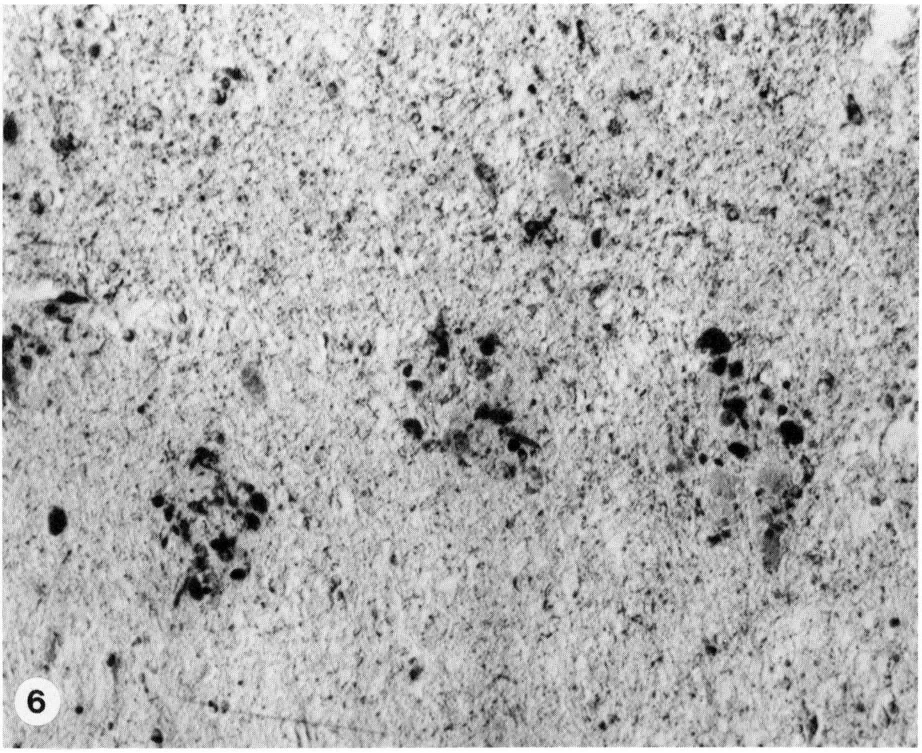

FIGURE 6 Formalin-fixed, paraffin-sectioned AD hippocampus was immunohistochemically labeled with the anti-PHF antibody. The degenerating neurites of the NP are labeled, but not the amyloid core.

Several laboratories have also produced monoclonal antibodies to PHF (26-28). These antibodies are specific to the PHF and should complement the polyclonal antibodies in the immunological studies of the PHF.

THE NEURITIC PLAQUE

Cellular Pathological Findings

The NP consists of degenerating neuronal processes associated with extracellular amyloid (29). The "immature" plaque is made up of abnormal neuronal processes and little amyloid. The "mature" or "classic" plaque is composed of degenerating neurities, which contain PHF, surrounding a central core of amyloid. The "end-stage" or "burned out" plaque is made up almost exclusively of the amyloid core that remains after the neurities have completely degenerated. The NP occur in specific brain regions. They are greatest in the temporal neocortex and are also present in significant numbers in other areas of the neocortex, especially frontal and parietal regions. Our preliminary evaluations showed that end-stage plaques seem to predominate in the calcarine (visual) cortex.

The amyloid core is composed of individual amyloid fibrils (AF) that are randomly oriented. The ultrastructure of the AF has not been investigated to the same degree as the PHF. Several laboratories have reported the AF to be composed of straight fibrils that vary from 5 to 12 nm (30,31). Others have reported the AF to be 4-8 nm in diameter, with a narrowing every 30-40 nm and apparently composed of two 4 nm filaments (32). A most recent study that uses quick freezing of the specimens and carbon-platinum replicas reveals that the AF are

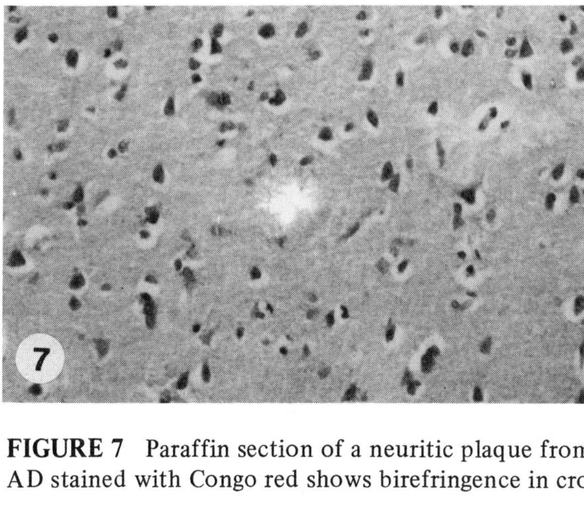

FIGURE 7 Paraffin section of a neuritic plaque from the calcarine cortex in AD stained with Congo red shows birefringence in cross-polarized light.

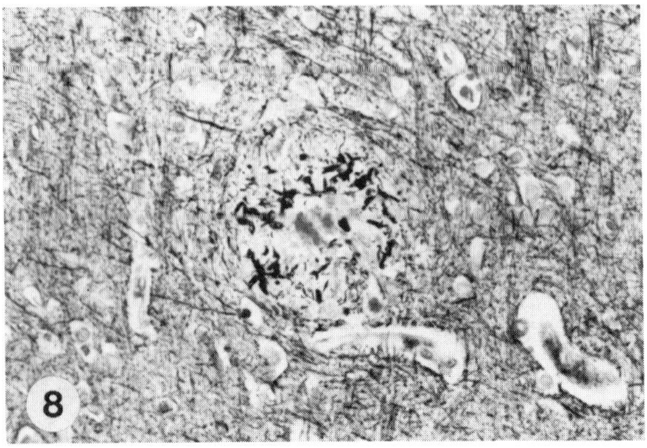

FIGURE 8 Paraffin section of an AD neuritic plaque. Neurites are apparent in this Sevier-Munger silver-stained preparation. An amorphous core of amyloid is present in the center of the plaque.

6-11 nm fibrils that are randomly oriented, but tend to form bundles (33). The AF consist of paired filaments and have a beadlike structure (33). Replicas of transverse sections indicate that the AF is a hollow fibril made up of six subunits (33). X-ray diffraction studies of the AF have shown that they have a beta-pleated structure (12) that causes the amyloid cores to display Congo red birefringence in cross-polarized illumination (Fig. 7). NP can also be silver stained,

Isolation of Amyloid

The AF, like the PHF, are uniquely insoluble in a variety of chaotropic salts and resistant to proteases. The first isolations used protease treatment and differential centrifugation (34). These isolations were modified to include high salt extractions to solubilize tissue further (35,36), although in our hands, we have found them highly contaminated with lipofuscin. A recent isolation procedure that uses boiling in SDS and sucrose density centrifugation (30) gives a highly purified core preparation (Fig. 9). The isolated cores can then be further purified by FACS to give a homogeneous preparation for analysis. These cores have been solubilized in formic acid to give a 4 kd peptide that has been partially sequenced (36).

AF are also found in the cerebral vessels in the form of cerebrovascular amyloid (CVA). The CVA has been isolated by solubilization in guanidine hydrochloride and separated by chromatography (37). The protein has been partially sequenced and at present it does not match any known cellular protein and shows

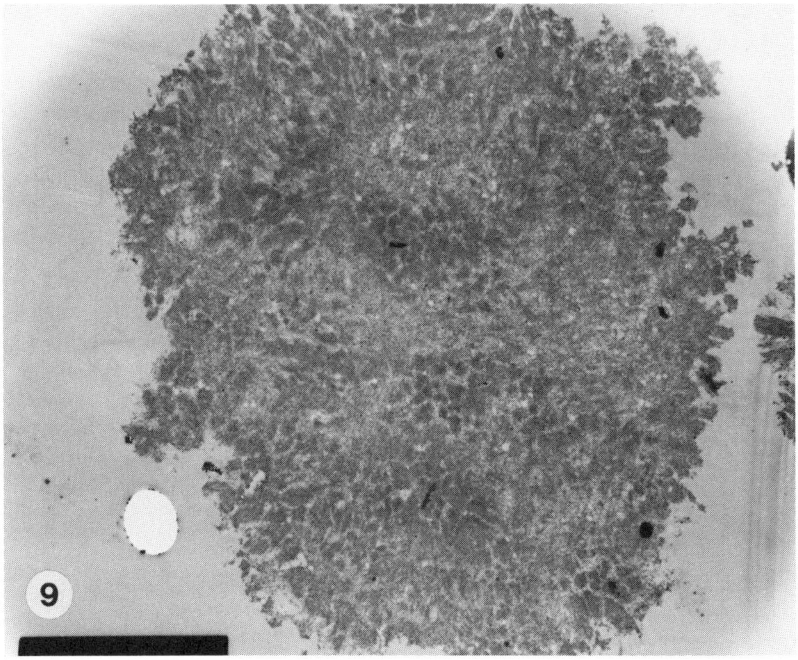

FIGURE 9 Electron microscopy of purified amyloid cores. Amyloid cores were isolated by the SDS-boiling procedure (30), fixed, embedded in Medcast, and sectioned. The sections were stained with uranyl acetate and lead citrate.

no homology with the scrapie prion, an amyloidlike material associated with Creutzfeldt-Jakob disease (36). Sequencing of the amyloid core protein gives an identical sequence to that of CVA. Since they appear to be homologous proteins and cores are often in close proximity to vessels (33), amyloid may arise from a protein of blood origin that infiltrates the vessels and is secreted into areas of core formation.

Antibodies to Amyloid

Polyclonal antibodies have been produced to the amyloid cores. This antiserum immunohistochemically labels the amyloid cores and the CVA in vessels (30,36). Antibodies have been made to a synthetic peptide that corresponds to the N-terminal amyloid sequence (36,38) and it has been found also to label the amyloid cores and CVA. Monoclonal antibodies to the synthetic sequence have also been produced (39). Since amyloid has been reported to share some epitopes with the NFT (36), the use of these antibodies in the study of AF and PHF should be useful. We are currently working to develop antibodies to both the intact amyloid protein isolated from the cores and to a synthetic peptide that includes the first 14 amino acids of the N-terminal sequence.

THE PICK BODY

Cellular Pathological Findings

The Pick body (PB) is a neuronal inclusion that consists of numerous straight fibrils randomly oriented in the cytoplasm. The fibrils are 15 nm in diameter and occur in specific areas of the brain, such as the dentate gyrus of the hippocampus. They are argentophilic (Fig. 10a), but do not show Congo red birefringence.

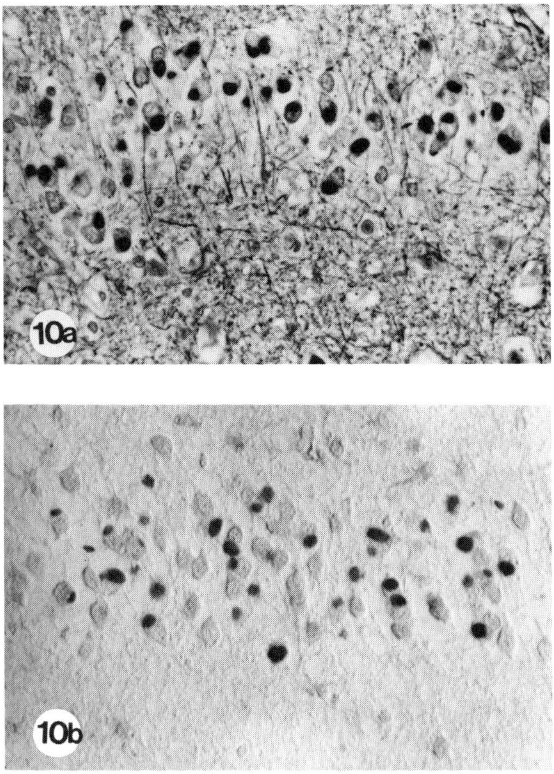

FIGURE 10 Formalin-fixed paraffin sections of PD hippocampus showing (a) argentophilic staining of PB by the Sevier-Munger method, and (b) immunoreactivity with antiserum to AD PHF.

The PB are characteristic of Pick's disease (PD), another form of degenerative dementia with clinical features similar to those of AD.

Isolation of Pick Fibrils

The PB have been found to cross-react immunohistochemically with the anti-PHF serum. Paraffin sections of hippocampus from PD show strong immunoreactivity with antiserum to Alzheimer PHF (Fig. 10b). This immunoreactivity is eliminated by first absorbing the PHF antiserum with unfixed AD brain homogenates, but not by preabsorption with normal brain. Similarly, preabsorption of the antiserum with PD brain completely neutralizes PHF immunoreactivity in paraffin sections of AD brain (23). These results suggest significant antigenic similarities, if not immunologic identity, between PB and Alzheimer NFT.

These antigenic similarities led us to investigate their biochemical properties. We found them to be the same as the PHF, that is, insoluble in strong chaotrophic

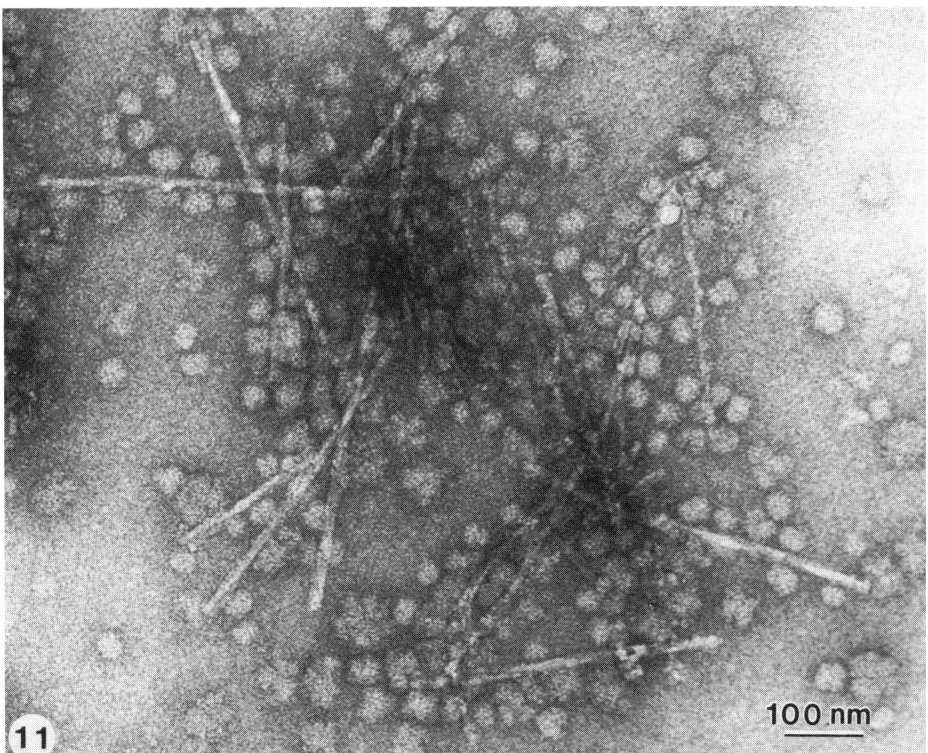

FIGURE 11 Isolated Pick fibrils negatively stained with 1% uranyl formate.

salts. Thus, the same SDS-boiling procedure that is used to isolate the PHF we used to isolate the PF (Fig. 11) (40). The isolated fibrils are 15 nm as observed in situ and may be composed of protofilaments since some splitting of the fibrils has been observed. The isolation of these fibrils will allow their ultrastructural characterization and antibodies can be made so they can be immunologically characterized and further compared to the PHF.

CLINICAL AND RESEARCH APPLICATIONS

Since there is much research to be done on the PHF and NP, highly specific antibodies, both polyclonal and monoclonal, will be of great value to the researcher. More work could be done, for example by colocalizing abnormal proteins to neurotransmitter-specific cell types in the areas that are most prone to degenerate. The antibodies could also be used to test other fibrous inclusions such as those that occur in normal aging, Down's syndrome, and progressive supranuclear palsy to determine if they share epitopes with the fibrous lesions of AD.

Isolation of mRNA from AD brains will allow in vitro translation studies in which the protein product can be immunoprecipitated and visualized by gel electrophoresis. The mRNA can be used to construct recombinant DNA libraries where the genes are expressed, and clones expressing the genes for PHF and amyloid can be identified by these antibodies. These genes could then be tested to see if a restriction fragment length polymorphism exists that is linked to AD and would serve as a basis for an early diagnosis, as is currently being done for Huntington's disease (41).

The antibodies could also serve as a direct diagnostic tool if a marker protein could be identified in the blood or CSF. There has been a report of NFT-like or amyloidlike material in the CSF (42) and a report of an antibody that reacts with a protein in the CSF of AD patients (43). Much more work will have to be done before these can be declared diagnostic, and other markers will also surely be found.

Finally, there remain AD-specific proteins yet to be identified, but that may prove to be highly valuable in AD research. One such protein may have been identified by making a monoclonal antibody to AD brain. This monoclonal antibody designated Alz-50 has been found to immunolabel some NFT and specifically label a unique protein by protein blotting (44). Another monoclonal library made to cell membranes of hypoglossal nuclei from normal human brain has produced a monoclonal antibody that suggests that AD astrocytes are antigenically different from normal controls (45).

The use of the existing antibodies to AD proteins and development of antibodies to as yet anonymous proteins will allow us to locate the primary defect of AD and, we hope, provide a method of specific early diagnosis.

NOTE ADDED IN PROOF

There have been reports of neurofibrillary tangles containing contaminating proteins, such as the microtubule-associated protein tau, ubiquitin, and A4 amyloid; and antisera to these preparations contain contaminating antibodies to the same. However, under optimal working dilutions, our PHF antiserum does not react with these contaminants and appears to be monospecific to the PHF core protein (Sparkman and White, manuscript submitted for publication).

REFERENCES

1. Heston, L.L. (1983). Dementia of the Alzheimer type: A perspective from family studies. In: *Banbury Report 15*, R. Katzman (Ed.), New York, Cold Spring Harbor Laboratory, pp. 183-191.
2. Matsuyama, S.S. (1983). Genetic factors in dementia of the Alzheimer type. In: *Alzheimer's Disease, The Standard Reference*, B. Reisberg (Ed.) New York, The Free Press, pp. 155-160.
3. Heyman, A., wilkinson, W.E., Hurwitz, B.J., Schmechel, D., Sigmon, A.H., Weinberg, T., Helms, M.J., and Swift, M. (1983). Alzheimer's disease: Genetic aspects and associated clinical disorders. *Ann. Neurol.* 14: 507-515.
4. Breitner, J.C.S., Folstein, M.F., and Murphy, E.A. (1986). Familial aggregation in Alzheimer dementia–I. A model for the age-dependent expression of an autosomal dominant gene. *J. Psychiatr. Res.* 20: 31-43.
5. Heston, L.L. (1982). Alzheimer's dementia and Down's syndrome: Genetic evidence suggesting an association. *Ann. N.Y. Acad. Sci.* 396: 29-37.
6. Oliver, C., and Holland, J. (1986). Down's syndrome and Alzheimer's disease: A review. *Psychol. Med.* 16: 307-322.
7. Terry, R., and Katzman, R. (1983). Senile dementia of the Alzheimer type: Defining a disease. In: *The Neurology of Aging*, R. Katzman and R. Terry (Eds.) Philadelphia, F.A. Davis, pp. 51-84.
8. Ball, M.J. (1982). Alzheimer disease–a challenging enigma. *Arch. Pathol. Lab. Med.* 106: 157-162.
9. Iqbal, K., and Wisniewski, H.M. (1983). Neurofibrillary tangles. In: *Alzheimer's Disease, The Standard Reference*, B. Reisberg (Ed.) New York, The Free Press, pp. 48-56.
10. White, C.L. III, Sparkman, D.R., and Gause, J.M. (1985). Distribution of paired helical filament immunoreactivity in Alzheimer-type dementia. *J. Neuropathol. Exp. Neurol.* 44: 368.
11. Terry, R.D., Gonatas, N.K., and Weiss, M. (1964). Ultrastructural studies in Alzheimer's presenile dementia. *Am. J. Pathol.* 44: 269-297.
12. Kirschner, D.A., Abraham, C., and Selkoe, D.J. (1986). X-ray diffraction from intraneuronal paired helical filaments and extraneuronal amyloid fibers in Alzheimer disease indicates cross-8 conformation. *Proc. Natl. Acad. Sci. USA* 83: 503-507.
13. Sevier, A.C., and Munger, B.L. (1965). A silver method for paraffin sections of neural tissue. *J. Neuropathol. Exp. Neurol.* 24: 130-135.

14. Selkoe, D.J., Ihara, Y., Abraham, C., Rasool, C.G., and McCluskey, A.H. (1983). In: *Banbury Report 15*, R. Katzman (ed.) New York, Cold Spring Harbor Laboratory, pp. 125-135.
15. Ihara, Y., Abraham, C., and Selkoe, D.J. (1983). Antibodies to paired helical filaments in Alzheimer's disease do not recognize normal brain proteins. *Nature* 304: 727-730.
16. Iqbal, K., Zaidi, T., Thompson, C.H., Mertz, P.A., and Wisniewski, H.M. (1984). Alzheimer paired helical filaments: Bulk isolation, solubility, and protein composition. *Acta Neuropathol.* 62: 167-177.
17. Miller, C.C.J., Haugh, M., Anderton, B.H., Hudson, L., and Murphy, J. (1986). Neurofibrillary tangles from Alzheimer's disease brain purified using a cell sorter. *Neurosci. Lett.* 63: 247-252.
18. Hussey, S., Yates, C.M., and Fink, G. (1986). Fluorescence activated cell sorting (FACS) as a separation method for neurofibrillary tangles in Alzheimer's disease. *J. Neurosci. Methods* 16: 1-8.
19. Brion, J.P., Couck, A.M., Passareiro, E., and Flament-Durand, J. (1985). Neurofibrillary tangles of Alzheimer's disease: An immunohistochemical study. *J. Submicrosc. Cytol.* 17: 89-96.
20. Persuy, P., Defossez, A., Delacourte, A., Tramu, G., Bouchez, B., and Arnott, G. (1985). Anti-PHF antibodies: An immunohistochemical marker of the lesions of the Alzheimer's disease. *Virchows Arch.* (*Pathol. Anat.*) 407: 13-23.
21. Grundke-Iqbal, I., Iqbal, K., Tung, Y.C., and Wisniewski, H.M. (1984). Alzheimer paired helical filaments: Immunochemical identification of polypeptides. *Acta Neuropathol.* 62: 259-267.
22. Grundke-Iqbal, I., Iqbal, K., Tung, Y.C., Wang, G.P., and Wisniewski, H.M. (1985). Alzheimer paired helical filaments: Cross-reacting polypeptide/s normally present in brain. *Acta Neuropathol.* 66: 52-61.
23. White, C.L. III, Allison, P., Gause, J.M., Johnson, S.A., and Sparkman, D.R. (1985). Immunoreactivity of antiserum to Alzheimer paired helical filaments is neutralized by absorption with Pick disease brain. *Neurosci. Abstr.* 11: 168.
24. Rasool, C.G., and Selkoe, D.J. (1985). Sharing of specific antigens by degenerating neurons in Pick's disease and Alzheimer's disease. *N. Engl. J. Med.* 312: 700-705.
25. Yoshimura, N. (1984). Evidence that paired helical filaments originate from neurofilaments—electron microscopic observations of neurites in senile plaques in the brain in Alzheimer's disease. *Clin. Neuropathol.* 3: 22-27.
26. Wang, G.P., Grundke-Iqbal, I., Kascsak, R.J., Iqbal, K., and Wisniewski, H.M. (1984). Alzheimer neurofibrillary tangles: Monoclonal antibodies to inherent antigen(s). *Acta Neuropathol.* 62: 268-275.
27. Selkoe, D.J., Abraham, C., Rasool, C.G., McCluskey, A., and Duffy, L.K. (1986). Production and characterization of monoclonal antibodies to Alzheimer paired helical filaments. *Ann. N.Y. Acad. Sci.* 457: 774-778.
28. Yen, S.H., Crowe, A., and Dickson, D.W. (1985). Monoclonal antibodies to Alzheimer neurofibrillary tangles. I. Identification of polypeptides. *Am. J. Pathol.* 120: 282-291.

29. Wisniewski, H.M. (1983). Neuritic (senile) and amyloid plaques. In: *Alzheimer's Disease, The Standard Reference*, B. Reisberg (Eds.) New York, The Free Press, pp. 57-61.
30. Selkoe, D.J., Abraham, C.R., Podlisny, M.B., and Duffy, L.K. (1986). Isolation of low-molecular-weight proteins from amyloid plaque fibers in Alzheimer's disease. *J. Neurochem.* 46: 1820-1834.
31. Roher, A., Wolf, D., Palutke, M., and KuKuruga, D. (1986). Purification, ultrastructure, and chemical analysis of Alzheimer disease amyloid plaque core protein. *Proc. Natl. Acad. Sci. USA* 83: 2662-2666.
32. Merz, P.A., Wisniewski, H.M., Somerville, R.A., Bobin, S.A., Masters, C.L., and Iqbal, K. (1983). Ultrastructural morphology of amyloid fibrils from neuritic and amyloid plaques. *Acta Neuropathol.* 60: 113-124.
33. Miyakawa, T., Katsuragi, S., Watanabe, K., Shimoji, A., and Ikevchi, Y. (1986). Ultrastructural studies of amyloid fibrils and senile plaques in human brain. *Acta Neuropathol.* 70: 202-208.
34. Allsop, D., Landon, M., and Kidd, M. (1983). The isolation and amino acid composition of senile plaque core protein. *Brain Res.* 259: 348-352.
35. Candy, J.M., Ckinowski, J., Perry, R.H., Perry, E.K., Fairbairn, A., Oakley, A.E., Carpenter, T.A., Atack, J.R., Blessed, G., and Edwardson, J.A. (1986). Alumino silicates and senile plaque formation in Alzheimer disease. *Lancet* 1: 354-356.
36. Masters, C.L., Simms, G., Weinman, N.A., Multhaup, G., McDonald, B.L., and Beyreuther, K. (1985). Amyloid plaque core protein in Alzheimer disease and Down syndrome. *Proc. Natl. Acad. Sci. USA* 82: 4245-4249.
37. Glenner, G.C., and Wong, C.W. (1984). Alzheimer's disease: Initial report of the purification and characterization of a novel cerebrovascular amyloid protein. *Biochem. Biophys. Res. Commun.* 120: 885-890.
38. Wong, C.W., Quaranta, V., and Glenner, G.C. (1985). Neuritic plaques and cerebrovascular amyloid in Alzheimer disease are antigenically related. *Proc. Natl. Acad. Sci. USA* 82: 8779-8732.
39. Allsop, D., Landon, M., Kidd, M., Lowe, J.S., Reynolds, G.P., and Gardner, A. (1986). Monoclonal antibodies raised against a subsequence of senile plaque core protein react with plaque cores, plaque periphery and cerebrovascular amyloid in Alzheimer's disease. *Neurosci. Lett.* 68: 252-256.
40. Sparkman, D.R., Johnson, S., Hammon, K., Allison, P., and White, C.L. III. (1987). Isolation of the insoluble straight fibrils of Pick's disease. *J. Neurol. Sci.* 80: 173-184.
41. Gusella, J.F., Wexler, N.S., Conneally, P.M., Naylor, S.L., Anderson, M.A., Tanzi, R.E., Watkins, P.C., Ottina, K., Wallace, M.R., Sakaguchi, A.Y., Young, A.B., Shoulson, I., Bonilla, E., and Martin, J.B. (1983). A polymorphic DNA marker genetically linked to Huntington's disease. *Nature* 306: 234-238.
42. Townsend, L.E., Gilroy, J., LeWitt, P.A., Wolfe, D.E., Pomara, N., and Weintraub, J. (1986). Cerebrospinal fluid proteins in the diagnosis of Alz-

heimer's disease. 38th Annual Meeting of the American Academy of Neurology, New Orleans, Louisiana, 1986.
43. Sirkin, B. (1986). Monoclonal antibody test developed for diagnosing Alzheimer's disease. *Genet. Engin. News* 6: 38.
44. Wolozin, B.L., Pruchnicki, A., Dickson, D.W., and Davies, P. (1986). A neuronal antigen in the brains of Alzheimer patients. *Science* 232: 648-232.
45. Yates, C.M., Laszlo, I., Fink, G., Hastings, I., Boyd, J., and James, K. (1986). Monoclonal antibodies to human hypoglossal nucleus which stain neurons and astrocytes in normal brains and brains from cases of Alzheimer-type dementia. *Neuroscience* 18: 183-191.

18

Plasma and Cerebrospinal Levels of Methionine-Enkephalin in Senile Dementia of the Alzheimer's Type

JIMMIE L. VALENTINE, NICHOLAS P. PLOTNIKOFF, JONATHAN BENNETT, MARION S. PATTEN, CAROL S. CROMER, and RALPH W. RICHTER / *Oral Roberts University, School of Medicine, City of Faith Medical and Research Center, Tulsa, Oklahoma*

INTRODUCTION

Alzheimer's disease is generally thought to be responsible for 50-75% of all cases of progressive dementia (1), although one series reported a level as high as 84% (2). An earlier age at onset of dementia symptoms, especially aplasia, has been associated with familial Alzheimer's disease in some studies (3) but not all (2). At present, diagnosis of Alzheimer's disease remains a combined clinicopathological diagnosis and the relationship between neuropsychological, neuroradiological, and neuropathological indices of the disease is not well understood (4).

In 1983, 2-3 million Americans 65 years and older suffered from dementia (5, 6). This was approximately 15% of the population over 65 years of age. For people with clinical signs of dementia, 55% had Alzheimer's disease or senile dementia of the Alzheimer's type, 15% were affected by multi-infarct dementia, and 22% by a combination of the two (7). Alzheimer's disease claims more than 120,000 lives a year, making it the fourth leading cause of death among the elderly, after heart disease, cancer, and stroke (6,8). The clinicopathological diagnosis of Alzheimer's disease requires the demonstration in life of the presence of dementia and the finding of typical pathological features, such as neurofibrillary tangles and neuritic plaques either by biopsy of the cerebral cortex or by postmortem examination of the cerebral cortex and hippocampus (5). Clinicians lack specific biological markers of the disease and can only approximate the true diagnosis. For this reason many diagnoses of Alzheimer's disease are listed as senile dementia of the Alzheimer's type.

CHARACTERISTICS OF ALZHEIMER'S DISEASE

Gross Pathological Changes

Alzheimer's disease is characterized by progressive abnormalities of memory, behavior, and cognition (9). Clinically, a diffuse slowing of the electroencephalogram and a decrease in cerebral flow can be measured. There is a loss of neurons, particularly in regions essential for memory and cognition (6). Neurofibrillary tangles accumulate adjacent to and within blood vessels and there are scattered foci of cellular debris and amyloid called neuritic plaques (5). There is also a significant loss of neurons in certain more primitive regions at the base of the brain, with consequent reduction in the amount of neurotransmitters. Plaques and tangles are also found in the basal nucleus of Maynert, amygdala, hippocampus, parahippocampic gyrus, hypothalamus, and the pontine tegmentum. Symptoms involving the highest cognitive functions, including memory, judgment, orientation, and speech, imply a widespread disorder of neocortex in frontal, temporal, and parietal regions, as well as of the limbic system (10).

Changes in Central Cholinergic and Adrenergic Systems

In addition to neuronal loss from the neocortex, a significant diminution in the number of neurons in the basal nucleus of Meynert occurs. These neurons are cholinergic and constitute a major cholinergic input into the cortex. Postmortem studies report lower levels of acetylcholine (10) and choline acetyltransferase (10-15). There is also a decrease in the noradrenergic locus ceruleus cortical tissue, causing a deficiency in norepinephrine as evidenced by a postmortem decrease in norepinephrine (10). A 25% decrease in norepinephrine has been found in the hypothalamus (16) and neurochemical studies have also found a decrease of this adrenergic amine in the caudate nucleus and cerebral cortex, as well as a decrease in dopamine-beta-hydroxylase in the cerebral cortex (17,18). 3-Methoxy-4-hydroxylphenylglycol (a metabolite of norepinephrine) is increased in several areas of the brain in which norepinephrine is decreased (18). Since central nervous system noradrenergic pathways appear to be involved in the cognitive function and motor activity, abnormal adrenergic activity might be related to behavior abnormalities of Alzheimer's disease. Other research (19) has shown that 5-hydroxytryptamine (serotonin) and norepinephrine decreased in all areas of the brain and dopamine and homovanillic acid decreased in the caudate nucleus of patients with Alzheimer's disease.

Changes in Neurotransmitters

Alzheimer's disease involves the death of certain groups of neurons that seem to be, inter alia, cholinergic cells with endings in the cerebral cortex and the norepinephrine cells whose bodies are to be found in the locus ceruleus (10,17). The principal transmitters affected in Alzheimer's disease appear to be acetylcholine and norepinephrine, but this raises the question of what other neurotransmitters may be involved. Altered levels of some peptides are seen in the brain of demented patients. Neuropeptides that have been measured in Alzheimer's disease include choleocystikinin (CCK) markers of cortical cells, vasointestinal peptide (VIP), beta-endorphin, and somatostatin, all of which may function as neurotransmitters or neuromodulators. Levels of CCK and VIP were unchanged (14,15,23), whereas those of beta-endorphin, somatostatin, and substance P were decreased (15,21, 22) in Alzheimer's disease. This pattern of neurotransmitter abnormalities indicated predominant damage to the diffuse ascending cholinergic system, with relative preservation of certain populations of intrinsic cortical cells (15).

Role of Neuropeptides

Neuropeptides may have a physiological role as neurotransmitters or neuromodulators (21-25). Two main functions have been suggested for endogenous opiates: (a) to act as hormones, transported to their target organs by the cerebrospinal fluid and blood system, or (b) to act as neurotransmitters that are liberated from nerve terminals and bind to the immediate post synaptic membrane (25-27). Also, a peripheral role as immunomodulators has been suggested (28,29). Some peptides can be shown to coexist with classic neurotransmitters, for example, substance P and thyrotropin-releasing hormone (TRH) within some of the 5-hydroxytryptamine-containing neurons of the medulla oblongata (13), or methionine-enkephalin within the chromatin granules of the adrenal gland (30). The serotonergic neurons in the nucleus raphae dorsalis and paragigantocellularis of the cat have been reported to contain enkephalin (31).

PENTAPEPTIDES

Two endogenous pentapeptides, methionine-enkephalin and leucine-enkephalin, were first isolated and characterized from porcine and bovine brain (32). The methionine-enkephalin sequence, Try-Gly-Gly-Phe-Met-OH, is contained in the carboxy terminal fragment of a pituitary hormone beta-lipotropin that also contains beta-endorphin, but the major precursor for methionine-enkephalin is proenkephalin A (33). Proenkephalin A contains four copies of methionine-enkephalin and one copy of leucine-enkephalin. Proenkephalin B (also termed prodynorphin) contains three copies of leucine-enkephalin in addition to several larger opioid peptides that have been isolated from porcine pituitary and brain (34).

Anatomical Location

Enkephalin-containing neurons have been demonstrated in every major region of the brain except the neocortex. Enkephalin-containing neurons and their terminals (and receptors) are located in areas such as the periaqueductal gray, raphe magnus, trigeminal nucleus, and laminae I and II of the spinal cord, where they could modulate the passage of sensory information concerned with pain perception (34). Since high densities of enkephalin nerve terminals are also found in areas such as the globus pallidus, hypothalamus, stria terminalis, and locus cereleus, the enkephalins may be involved in extrapyramidal motor function, mood, and behavior (34). Their location in the median eminance could result in regulation of neuroendocrinological functions. Enkephalins possibly increase the release of oxytocin and vasopressin, suggesting a modulatory role for opiate peptides in the neurohypophysis (35). Opiate receptors and enkephalins have been demonstrated in brain regions where neither stimulation nor morphine causes analgesia, and morphine and enkephalins depress cell firing in these regions (24). If enkephalins are active neurohumoral transmitters or modulators, they probably have roles beyond that in pain perception. There are more than 20 separate enkephalin regions, with the highest concentrations occurring in the globus pallidus, striatum, hypothalamus, midbrain, and brain stem nuclei, and the dorsal horn of the spinal cord (36).

Role as Neurotransmitters

Enkephalins may be inhibitory neurotransmitters in particular brain regions (24, 34). Opiates may act by impairing Na^+ influx at the postsynaptic membrane caused by excitatory neurotransmitters such as glutamate and acetylcholine (24). The opiates depress the release of acetylcholine or norepinephrine from many central or peripheral sites (24,37-38). Methionine-enkephalin is degraded very rapidly when administrated either intravenously or directly into the brain. The plasma half-life is about 40 sec and the analgesic activity about 3 min when administrated directly into the brain (39). This short half-life would tend to limit the role of enkephalins as major hormones, although they could express themselves in remote locations if protected either by being a part of a larger molecule or by forming a stable complex in blood or the cerebrospinal fluid (31). Because of its location in the hypothalamus and pituitary and its relatively longer duration of action, a hormonal role for the active pentapeptide, methionine-enkephalin, is a more reasonable possibility. Of the endogenous opiates that have been described to date, the enkephalin pentapeptides are being seriously considered as having a neurotransmitter role.

Association with Hormones

Enkephalins that arise from both proenkephalin and prodynorphin are closely associated intracellularly with other hormonal agents, for example, proenkephalin and its correspondent peptides are present in adrenal chromaffin granules and are released along with epinephrine during exocytosis (30). Recently, the presence of methionine-enkephalin has also been demonstrated in the islets of Langerhans in the pancreas (40). In sympathetic nerves these enkephalin precursors are localized along with the norepinephrine in the secretory granules from which they are simultaneously released during sympathetic stimulation. Alternatively, these peptides act in concert with an associated hormonal agent and modulate its effects at the same end organ. There are close anatomical and biochemical correlations between the dopaminergic and peptidergic systems in the substatia nigra and striatum. Methionine-enkephalin seems to modulate the synthesis and the release of dopamine from nerve endings and also affects the sensitivity of postsynaptic dopaminergic receptors. The presence of so many peptides, so widely distributed, and coded for by at least three distinct genes, argues for a much broader role for opioid peptides than simply the modulation of pain (34,35).

Methionine-enkephalin, as well as somatostatin, vasointestinal peptide, and choleocystikinin, is found in the hypothalamus. The influence of the hypothalamus on intelligence and memory is unknown but it has close connections with the amygdala, hippocampus, limbic system, and mamillary bodies, all of which play a major part in memory, emotion, and behavior (10). These hypothalamic peptides may have an influence on memory either through their hypothalamic role or via their distribution in other areas of the cerebrum, or as a modulator of other neurotransmitters, such as acetylcholine. This relationship between peptides, memory, and neurotransmitters (especially acetylcholine and norepinephrine) presents a possible role for neuropeptides in Alzheimer's disease.

Recently, reports have appeared that document changes in the immune system of Alzheimer's patients that are very different from those observed in normal aging (41,42). Also it has recently become apparent that many of the neuropeptides are functioning as neuroimmunomodulators (28,29). This provides other evidence that the neuropeptides may be involved in Alzheimer's disease, since an imbalance in these neuropeptides would affect the immune system.

RATIONALE FOR ANALYSIS OF METHIONINE-ENKEPHALIN IN ALZHEIMER'S DISEASE PATIENTS

It would be important to differentiate Alzheimer's disease clinically from other similar diseases such as multi-infarct dementia, severe depression, nutritional deficiencies, or Pick's disease. The occurrence of these diseases often increases with advancing age and thus any potential biochemical marker(s) for Alzheimer's disease must be compared with an age-matched group as well as with a younger population. Evidence cited above that methionine-enkephalin may be a neurotransmitter prompted us to examine its levels in blood plasma of young and aged volunteers as well as in patients with senile dementia of the Alzheimer's type. In addition, a few patients' cerebrospinal fluid levels of methionine-enkephalin were examined, and in two patients simultaneous determinations of blood plasma and cerebrospinal fluid levels were made.

METHODS

Patients with diagnosed senile dementia of the Alzheimer type (SDAT) were identified in several institutions. Informed consent was obtained from all participants or a responsible relative.

Specimen Collection

A total of 14 patients with SDAT and 5 age-matched controls had blood specimens drawn for analysis of methionine-enkephalin levels. All were residents of the Family Life Enrichment Centers, Incorporated, a skilled nursing facility in High Schoals, Georgia. Cerebrospinal fluid levels for SDAT were obtained from patients in St. Johns Medical Center in Tulsa, Oklahoma. Normal volunteers used in the blood plasma determinations were laboratory and staff personnel at the City of Faith Medical and Research Center in Tulsa, Oklahoma. Cerebrospinal fluid used as age-matched controls was obtained from patients at the latter institution who were undergoing a routine lumbar puncture and in whom no clinical laboratory abnormalities had been determined.

Cerebrospinal Fluid

Lumbar punctures were made using aseptic conditions and 1.5 ml aliquots of CSF frozen at $-20^{\circ}C$ until analyzed. Bloody or opaque specimens were not used.

Serum

Blood specimens were obtained via venipuncture of an antecubital vein on the forearm and collected in a commercial vacuum tube (Lavender top Vacutainer, Becton Dickinson, Rutherford, NJ) containing EDTA. The blood specimen was gently mixed and immediately placed on ice, then centrifuged at 2800 rpm at $4^{\circ}C$ for 15 min. Plasma was removed and individual 1.5 ml aliquots frozen at $-20^{\circ}C$ until analyzed.

Analysis of Specimens

Blood plasma or cerebrospinal fluid (1 ml) was analyzed for its content of methionine-enkephalin using a commercially available radioimmunoassay kit (Immuno Nuclear Corporation, Stillwell, MN). This procedure uses chromatographic separation on ODS silica columns (Sep-pak ODS silica, Millipore Corporation, Milford, MA) and a second antibody precipitation of bound radiolabeled methionine-enkephalin. Standards of 500, 250, 150, 100, 50, 25, 12.5, 6.25, and 0 pg/ml were processed during each analysis and used to prepare a standard logit-log curve.

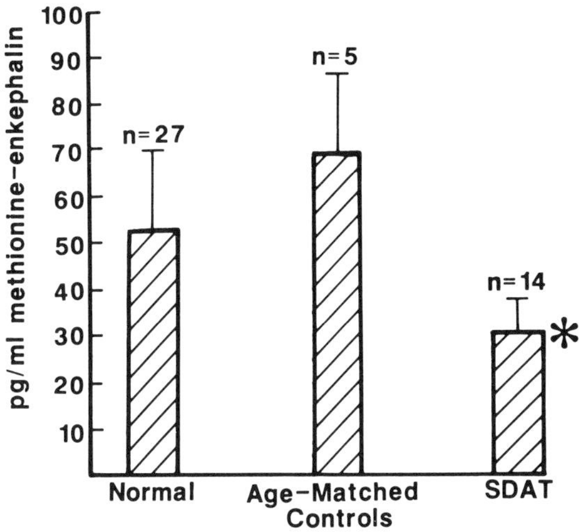

FIGURE 1 Plasma levels of 14 SDAT nursing home patients compared to 5 age-matched controls in the same environment and 27 normal volunteers ages 21-59 (*$p<0.05$).

RESULTS

Blood plasma specimens from a total of 27 volunteers ages 21-59 were analyzed for the level of methionine-enkephalin, and gave a mean of 53±17.4 pg/ml. This level was not significantly different from the mean of 70±15.7 pg/ml found in the plasma of five nursing home patients with a mean age of 87±6.7 years. Significantly different from either of these groups were the plasma samples from 14 SDAT nursing home patients, who had a mean of 31±7.5 pg/ml and a mean age of 84±7.5 years. These results are shown in Figure 1. The ages of the two groups were not significantly different.

Cerebrospinal fluid levels of methionine-enkephalin were found to be 58±26.9 pg/ml in a set of six age-matched controls with a mean age of 73±12.2 pg/ml. This was significantly different from the CSF levels of five patients (30±15.7 pg/ml) diagnosed as having SDAT and with a mean age of 66±11.2 years. These results are shown in Figure 2. The ages of the two groups were not significantly different. Two patients with SDAT had blood and cerebrospinal fluid obtained at the same time. The plasma level was found to have a mean of 27±1.4 pg/ml; the CSF was essentially identical at 30±9.9 pg/ml (not significantly different) (Fig. 3).

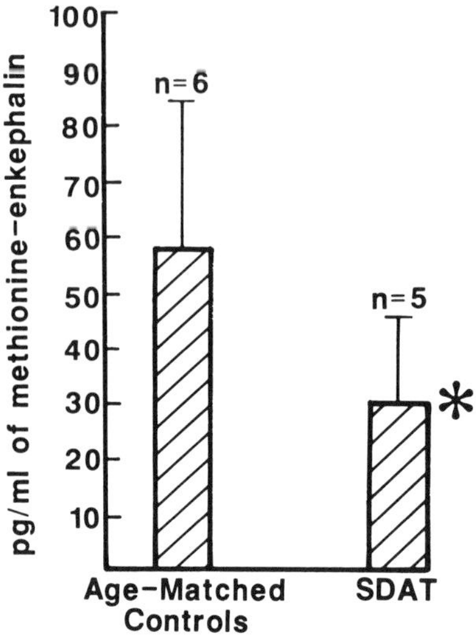

FIGURE 2 Cerebrospinal fluid levels of methionine-enkephalin in five patients diagnosed as having SDAT compared to six age-matched controls undergoing lumbar spinal puncture for medical diagnosis. The controls had normal biochemical parameters determined and nonpathological findings (*$p < 0.05$).

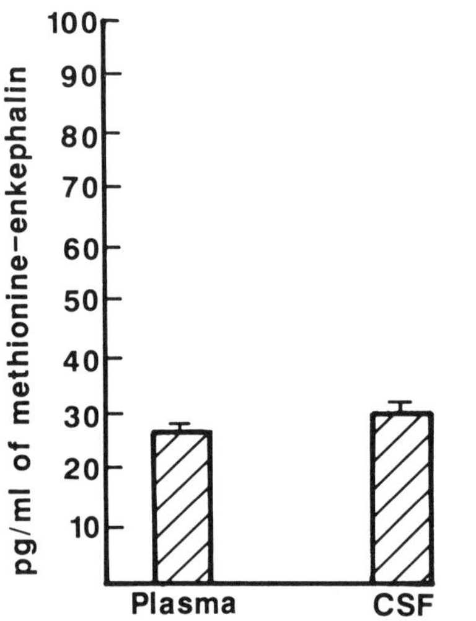

FIGURE 3 Comparison of the blood plasma and cerebrospinal fluid levels of methionine-enkephalin in two patients with simultaneous specimen collections of each body fluid.

DISCUSSION

The measurement of methionine-enkephalin in the blood plasma and cerebrospinal fluid of patients with senile dementia of the Alzheimer's type appears to be promising, although more studies with many more patients need to be carried out. The finding that plasma levels as well as cerebrospinal fluid levels of methionine-enkephalin were depressed in patients with SDAT may be related to the depletion of this potential neurotransmitter during progression of the disease. The investigation of neurotransmitter levels and/or their metabolites could become a promising approach to the diagnosis of Alzheimer's disease. Literature was cited above reporting decreased levels of acetylcholine, norepinephrine, dopamine, gamma-aminobutyric acid, and 5-hydroxytryptamine. Particularly interesting was the finding that plasma and CSF levels of methionine-enkephalin were essentially identical in SDAT. This may infer that some deterioration of the blood-brain barrier may also occur in SDAT, since most studies have shown that methionine-enkephalin does not cross the blood-brain barrier (7). Likewise, the finding by others (23) that beta-endorphin levels are also lower in SDAT and multi-infarct dementia patients adds support to the theory of a depressed endogenous opiate system in persons so affected.

A close relationship has been reported between CSF and plasma norepinephrine levels (43). This relationship is difficult to explain given that it is very unlikely that norepinephrine crosses the blood-brain barrier. One possible explanation for the close relationship between CSF and plasma norepinephrine levels is that common mechanisms regulate noradrenergic outflow in the CNS and the periphery, functionally linking the CNS noradrenergic systems and the peripheral sympathetic nervous system (44). The blood-brain barrier is also basically impenetrable to methionine-enkephalin, as it is to norepinephrine and other neurotransmitters (45). Some common mechanism may regulate the levels of methionine-enkephalin centrally and peripherally, as is the case with norepinephrine. Also it is possible that methionine-enkephalin communicates through the choroid plexus and hypothalamus (46). Enkephalins are also localized in areas of the forebrain where the blood-brain barrier is permeable to certain substances in the subfornical organ and the organum vasculosum lamina terminalis (47).

Reasons for the lower levels of methionine-enkephalin in our study are unknown. Methionine-enkephalin can be hydrolyzed by purified acetylcholinesterase (48). In Alzheimer's disease the level of acetylcholinesterase in the CSF has been reported to be both decreased (49) and unchanged (50). Other enzymes, termed enkephalinases, have been reported in various brain homogenates (51-53). If the levels of any of these enzymes were increased in Alzheimer's disease, this could explain the decreased levels of methionine-enkephalin. To date this has not been demonstrated.

The interrelationship between neurotransmitter pathways and neurotransmitters themselves continues to become of greater importance. There is decreased activity of GABAnergic, dopaminergic, noradrenergic, and serotonergic systems in patients with dementia, especially Alzheimer's disease (54). Our report is the first to show an apparent decrease in methionine-enkephalin in both the plasma and CSF of patients with senile dementia of the Alzheimer's type. Such a decrease in this possible neurotransmitter may in turn affect other neurotransmitters. For example, it has been previously reported that methionine-enkephalin interacts with endogenous opiate receptors in the brain to modulate the release of acetylcholine from cholinergic neurons (37) and that methionine-enkephalin inhibits dopamine and norepinephrine release (55,56). These facts all point out that the relationships between the enkephalins and the classic neurotransmitters are not by any means completely defined in the normal person and even less so in those with senile dementia of the Alzheimer's type.

CONCLUSIONS

Our preliminary studies showed that blood plasma levels of methionine-enkephalin are significantly depressed in patients with senile dementia of the Alzheimer's type when compared to age-matched controls with no signs of dementia. The studies also suggest that some increase in the plasma levels of methionine-enkephalin occurs as part of the natural aging process, since these age-matched controls were different from the levels found in a younger normal population. The studies of methionine-enkephalin levels in the cerebrospinal fluid of the senile dementia of the Alzheimer's type again suggested in a preliminary fashion that a significant depression occurred compared to patients without dementia.

REFERENCES

1. Mortimer, J.A., Schuman, L.M., and French, L.R. (1981). Epidemiology of dementing illness. In: *Epidemiology of Dementia*, J.A. Mortimer and L.M. Schuman (Eds.) Oxford. Oxford University Press, pp. 3-24.
2. Chui, H.C., Teng, E.L., Henderson, H.W., and Moy, A.C. (1985). Clinical subtypes of dementia of the Alzheimer type. *Neurology* 35: 1544-1550.
3. Folstein, M.F., and Breitner, J.C.S. (1981). Language disorder predicts familial Alzheimer's disease. *John Hopkins Med. J.* 149: 145-147.
4. Khachaturian, Z.S. (1985). Diagnosis of Alzheimer's disease. *Arch. Neurol.* 42: 1097-1105.
5. Terry, R., and Zatzman, R. (1983). Senile dementia of the Alzheimer type. *Ann. Neurol.* 14: 497-506.
6. Wurtman, R. (1985). Alzheimer's disease. *Sci. Am.* 252: 62-66, 71-74.
7. Wisniewski, H., and Kozlowski, P. (1982). Evidence for blood-brain-barrier changes in senile dementia of the Alzheimer type (SDAT). *Ann. N.Y. Acad. Sci.* 396: 119-129.
8. Roach, M. (1985). Reflection in a fatal mirror. *Discover* 6: 76-85.

9. Sandyk, R., and Snider, S. (1985). CSF met-enkephalin levels in Parkinson's disease. *Neurology* 35: 776-777.
10. Marchbanks, R. (1982). Biochemistry of Alzheimer's dementia. *J. Neurochem.* 39: 9-15.
11. Oram, J., Edwardson, J., and Millard, P. (1981). Investigation of cerebrospinal neuropeptides in idiopathic senile dementia. *Gerontology* 27: 216-223.
12. Wortis, J. (1983). Alzheimer's disease and the new neuroscience. *Biol. Psychiatry* 18: 847-848.
13. Soininen, H., Jolkkone, J., Reinikainen, K., Halonen, T., and Riekkinen, P. (1984). Reduced cholinesterase activity and sometostatin-like immunoreactivity in the cerebrospinal fluid of patients with dementia of the Alzheimer type. *J. Neurosci.* 63: 167-172.
14. Rossor, M., Fahrenkrug, J., Emso, P., Mountjoy, C., Iversen, L., and Roth, M. (1980). Reduced cortical choline acetyltransferase activity in senile dementia of Alzheimer type is not accompanied by changes in vasoactive intestinal polypeptide. *Brain Res.* 201: 249-253.
15. Rossor, M.N. (1982). Neurotransmitters and CNS disease. *Lancet* 2: 1200-1204.
16. Yates, C., Simpson, J., Gordon, A., Maloney, A., Allison, Y., Ritchie, I., and Urquhart, A. (1983). Catecholamines and cholinergic enzymes in pre-senile and senile Alzheimer's-type dementia and Down's syndrome. *Brain Res.* 280: 119-126.
17. Miyata, S., Nagata, H., Yamao, S., Nakamura, S., and Kameyama, M. (1984). Dopamine-beta-hydroxylase activities in serum and cerebrospinal fluid of aged and demented patients. *J. Neurol. Sci.* 63: 403-406
18. Raskind, M., Peskind, E., Halter, J., and Jimerson, D. (1984). Norepinephrine and MHPG levels in CSF and plasma in Alzheimer's disease. *Arch. Gen. Psychiatry* 41: 343-346.
19. Gottfries, C., Adolfsson, R., Aquilonius, S., Carlsson, A., Eckernas, S., Nordberg, A., Oreland, L., Svennerholm, L., Wiberg, A., and Winblad, B. (1983). Biochemical changes in dementia disorders of Alzheimer type (AD/SDAT). *Neurobiol. Aging* 4: 261-271.
20. Perry, R., Dockray, G., Dimaline, R., Perry, E., Blessed, G., and Tomlinson, B. (1981). Neuropeptides in Alzheimer's disease, depression and schizophrenia. A postmortem analysis of vasoactive intestinal peptide and cholecystonia. *J. Neurol. Sci.* 51: 465-472.
21. Wikkelso, C., Blomstrand, C., and Nordquist, P. (1981). Cerebrospinal fluid investigations in multi-infarct dementia and senile dementia. *Acta Neurol. Scand.* 64: 1-11.
22. Beal, M., Mazurek, M., Tran, V., Chattha, G., Bird, E., and Martin, J. (1985). Reduced numbers of somatostatin receptors in the cerebral cortex in Alzheimer's disease. *Science* 229: 289-291.
23. Sulkava, R., Erkinjuntti, A., and Laatikainen, T. (1985). CSF beta-endorphin and beta-lipotropin in Alzheimer's disease and multi-infarct dementia. *Neurology* 35: 1057-1058.
24. Frederickson, R. (1977). Enkephalin pentapeptides. A review of current evidence for a physiological role in vertebrate neurotransmission. *Life Sci.* 21: 23-42.

25. Uzumaki, U., Govoni, S., Faccini, E., Pasinetti, G., Missale, C., and Trabucchi, M. (1984). Neuropeptidergic inhibitory regulation of met-enkephalin immunoreactive material release from rat spinal cord in vitro. *Peptides* 5: 849-852.
26. Kasakov, L., and Venkov, L. (1983). The effect of enkephalins on the acetylcholinesterase activity in rat brain synaptosomes. *Cell. Mol. Biol.* 29: 153-157.
27. Sarne, Y., Azov, R., and Weissman, B. (1978). A stable enkephalin-like immunoreactive substance in human CSF. *Brain Res.* 151: 399-403.
28. Chaminade, M., Foutz, A.S., and Rossier, J. (1983). Co-release of enkephalins and precursors with catecholamines by the perfused cat adrenal in situ. *Life Sci.* 33 (Supp I): 21-24.
29. Wybran, J. (1985). Enkephalins and endorphins as modifiers of the immune system: Present and future. *Fed. Proc.* 44: 92-94.
30. Plotnikoff, N.P., Murgo, A.J., Miller, G.C., Corder, C.N., and Faith, R.E. (1985). Enkephalins: Immunomodulators. *Fed. Proc.* 44: 118-122.
31. Glazer, E., Steinbusch, H., Verhofstad, A., and Basbaun, A. (1981). Serotonergic neurons in nucleus raphe dorsalis and paragigantocellularis of the cat contain enkephalin. *J. Physiol.* (Paris) 77: 241-245.
32. Hughes, J., Smith, T.W., Kosterlitz, H.W., Fothergill, L.A., Morgan, B.A., and Morris, H.R. (1975). Identification of two related pentapeptides from the brain with potent opiate agonist activity. *Nature* 258: 577-580.
33. Undenfriend, S., and Kilpatrick, D. (1983). Biochemistry of the enkephalin-containing peptides. *Arch. Biochem. Biophys.* 221: 309-323.
34. Hokfelt, T., Vincent, S.R., Dalsgaard, C.J., Herrera-Marschitz, M., Ungerstedt, U., Schultzberg, M., Christensson, I., and Terenius, L. (1984). Some aspects on distribution and role of opioid peptides in the central and peripheral nervous system. In: *Central and Peripheral Endorphins: Basic and Clinical Aspects*, E. Muller and A. Genazzani (Eds.) New York, Haven Press, pp. 1-16.
35. Emson, P. (1979). Peptides as neurotransmitter candidates in the mammalian CNS. *Prog. Neurobiol.* 13: 61-116.
36. Beaumont, A., and Hughes, J. (1979). Biology of opioid peptides. *Annu. Rev. Pharmacol. Toxicol.* 19: 245-267.
37. Jhamandas, K., and Elliott, J. (1980). Investigation of action of enkephalin on the spontaneous and evoked release of acetylcholine from rat cortical and striatal slices. *Br. J. Pharmacol.* 71: 211-217.
38. Pezzoli, G., Panerai, A., Di Giulio, A., Longo, A., Passerini, D., and Carenzi, A. (1984). Methionine-enkephalin, substance P and homovanillic acid in the CSF of parkinsonian patients. *Neurology* 34: 516-519.
39. Kastin, A.J., Nissen, C., Schally, A.V., and Coy, D.H. (1976). Blood-brain-barrier half-time disappearance, and brain distribution for labeled enkephalin and a potent analog. *Brain Res. Bull.* 1: 583-589.
40. Timmers, K.I., Voyles, N.R., King, C., Wells, M., Fairtile, R., and Recant, L. (1986). Opioid peptides in rat islets of Langerhans: Immunoreactive met- and leu-enkephalins and BAM-22P. *Diabetes* 35: 52-57.

41. MacDonald, S.M., Goldstone, A.H., Morris, J.E., Exton-Smith, A.N., and Callard, T.E. (1982). Immunological parameters in the aged and in Alzheimer's disease. *Clin. Exp. Immunol.* 49: 123-128.
42. Skias, D., Bania, M., Reder, A.T., Luchins, D., and Antel, J.P. (1985). Senile dementia of Alzheimer's type (SDAT): Reduced $T8^+$ cell-mediated suppressor activity. *Neurology* 35: 1635-1638.
43. Ziegler, M., Lake, C., Wood, J., Brooks, B., and Ebert, M. (1977). Relationship between norepinephrine in blood and CSF in the presence of a blood-CSF barrier for norepinephrine. *J. Neurochem.* 28: 677-679.
44. Wood, P., Etienne, P., Lal, S., Gauthier, S., Cajal, S., and Nair, N. (1982). Reduced lumbar CSF somatostatin levels in Alzheimer's disease. *Life Sci.* 31: 2073-2079.
45. Pardridge, W., and Mietus, L.J. (1981). Enkephalin and blood-brain-barrier: Studies of binding and degradation in isolated brain microvessels. *Endocrinology* 109: 1138-1143.
46. Cornford, E., Braun, L., Crane, P., and Oldendorf, W. (1978). Blood-brain-barrier restriction of peptides and the low uptake of enkephalins. *Endocrinology* 103: 1297-1303.
47. Wamsley, J., Young, W., and Kuhar, M. (1980). Immunohistochemical localization of enkephalin in rat forebrain. *Brain Res.* 190: 153-174.
48. Chubb, W., Ranier, E., White, G., and Hodgson, A. (1983). The enkephalins are amongst the peptides hydrolyzed by purified acetylcholinesterase. *Neuroscience* 10: 1369-1377.
49. Deutsch, S., Mohs, R., Levy, M., Rothpearl, A., Stockton, D., Horvath, T., Coco, A., and Davis, K. (1983). Acetylcholinesterase activity in CSF in schizophrenia, depression, Alzheimer's disease and normals. *Biol. Psychiatry* 18: 1363-1373.
50. Bisso, G.M., Masullo, C., Michalek, H., Silveri, M.C., and Pocchiari, M. (1986). Molecular forms of cholinesterases in CSF of Alzheimer's disease/senile dementia of Alzheimer type patients and matched neurological controls. *Life Sci.* 38: 561-567.
51. Coletti-Previero, M.-A., Mattras, H., Descomps, B., and Previero, A. (1981). Purification and substrate characterization of a human enkephalin-degrading aminopeptidase. *Biochem. Biophys. Acta* 657: 122-127.
52. Dupont, A., Cusan, L., Garon, M., Alvarado-Urbina, G., and Labrie, F. (1977). Extremely rapid degradation of [3H] methionine-enkephalin by various rat tissue in vivo and in vitro. *Life Sci.* 21: 907-914.
53. Hambrook, J., Morgan, B.A., Rance, M.J., and Smith, C.F.C. (1976). Mode of deactivation of the enkephalins by rat and human plasma and rat brain homogenates. *Nature* 262: 782-783.
54. Miyata, S., Yamao, S., Nakamura, S., Udaka, F., and Kameyama, M. (1981). Alterations in neurotransmitter in multi-infarct dementia and senile dementia of Alzheimer's type. *Rinsho Shinkeigaku* 21: 491-497.
55. Taube, H., Borowski, E., Endo, T., and Starke, K. (1976). Enkephalin a potential modulator of noradrenaline release in rat brain. *Eur. J. Pharmacol.* 38: 377-380.

56. Loh, H., Brase, D., Sumpath-Khanna, S., Jeffery, B., Way, E., and Li, C. (1976). Beta-endorphin in vitro inhibition of striatal dopamine release. *Nature* 264: 567-568.

19

Brain Imaging and Related Technology in the Diagnosis of Alzheimer's Disease

WILLIAM S. YAMANASHI, NABIL A. YASSA, and PATRICK D. LESTER / *City of Faith Medical and Research Center, Tulsa, Oklahoma*

NEAL R. CUTLER / *Center for Aging and Alzheimer's, Beverly Hills, California*

JOHN ROSS-DUGGAN / *Orlando Diagnostic Clinic, Orlando, Florida*

INTRODUCTION

The recent development of imaging modalities such as positron emission tomography (PET), single photon emission computed tomography (SPECT), and magnetic resonance imaging (MRI) have resulted in some optimism in the early diagnosis of senile dementia of Alzheimer's type (SDAT) (1-3). The advantage of PET, SPECT, and MRI over conventional computed tomography (CT) is that the imaging of these modalities reflect metabolic and physiological changes to some degree (4,5). However, despite the advent of these new imaging modalities, the unequivocal diagnosis of SDAT prior to autopsy remains one of exclusion. This is in part due to the multiplicity of causative factors that may contribute to the symptomatic manifestations of the senile plaque and neurofibrillary tangles first observed by Alzheimer in 1907 (6). Some of these postulated factors include age, head trauma, genetics, slow virus, immune defects, toxic levels of aluminum and silicone in the brain, amyloid deposition, and altered enzyme levels (7-15).

Scanning with CT reveals density difference in tissue. The use of MRI reveals relaxation times of protons, principally those contained in tissue water. The PET technique detects the dual photon emission following positron electron annihilation, while SPECT detects the presence of gamma ray emitters in the brain. Isotopes containing either of the latter two types of emitters may be incorporated into a variety of radiochemicals that reach the brain, yielding an in vivo autoradiographic picture.

Macroscopic morphologic changes in SDAT, especially atrophy with decrease in the volume of the gray matter, are accompanied by widening of sulci, shrinkage of gyri, and increase in the ventricular volume and can be detected equally well by either CT or MRI. These atrophic changes, however, may be seen in usual age-related or non-SDAT dementia and are not specific for Alzheimer's type dementia. Also, the cortex does not shrink at the early stages but seems to be replaced by gliosis. The atrophy thus should not be expected to parallel gradually the worsening of symptoms or metabolic decrement until late in the disease. This should apply also to the atrophy that can be visualized on CT scans or MRI pictures; also atrophy and degenerative processes do not proceed at the same pace in all areas of the cortex (16).

In the past years various biochemical makers for SDAT have been claimed, some of which are associated with neuritic plaques and neurofibrillary tangles while others are monoclonal antibodies or soluble proteins (17-19). Authenticity of these markers is still controversial due mainly to the unresolved issue of clinical subtypes of SDAT. Combined criteria of *DSM-III* (for primary progressive dementia), Hachinske ischemia score of 4 or more, age of onset, aphasia, motor disorder, and family history based on total of 173 subjects indicate that familial SDAT affects a significant percentage of the population of demented patient (44.8%). This group is associated with earlier onset and language disorder (21), and can be distinguished from those with nonfamilial or sporadic SDAT. While the biochemical and molecular genetic data are being assessed to refine the definition of the disease, the familial subpopulation of SDAT is becoming an important factor in the understanding, diagnosis, and, it is hoped, treatment of this disease. We will review briefly here the imaging modalities, CT, PET, SPECT, and MRI and present preliminary MRI examples of familial SDAT patients. Finally, we will discuss in vivo MR spectroscopy, a technique that compensates for some of the limitations of current proton MRI, including the less than ideal tissue specificity, and that may provide more physiological and metabolic data at the molecular level.

IMAGING MODALITIES, PARAMETERS, STRENGTHS, AND LIMITATIONS IN THE DIAGNOSIS OF SDAT

In general, CT and SPECT nuclear brain scans as well as PET and MRI are considered complementary in the diagnosis of SDAT. History, clinical tests, and laboratory data are necessary for the presumptive diagnosis. Noninvasive brain scans rather than cortical biopsy would be the obvious choice for diagnostic testing due to the risk of biopsy. Since the neuropathological changes in SDAT are most marked in the region of the angular and the inferior and middle temporal gyri, as well as the amygdala, hippocampus, and the parahippocampal gyri in the medial temporal region, one would especially look for changes in these regions (21). The CT scan is not useful in the specific diagnosis of SDAT but it is helpful in the detection of associated gross atrophic changes. The MRI, PET, and SPECT techniques are potentially capable of detecting physiological or metabolic changes in SDAT, but their use is still in the early stages of development.

Computed Tomography

Computed tomographic scans differentiate tissue by the absorption of x-ray photons. Images are usually obtained in axial sections with a spatial resolution of approximately 1 mm. Contributing to the strength of this modality are its fast scan time; superior contrast of hard to soft tissue, such as organically bound iodine; and the availability of radioopaque contrast-enhancing agents. The limitation of the CT scan is that contrast between soft tissues is significantly inferior to that of MRI. A CT scan is of the great value in indicating the absence of other dementing illnesses; it cannot be relied on to confirm the diagnosis of SDAT. Atrophy may be seen on CT to be dominant in the anterior and medial portions of the temporal lobes with widening of the suprasellar and adjacent cisterns, and with enlargement of the temporal horns of the lateral ventricles (22). The widening of the temporal horns occurs anteriorly and posteriorly, the latter resulting from the temporal lobe white matter atrophic changes as well as atrophy within the hippocampus. The widening of the sylvian fissures anteriorly in patients with SDAT is also seen in the aging brain, but is more prominent in SDAT. This, along with a greater degree of widening of the temporal horns, may help to differentiate SDAT from other dementia by CT, but generally this distinction is not possible. A CT scan reveals reduced density in the medial temporal lobe, anterior frontal lobe, and the head of the caudate in Alzheimer's disease (23).

Familial SDAT does have an earlier onset and may progress faster once symptoms develop. A CT scan may distinguish familial SDAT from other causes of dementia such as hydrocephalus, where there is not cortical atrophy, Creutzfelt-Jakob disease, which involves rapidly progressive atrophy, and Huntington's chorea, with basal ganglia involvement and atrophic changes in the anterior portion of the lateral ventricle and caudate nuclei. Postsubarachnoid hemorrhage due to aneurysm or arteriovenous malformation (AVM) is normally distinguishable due to extensive hemorrhaging and vascular predominance, respectively. Pick's disease involves the superior temporal gyrus and the frontal lobe, but early cases are difficult to differentiate from SDAT on the basis of CT scans alone.

Positron Emission Tomography

Positron emission tomography (PET) provides dynamic images of the brain's metabolism and permits study of the brain's chemistry in living beings. Used alone or as a complement to other imaging techniques, it may be the best technique presently available for obtaining a differential diagnosis, for early detection of the dementing disorders, and to further our understanding of normal aging and the underlying disease mechanisms in pathological conditions. The resolution of PET will always be poor compared with CT or MRI scanning, due to the distance traveled through tissue by emitted positrons before electron-positron annihilation. Most studies are directed at blood flow or energy metabolism measuring glucose or oxygen consumption (24).

The PET technique has been used with a labeled glucose analogue [^{18}F] 2-fluoro-2-deoxy-D-glucose (FDGL) to study glucose metabolism in dementia noninvasively (25).

Based on an autoradiographic technique developed by Sokoloff et al. (26), PET permits noninvasive in vivo assessments of cerebral metabolism and cerebral blood flow (CBF). It was first applied as an in vivo autoradiographic technique to measure the local cerebral metabolic rate for glucose LCMR-gl in humans using FDGL as the tracer (26). In order to assess the functional implications of age-related and disease-related neurochemical, morphometric, and anatomical decrements in SDAT and other dementias, tracers such as FDGL and oxygen 15 (^{15}O) have since been used to study CBF and cerebral metabolic rates in defined anatomic regions of interest. The brain accounts for about 25% of total body oxygen consumption at rest. Glucose and O_2 are the major substrates for brain oxidative metabolism. The cerebral metabolic rate of oxygen (CMR-O_2) and (CMR-glc), therefore, have been the principal in vivo "markers" of SDAT assessed in PET studies of brain function.

Cortical local cerebral metabolic rate for glucose (LCMR-gl), as calculated with PET, would appear to be far more revealing than MRI or CT scans of the pathological changes that take place in dementia. LCMR-gl is highly correlated with dementia, and also has a regional correlation with the type of psychological deficit present. Patients with SDAT showed significant hypometabolism and greater asymmetry than controls in the temporal, frontal, parietal, and occipital regions but not in the precentral gyrus, basal ganglia, thalamus, or cerebellum (27,28).

In studies of glucose metabolism, FDGL is used to determine LCMR-gl in various brain regions. Several studies have confirmed that the LCMR-gl is reduced in a number of cortical areas in senile dementia compared with age-matched controls (26).

In studies of oxygen metabolism and blood flow, correlation have been found between regional cerebral metabolic rate for oxygen. However, focal flow metabolism mismatches have been found in certain disease states, particularly stroke. Fracbkowick et al., using continuous inhalation of ^{15}O-labeled CO_2 and O_2, showed a highly similar decrease in CMR-O_2 with age in grey but not white matter in 14 normals aged 26-74 years (28). Previous studies of regional changes in cerebral blood flow or metabolism with radiopharmaceuticals have used one of several methods: xenon 133 or the positron emitter (FDGL to study the regional metabolism of glucose and [^{11}C] L-methionine to examine protein synthesis. The ^{133}Xe technique requires specialized imaging equipment if it is to be used for tomography, while the positron emitters require a cyclotron for production as well as dedicated imaging equipment. [^{125}I] isopropylamphetamine (IMP) requires only standard nuclear medicine imaging facilities (28). When used in measuring regional cerebral blood flow in patients with SDAT, IMP showed bilateral reduction in uptake in the temporoparietooccipital region. The IMP images of patients with multiple-infarct dementia varied from normal to marked focal deficits. In both Korsakoff's psychosis and Huntington's chorea the IMP uptake pattern and the NMR study were normal. Imaging with IMP is a sensitive indicator of cortical abnormality in SDAT; however, multiple-infarct dementia gives a similar radionuclide appearance. The differentiation between the two classes is improved by considering the radionuclide findings in tandem with the MRI findings (28).

Brain Metabolism in Normal Aging and Alzheimer's Disease

Changes that may accompany the normal aging process have been assessed in several cross-sectional studies of healthy individuals. As shown in studies using CBF and CMR-O_2, FDGL PET studies (29,30), and in several studies based on measurements of LCMR-gl (31,32), brain metabolism appears to be age-invariant. This age invariance persists despite morphological changes and neurochemical alterations that may occur with age, possibly because of compensatory processes in the brain (33). Three groups, however, have reported reduced CMR-O_2 in the elderly (34,35), although it is not clear that these studies were controlled for vascular atherosclerotic changes or hypertension, which may account for reduced cerebral metabolism. Several abnormalities were reported to be related to the severity of dementia and appear to correlate with regional cortical neuronal loss and glial proliferation (36). One group has reported that CMR-glc is low in even the early stages of SDAT, most prominently in the parietotemporal cortex. In multiple-infarct dementia (MID) it is reduced primarily in the small, multifocal infarcts (37). On the basis of prior work (30) and several reports discussed below (38-41), we have concluded that global whole-brain metabolism remains unchanged in patients with SDAT of mild severity, although there are regional metabolic changes in the perietal lobe. There are significant reductions throughout the brain in the later, more severe stages of the disease (see Fig. 1). The initial reductions in the parietal lobe precede neuropsychological changes.

Relation of CMRglc Measures to Neuropsychological Changes in Alzheimer's Disease

In patients with SDAT of varying degrees of severity, reductions in LCMR-gl occur primarily in the parietal, temporal, and frontal lobes (29,42-44). In mild SDAT, a change or reduction in LCMR-gl has been shown in the temporal lobe (34,42-45) or the parietal lobe (41). In the severe or late form of SDAT, the

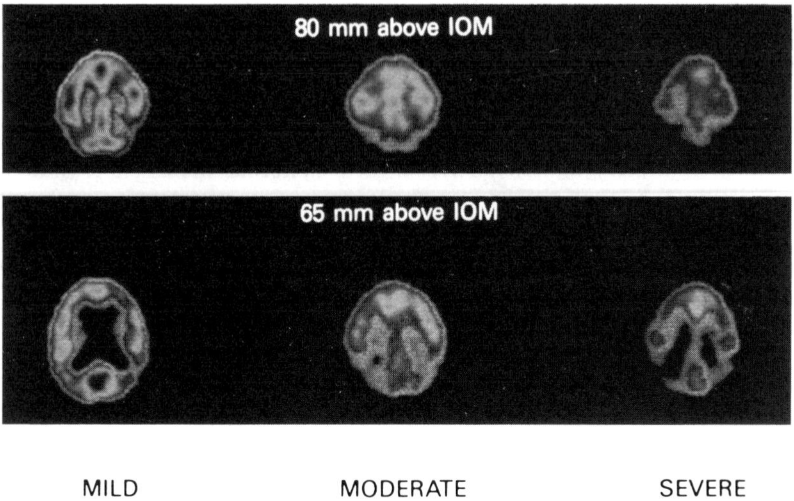

FIGURE 1 PET scans at the 80 and 65 mm level above the inferior orbitomeatal (IOM) line. Patients with presumptive Alzheimer's disease with mild, moderate, and severe forms of the disease are shown.

greatest reduction in metabolism was the frontal lobes, according to one report (44), although others have later shown metabolic decrements throughout the brain (22,44,46). Cutler and colleagues have found reductions primarily in the parietal lobe of patients with mild to moderate SDAT (41,47,48). It appears reasonable that among the parietal, temporal, and frontal lobes, different lobes may be affected more significantly at different stages of disease.

A recent study (30) evaluated PET measurements of LCMR-gl only and in comparison with the results of neuropsychological performance measures (49-52). The study included 50 vigorously selected subjects: 21 patients with SDAT and 29 controls. Neuropsychological and cognitive testing was done in patients with mild or moderate SDAT and, insofar as testing was possible, in those with severe SDAT. Compared with control subjects, the SDAT patients showed significantly impaired performance, including marked intellectual and memory dysfunction. The PET technique was used to evaluate LCMR-gl in the parietal, frontal, temporal, and occipital lobes. We initially found no significant reductions in lobar metabolism in the mild or moderate SDAT patients compared to controls, perhaps because of intersubject variation in LCMR-gl (+20-25%). In contrast, patients with severe SDAT showed significant decrements ($p<0.05$) in all but the occipital lobe (32). Normalizing LCMR-gl to the mean CMR-glc (LCMR-gl / sensorimotor CMR-glc.

at each of the four lobes) to increase the sensitivity of PET to smaller differences yielded significant coefficient variant deficits in the parietal lobes (52) in the mild to moderate SDAT group, and significant coefficient variant deficits in the parietal and temporal lobes in the severely affected group. As assessed by ratio analysis, therefore, intellectual deficit in even mild to moderate cases of SDAT is accompanied by selected changes in cortical LCMR-gl.

Based on comparisons of PET and psychological data, McGeer et al. (53) have shown that decrements in cortical LCMR-gl become more pronounced, and the number of cortical regions involved may increase, as SDAT progresses clinically. Indeed, Haxby and Rapoport (54) have delineated three areas in which metabolic alterations observed in patients with SDAT have been shown to be related to the severity of their associated neuropsychological deficits: (a) reduction in the CMR-glc of whole brain is related to the overall severity of dementia; (b) LCMR-gl shows relatively greater reductions in the association cortices than in the primary sensory and motor cortices, accounting for the preferential impairment of higher cognitive function in relation to sensory and motor function; (c) LCMR-gl in the association cortices shows a greater left-right asymmetry in SDAT patients than in controls. Several studies have shown that the reduction in CMR-glc observed in patients with mild to moderate SDAT is asymmetrical (38,39,54-57), and that this metabolic asymmetry correlates with asymmetries in neocortically mediated neuropsychological function (38,39,54,56). Both Foster et al. (56) and Haxby and Rapoport (54) report that greater metabolic asymmetry is reflected in increased neuropsychological impairment of language or visual-spatial function, depending on whether the lower LCMR is in the right or left cerebral hemisphere, respectively. Two studies in this area suggest a possible neurodiagnostic marker of SDAT. Haxby et al. (38) found a correlation between decrements in resting LCMR-gl in the parietal association cortex and increased left-right metabolic asymmetry in their patients with SDAT of moderate degree, but those with mild dementia who had the same metabolic deficit showed no neuropsychological deficit. Rapoport et al. (39) also reported and extended earlier reports (30,31,47,49) of LCMR-gl decrements in parietal lobe and left-right neocortical metabolic asymmetries in SDAT patients with mild dementia who had no measurable cognitive decrements; their patients with SDAT of moderate degree showed similar metabolic changes accompanied by corresponding language or visual-spatial deficit. The left-right metabolic asymmetries corresponded with reduced metabolic rates in homologous right and left regions, suggestive of functional disconnection of neocortical association areas. Autopsy findings showed correlation of these regions with those showing neuropathological changes typical of SDAT (39). These findings suggest that metabolic dysfunction measurable by PET in the association neocortex may foreshadow neuropsychological involvement.

Such a notion is consistent with our observations of a patient who had documented familial SDAT (31,47,49). This patient, who noticed the first signs of dementia 5 years ago, has undergone serial assessments of CMR-glc and cognitive function during the past 2-1/2 years. For the first 1-1/2 years, essentially no change was evident from severity scales and cognitive tests of parietal lobe function despite reductions in LCMR-gl, particularly in the parietal lobe, over the same period of time. Neuropsychological testing showed that both short-term and long-term memory were significantly impaired, but there were no changes in parietal lobe functions such as naming, arithmetic, or visual-spatial construction.

Work in this area and reports by other investigators suggest that PET measurements of LCMR-gl at the parietal lobe more sensitively indicate cognitive changes in SDAT than do neuropsychological or cognitive tests of function in this region (41). The apparently early presence of metabolic decrements in the parietal lobe, some time before testing identifies neuropsychological deficits, implies that there exists a "threshold" of metabolic deficit or damage to brain (40) that must be exceeded before individuals with SDAT can be identified on the basis of neuropsychological testing. With refinement, PET used in combination with neuropsychological measures may afford reliable assessments of specific alterations of cerebral function during the course of SDAT.

Neurotransmitter Systems

Using PET, it appears to be possible to assess the state of neurotransmitter receptors, including dopamine, serotonin, muscarinic cholinergic, opiate, and benzodiazepine receptors, in different regions of the brain (58). Moreover, PET can be used to trace neurotropic drugs in the biological system, providing information with which to correlate the physiological distribution with the effects of such drugs in the treatment of nervous or mental disorders such as SDAT (58). Determinations of the involvement, or lack of involvement, of various neurotransmitter systems in SDAT are being made with radiotracers and PET, and using a specific radiotracer of the cholinergic system with single-photon emission computed tomography (SPECT) (59). The MRI studies of the cholinergic system in SDAT are discussed below.

The PET studies of dopamine receptors with 3-N [^{11}C]methylspiperone have shown normal caudate/putamen uptake in SDAT patients (60,61), suggesting a lack of dopaminergic involvement in SDAT. However, the finding that a significant reduction in dopamine receptors occurs during the period between the ages of 19 and 73 years, and to a greater degree in men than in women (58), suggests the need for studies to determine its relevance to the development, or perhaps differential diagnosis, of SDAT.

In a study mentioned earlier (59), the degree to which somatostatin-like immunoreactivity was reduced from normal levels in the CSF of patients with SDAT correlated with a decline in cortical LCMR-gl as determined by PET, as well as indices of intellectual decline; a close association between reduced CSF levels of someatostatin and reductions in CMR-glc in the parietal lobe was found.

Preliminary data with SPECT obtained using radiotracers that indicate reduced uptake in the temporal parietal lobe, such as the cholinergic tracer [^{123}I]3-quinuclidinyl-4-iodobenzolate with SPECT, may suggest further work to develop this tracer as a potential marker for SDAT. Evaluations of other transmitter systems require the development of new radiotracers, and additional studies using the available tracers of neurotransmitter systems are needed to map regions of the brain affected in SDAT and to disclose identifiable patterns for the various dementias.

Methodologic Concerns and Perspectives on Future Research

Several factors may alter LCMR-gl in patients with SDAT. In studies of the cerebral metabolism, these variables must be identified to permit thoughtful assessments of the validity of results and their specificity to various types and stages of dementia, and to allow for replication of studies with potential in vivo markers. Principal factors to be considered are the health and mental status of subjects, the influence of the subject's mental status, and the influence of visual, auditory, and somatosensory stimuli.

The inclusion and selection of control subjects according to the appropriate criteria of age and health status are of critical importance. For subjects with SDAT, or the dementia under study, the diagnostic criteria, age of onset, duration of illness, health status, and degree of severity of the disorder must be reported.

Brain atrophy, which is an important factor in calculating metabolic values in the brain, could account for the differences found in both normal aging and dementia (60,61). Failure of PET to show metabolic changes in the cortical regions associated with memory could be the result of methodological limitations of the technique, such as limited spatial resolution, a partial voluming effect, or errors in reconstruction (62,63), all of which must be taken into account in the performance of any PET study.

A crucial methodological factor in assessing the specificity of a proposed marker is the postmortem confirmation of SDAT. Whether neuropathological evidence corroborates or refutes findings obtained with PET, this technique should clarify many cerebral metabolic patterns to help characterize the heterogeneous disease process of SDAT. In order to establish the specificity of PET methodology and potential metabolic markers for SDAT, the metabolic patterns in SDAT must be assessed in relation to that in other types of dementia. One study of multi-infarct dementia (MID) with PET showed focal and asymmetrical metabolic reductions (64). Another showed LCMR-gl to be impaired in the early stages of SDAT, particularly in the parietal temporal cortex, whereas in MID it was reduced principally in the multifocal small infarcts (40). Further studies in patients with MID, as well as Huntington's disease, Creutzfeldt-Jakob disease, and Down's syndrome, may accelerate the findings of or perhaps establish the differential diagnosis of these disease processes.

As the resolution of PET scans is refined and as radioactive tracers and activation studies (65) continue to be developed, in vivo evaluation of the human brain in normal and in pathological conditions holds promise for the differential diagnosis of the dementias and definition of the mechanisms responsible for them.

Single Photon Emission Computed Tomography

This technique presents difficulties in the reconstruction of a three-dimensional brain image. For reasons of counting efficiency, most commonly used SP isotopes produce softer radiation than the 511 Kev photons of PET. They are therefore subject to greater scattering even if pinhole collimation can establish the path of a detected photon. Most studies have been done using helmets with multiple detectors as the recording system. Analyses of radiation from relatively large areas of the brain are then performed. Alzheimer's patients show a reduction in cerebral blood flow in parietal and occipital regions (66).

The SPECT technique is relatively new, similar to nuclear magnetic imaging, and based on gamma ray emission. A gamma-emitting isotope is injected into a patient and the emitted gamma rays (proportional to the local concentration of the isotope) are detected by a movable gamma detector, the position of which is changed sequentially, the composite signals assembled by a computer, and the image then reconstructed. The spatial resolution of this technique is approximately 5 mm. The advantage of SPECT is that it makes use of more stable isotopes so that metabolic and physiological information similar to that obtained from PET is obtainable without high cost. The limitation, similar to PET, is its low spatial resolution. With the use of inhaled ^{133}Xe, SPECT evaluation of SDAT showed reduction in gray matter blood flow greater than seen with normal aging. Use of [^{123}I]isopropylamphetamine showed a reduction in the cerebral perfusion in both the parietal and occipital regions. The significance of these findings specifically to SDAT is not known. There is a clear pattern of reductions in cortical rCBF measured using [^{99}Tc]hexamethyl-propyleneamineoxime (^{99}Tc-HM-PAO) and a tomographic gamma camera (66).

Magnetic Resonance Imaging

Magnetic resonance imaging (MRI) is based on nuclear spin density, and two types of nuclear magnetic relaxation times known as T1 and T2. Protons or hydrogen atoms in a patient align themselves along the direction of the magnetic field when the patient is placed in a strong magnet. When an oscillating magnetic field of the same precession (Lamor) frequency is applied, they become perturbed and lose their initial alignment with the magnetic field. After the cessation of the applied radiofrequency (RF) oscillating magnetic field, the protons return to their original equilibrium position (relaxation) and induce oscillating current in the receiving coil during relaxation. These are detected by an RF receiver. The spatial coordinates of RF-signal-emitting protons are determined by the small difference in either frequency or phase of such signal caused by the application of linear magnetic field gradients in x, y, or z direction. Images are obtainable in multiple slices and in three orthogonal orientations (axial, sagittal, and coronal) or oblique orientations without moving the patient, and with variable emphasis of soft tissue contrast (67). The resolution of a typical MRI in a clinical setting is approximately 1 mm. The two types of relaxation time are the time constant for magnetic nuclei to return to equilibrium with their molecular environment after the RF pulse excitation (T1), and the time constant for magnetic nuclei to return to equilibrium with each other (T2) (68). T1 and T2 of hydrogen atom nuclei differ in different molecular environments. More liquid-like tissues produce longer relaxation times, while more solid-like tissues have shorter relaxation times. Various tissues can be identified on the basis of differences in the ranges of T1 and T2. However, there is enough overlap of values between some tissues that there is often a limitation in specificity. Elevated T1 relaxation values suggestive of increased water content in white matter have been found with MR. T1 values increase with severity of dementia. T1 values observed clinically will depend on several factors. In the first place, total water content and water structure may interact in a complex way: generally speaking, the more free water, the higher the T1. While free lipid protons have a lower T1 than water protons, membrane lipids and proteins are too structured to give observable signals, but influence observed T1 by structuring adjacent water molecules. By and large the T1 data represent the state of protons in water and free lipids. The proton density values predominantly represent the proton concentration of water and free lipids, so that two tissues that have very different water/fat ratios may have the same proton density but different T1 values (69). Areas of hypodensity in cerebral white matter on CT were especially well visualized in the T2-weighted MRI images. Hypodense areas were seen in the white matter of patients with vascular dementias but not in those with primary degenerative dementias. Thus the presence or absence of white matter changes may be an important factor in the differential diagnosis of vascular dementia and primary degenerative dementia (70). The strength of MRI lies in its superior contrast resolution in soft tissue imaging, its capability to image at least three slice orientations (some imagers have additional oblique orientations), and the absence of ionizing radiation (71). The current limitations of MRI, especially of proton MRI, include the relative lack of tissue specificity, long scan time, and some motion and other technical artifacts (72). The possibility of eliminating some or most of these deficiencies is very good in the near future. Spin lattice relaxation times (T1) and proton density (PD) values in proton nuclear magnetic resonance (NMR) permit SDAT and multi-infarct dementia to be differentiated. Even though MRI is very sensitive to demyelination and detection of early multiple sclerosis, there has not been an extensive MRI study on SDAT. Preliminary studies have been reported (73,74) showing changes similar to changes

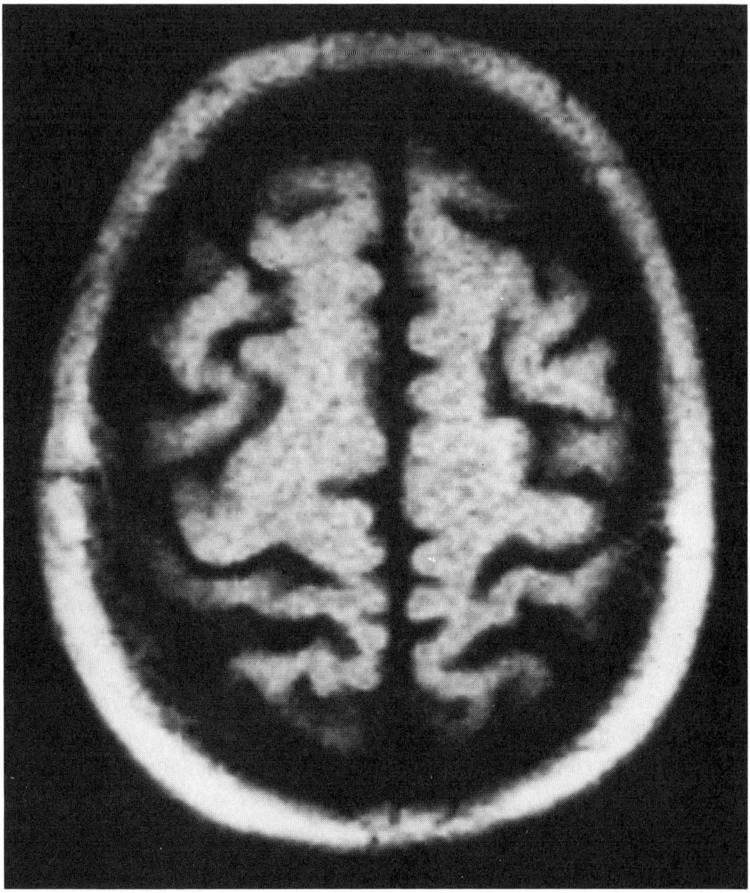

FIGURE 2 An MRI (1000/40) spin echo axial view through the cerebral cortex. The dark regions represent subarachnoid sulci filled with cerebral spinal fluid demonstrating moderate atrophic changes.

observed on CT, such as sulci widening, gyri shrinkage, and ventricular volume increase. Figures 1-5 illustrate some of these neuroanatomical and pathological features of SDAT observed with proton MRI at 0.5 Tesla. Work done at Aberdeen, Scotland, with several patients with presumed SDAT suggests that there are statistically significant differences in T1 and PD among normal, SDAT, and multi-infarct dementia (MID) patients (75). In a summarized and abbreviated form they are:

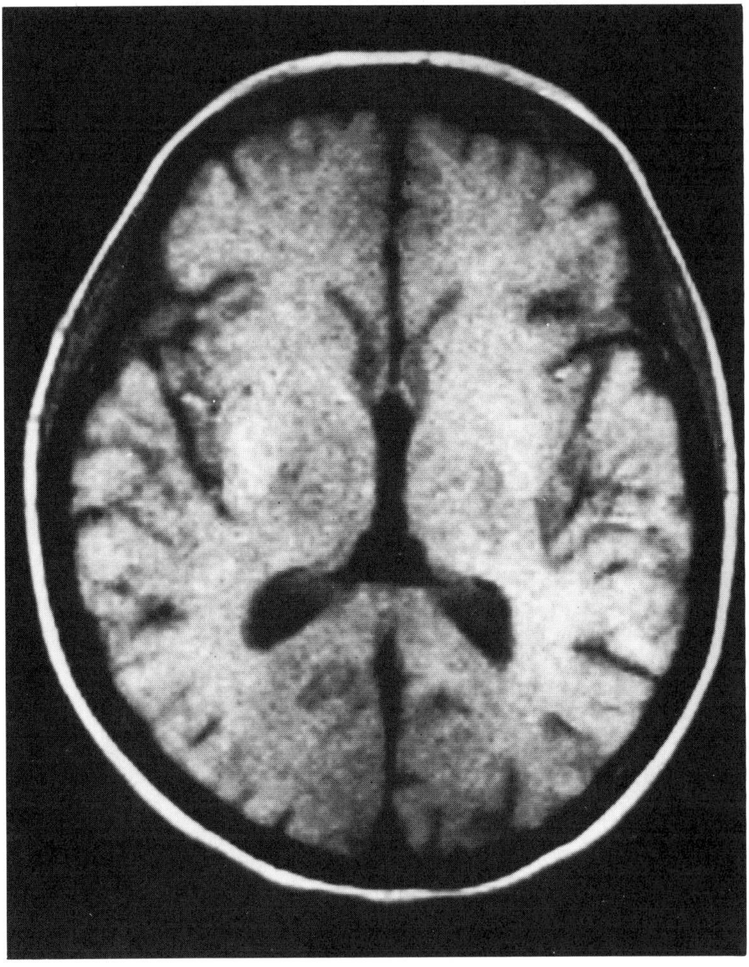

FIGURE 3 An MRI (1000/40) spin echo axial view. Mild dilatation of the third ventricle is present, probably representing parenchymal loss from the temporal lobes.

T1 (normal) < T1 (SDAT) < T1 (MID)
PD (normal) < PD (MID) < PD (SDAT)

Besson et al. related in vivo proton relaxation times measured by MRI and dementia. They reported that increases in T1 relaxation time (measured at 0.04 Tesla) in both cerebral gray and white matter were significantly related to severity of dementia, and could be used to identify patients with SDAT, vascular dementia, and

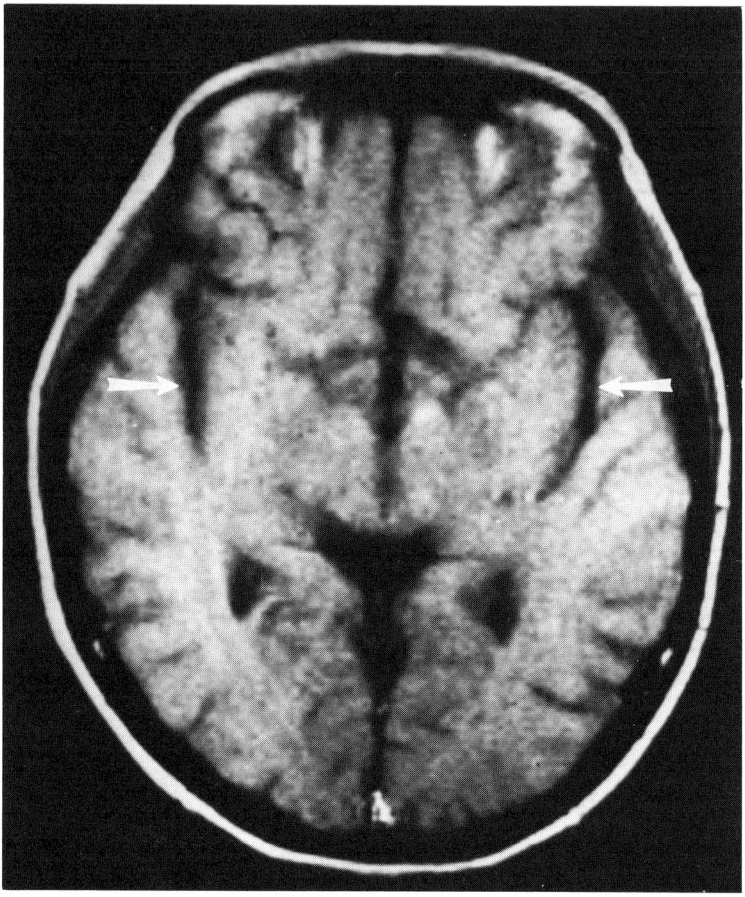

FIGURE 4 An MRI (1000/40) spin echo axial view. The prominent sylvian fissures (arrows) are filled with low-signal-intensity cerebral spinal fluid. This demonstrates bilateral temporal lobe atrophy.

normal nondemented control subjects. Magnetic resonance is superior to CT in displaying anatomical structures (such as the hippocampus and amygdala) that are affected in SDAT because differences in relaxation times are greater than differences in tissue density. Another advantage of MRI over CT is its superior ability to differentiate gray and white matter. Both MRI and CT are equivalent in detecting abnormalities in all four pairs of cortical brain regions, in subarachnoid spaces overlying these cortices, in basal ganglia, thalami, amygdalae, and posterior fossa. More abnormalities are detected on MRI than on CT images in subcortical

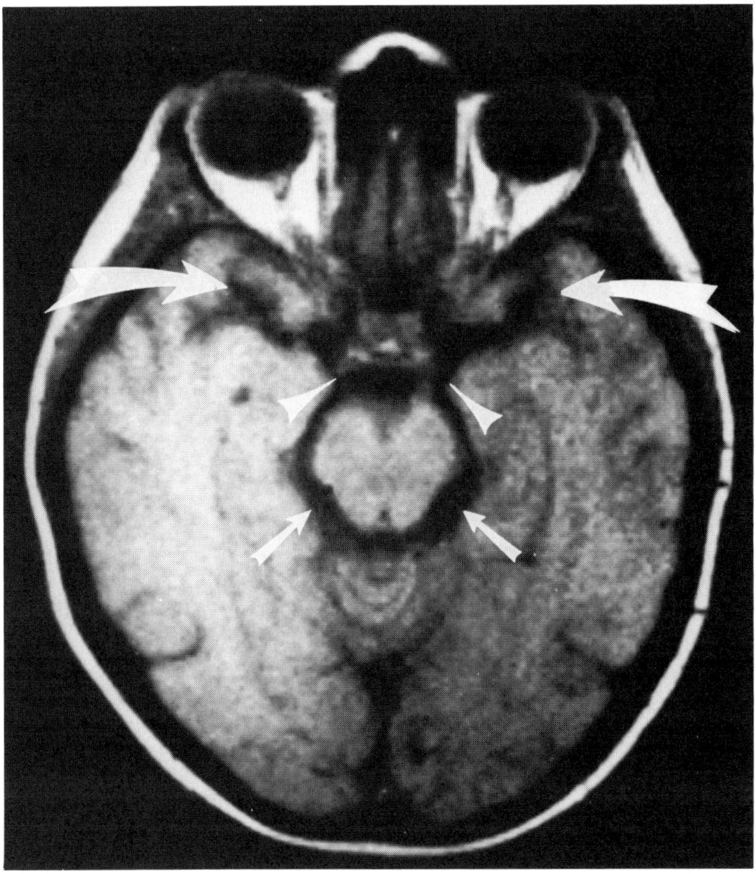

FIGURE 5 An MRI (1000/40) spin echo axial view. The perimesencephalic cistern (straight arrows) is prominant. There is also mild prominence of the suprasellar cistern (white arrowheads). Note the anterior temporal horns (curved white arrows).

periventricular white matter, hippocampus, sylvian fissures, and in lateral and third ventricles. The CT and MRI show equivalent linear measurements: qualitative ratings of lateral and third ventricle abnormality were greater for MR than for CT, suggesting that better tissue contrast and inclusion of coronal planes aid in the judgement of ventricular abnormality (75).

Despite these encouraging early results, other preliminary studies have not established any clear diagnostic advantages of proton MRI over CT, except for the former's multiplanar imaging and lack of ionizing radiation. It should be noted here that T1 values for a given tissue increase with increasing magnetic field but T2 values remain constant within the increasing magnetic field (76). Hence comparison of T1 values among imagers of different magnetic field strength has to be normalized. It is also known that T1 and T2 values computed from the pixel density have several error factors intrinsic to the technique (77). For this reason, general trends rather than absolute T1 and T2 values should be used.

RELATED NONINVASIVE TECHNOLOGY

Magnetic Resonance Spectroscopy

In analytical industrial chemistry, magnetic resonance spectroscopy (MRS) has been in use for many decades (78). An in vitro spectrometer typically used in an analytical laboratory uses small-bore vertical magnets of 1.5-7.1 Tesla, which are up to 14 times more powerful than many common imaging magnets. The variable for the preparation of chemical functional groups is the shift in the Lamor frequency or "chemical shift." In a molecular environment, each magnetic nucleus experiences the externally applied magnetic field through the local magnetic field induced by electrons in the nearby chemical bonding or nonbonding interactions (such as hydrogen bonding) (79). In a high-resolution analytical MRS, less than 0.1 parts per million (ppm) in frequency can be resolved so that functional groups such as CH3-, -CH2-, C=0, and -CH= can easily be differentiated. In addition each "chemically shifted" peak is further separated by spin-spin splittings from which the number of neighboring equivalent protons can be identified. Recently this analytical technique has been incorporated into in vivo spectrometers and spectrometer-imagers with the use of specialized receiving probes (or surface coils) (80). In addition to the proton ^{1}H, chemical shift imaging of ^{31}P, ^{23}Na, ^{19}F, and several other nuclei has been performed. The new generation of in vivo spectrometers or spectrometer-imagers uses either vertical or horizontal superconducting magnets and a medium-size bore to accomodate rabbits or small animals (dogs, pigs, etc.). Some commercial 1.5 Tesla MR imagers are equipped for limited-resolution in vivo spectroscopy but their usefulness in MRS diagnosis is yet to be established.

Many in vivo ^{31}P spectroscopy studies of metabolism, physiology, and pathology involving phosphates have been reported (81-83). Dynamic changes in relative concentration of inorganic phosphates, creatinine phosphates, sugar phosphates, phosphodiesters, and gamma-, alpha-, and beta-phosphate of ATP in several disease processes have been reported (84,85). Whether these higher field strength magnets will be safe and useful for determining biochemical changes in the brains of patients with SDAT remains to be determined.

Role of ^{31}P MRI in detecting alterations in phospholipid metabolism before an alteration in cellular structure becomes evident is questionable (86,87). Preliminary studies in SDAT have demonstrated elevated levels of phosphomonoesters and phosphodiesters in the areas of SDAT brain that exhibit neuropathological changes. Moreover, phosphomonoesters levels were also elevated in areas of SDAT brain that were devoid of neuropathological changes. These findings suggest that the phosphomonoester elevations in SDAT brain antedate changes in cellular morphology and structure. Abnormalities in protein kinase function could explain these findings, as well as the reported hyperphosphorylation of tau protein in SDAT brains. Recent studies from this laboratory suggest that aluminum could also be involved in the changes in phosphomonoesters and phosphodiesters (87,88).

Evoked Potentials

Evoked potentials, particularly the long latency event-related potentials, have been shown by several authors to be abnormal in demented subjects (89).

Patients with SDAT show abnormal visual-evoked potentials (90). SDAT disrupts the function of the central auditory nervous system as a result of temporal lobe pathological changes. Slow cortical and cognitive evoked potentials may be more sensitive to cortical auditory nervous system impairment in SDAT (91).

Biomagnetic Field Studies

Neuromagnetic studies may have a role in the future in the diagnosis of SDAT. Many sources of magnetically monitored alpha activity are located near or in the visual cortex and there are time series of the rhythm during periods of strong activity in which the oscillation period is constant and the magnetic field pattern remains stable. Biomagnetic measurements face the problem of environmental magnetic noise when applied to the weakest signals. Multiple SQUID sensors may act as a reference for subtracting a portion of this noise from the noisy signal itself (92).

In summary, gross anatomical changes in SDAT can be seen well by both CT and MRI, with MRI better able to delineate the differences in soft tissue contrast. Contributions to our understanding of abnormalities in brain metabolism and their relationship to SDAT should be expected in the future from multinuclear MRI, in vivo MRS, chemical shift imaging, PET, and SPECT.

REFERENCES

1. Friedland, R.P., Budinger, T.F., Koss, E., and Ober, B.A. (1985). Alzheimer's disease: Anterior-posterior and lateral hemisphere alterations in cortical glucose utilization. *Neurosci. Lett.* 53: 235-240.
2. Besson, J.A.O., Corrigan, F.M., Iljon Forman, E., Ashcroft, G.W., Eastwood, L.M., and Smith, F.M. (1983). Differentiating senile dementia of Alzheimer type and multi-infarct dementia by proton NMR imaging. *Lancet* 1:

3. Gemmel, H.G., Sharp, P.F., Evans, T.N.S., Besson, J.A.O., Lyall, D., and Smith, F.W. (1980). Single photon emission tomography with 1, 2, 3, I-isopropylamphetamine in Alzheimer's disease and multi-infarct dementia. *Arch. Neurol.* 37: 410-418.
4. Friedland, R.P., Budinger, T.F., Brand-Zawadzki, M., and Jaguest, W.J. (1984). The diagnosis of Alzheimer type dementia. *JAMA* 252: 2750-2752.
5. Chase, T.N., Foster, N.L., Feida, P., et al. (1984). Regional cortical dysfunction in Alzheimer's disease determined by positron emission tomography. *Ann. Neurol.* 15 (suppl): 5170-5174.
6. Alzheimer, A. (1907). *Allg. Z. Psychiatr. Grenzgeb* 64: 146-148.
7. Sajdel-Suldowska, E.M., and Marotta, C.A. (1984). Alzheimer's disease brain: Alterations in RNA levels and in a ribonnuclease-inhibitor complex. *Science* 225: 947-949.
8. Blessed, G., Tomlinson, B.E., and Roth, M. (1968). The association between quantitative measures of dementia and of senile change in the cerebral grey matter of elderly subjects. *Br. J. Psychiatry* 114: 797-811.
9. Gambetti, P., Shecket, G., Ghetti, B., Hirano, A., and Dahl, D. (1983). Neuro fibrillary changes in human brain, An immunocytochemical study with a neurofilament antiserum. *J. Neuropathol. Exp. Neurol.* 42: 69-79.
10. Bowen, D.M. (1983). Biochemical assessment of neurotransmitter and metabolic dysfunction and cerebral atrophy in Alzheimer's disease: Biological aspects of Alzheimer's disease. *Banbury Rep.* 15: 219-231.
11. Perl, D.P., and Brody, A.R. (1980). Alzheimer's disease: X-ray spectrometric evidence of aluminum accumulation in neurofibrillary tangle bearing neurons. *Science* 208: 297-299.
12. Glenner, G.G., and Wong, C.W. (1984). Alzheimer's disease: Initial report of the purification and characterization of a novel cerebrovascular amyloid protein. *Biochem. Biophys. Res. Commun.* 120: 885-890.
13. Davies, P., Katzman, R., and Terry, R.D. (1980). Reduced somatostatin like immunoactivity in cerebral cortex from cases of Alzheimer's disease and Alzheimer's senile dementia. *Nature* 228: 279-280.
14. Nikaido, T., Austin, J., Treub, L., et al. (1972). Studies in aging of the brain, II: Microchemical analyses of the nervous system in Alzheimer's patients. *Arch. Neurol.* 27: 548-554.
15. Crapper, D.R., Karlik, S., and deBoni, U. (1978). Aluminum and other metals in senile (Alzheimer's) dementia. In: *Alzheimer's Disease: Senile Dementia and Related Disorders*, vol. 7, R. Katzman, R.D. Terry and K.L. Bick (Eds.) pp. 471-487.
16. Brun, A., and Englund, E. (1986). Brain changes in dementia of Alzheimer's type relevant to new imaging diagnostic methods. *Prog. Neuropsychopharmacol. Biol. Psychiatry* 10: 297-308.
17. Miller, A.E., Neighbour, P.A., Katzman, R., Aaronson, M., and Lipkowitz, R. (1981). Immunological studies in senile dementia of the Alzheimer type: Evidence for enhanced supressor cell activity. *Ann. Neurol.* 10: 506-510.
18. Breenwald, B.S., Edasery, J., Mohs, R.C., Shah, N., Trigos, G.G., and Dan, K.L. (1985). Red blood cell choline: I. choline in Alzheimer's disease. *Biol. Psychiatry* 20: 367-374.

19. Wolozin, B.L., Pruchncki, A., Dikson, D.W., and Davies, P. (1986). A neuronal antigen in the brains of Alzheimer patients. *Science* 232: 648-650.
20. Ghui, H.C., Teng, E.L., Henderson, V.W., and Moy, A.C. (1985). Clinical subtypes of the Alzheimer type dementia. *Neurology* 35: 1544-1550.
21. LeMay, M. (1986). CT changes in dementing disease: A review. *Am. J. Neuroradiol.* 7: 841-853.
22. Friedland, R.P., Budinger, T.F., Brant-Zawadski, M., and Jagust, W.J. (1984). The diagnosis of Alzheimer-type dementia: A preliminary comparison of positron emission tomography and proton magnetic resonance. *JAMA* 252 (19): 2750-2752.
23. Benson, D.F. (1986). Neuroimaging and dementia. *Neurol. Clin.* 4(2): 341-353.
24. McGeer, P.L. (1986). Brain imaging in Alzheimer's disease. *Br. Med. Bull.* 42(1): 24-28.
25. Mcgeer, P.L., Kamo, H., Harrop, R., Li, D.K.B., Tuokko, H., McGeer, E.G., Adam, M.J., Ammann, W., et al. (1986). Positron emission tomography in patients with clinically diagnosed Alzheimer's disease. *Can. Med. Assoc. J.* 134: 597-607.
26. Sikoloff, L., Reivich, M., Kennedy, C., et al. (1977). The 14C-deoxyglucose method for the measurement of local cerebral glucose utilization: Theory, procedure and normal values in the conscious and anesthetized albino rat. *J. Neurochem.* 28: 897-916.
27. Luxenberg, J.S., May, C., Haxby, J.V., Grady, C., Moore, A., Berg, G., White, B.J., Robinette, D., and Rapoport, S.I. (1987). Cerebral metabolism, anatomy, and cognition in monozygotic twins discordant for dementia of the Alzheimer type. *J. Neurol. Neurosurg. Psychiatry* 50: 333-340.
28. Sharp, P., Gemmell, H., Cherryman, G., Besson, J., Crawford, T., and Smith, F. (1986). Application of iodine-123-labeled isopropylamphetamine imaging to the study of dementia. *J. Neurol. Med.* 27: 761-768.
29. Ferris, S.H., Deleon, M.H., Wolf, A.P., et al. (1983). Regional metabolism and cognitive deficits in aging and senile dementia. In: *Aging of the Brain*, Vol 22, D. Samuel, S. Algeri, S. Gershon, V.E. Grimm, and G. Toffano (Eds.) New York, Raven Press, pp. 133-142.
30. Cutler, N.R. (1986). Cerebral metabolism as measured with positron emission tomography (PET) and [18-F] 2-deoxy-d-glucose: Healthy aging, Alzheimer's disease and down syndrome. *Prog. Neuropsychopharmacol. Biol. Psychiatry* 10: 309-321.
31. Cutler, N.R., and Narang, P.K. (198X). Alzheimer's disease, dementia and Down syndrome: An evaluation using positron emission tomography (PET). *J. Mind Behav.* (in press).
32. Schlageter, N., Horowitz, B., Creasy, H., et al. (198X). Relation of measured brain glucose utilization and cerebral atrophy in man. *J. Neurol. Neurosurg. Psychiatry* (in press).
33. Buell, S.J., and Coleman, P.D. (1981). Quantitative evidence for selective dentritic growth in normal human aging but not in senile dementia. *Brain Res.* 21: 23-41.

34. Franckowiak, R.S., Lenzi, G.L., Jones, T., and Heather, J.D. (1980). Quantitative measurement of regional cerebral blood flow and oxygen metabolism in man using O-15 and positron emission tomography: theory, procedure and normal values. *J. Comput. Assist. Tomogr.* 4: 727-736.
35. Kuhl, D.E., Metter, E.J., Riege, W.H., and Phelps, M.E. (1982). Effects of human aging on patterns of local cerebral glucose utilization determined by the [18-F] fluorodeoxyglucose method. *J. Cereb. Blood Flow Metab.* 2: 163-171.
36. Frackowiak, R.S.J., Pozzillic, C., Legg, N.J., Doboulay, G.H., Marshall, J., Lenzi, G.L., and Jones, T. (1981). Regional cerebral oxygen supply and utilization in dementia: A clinical and psychological study with oxygen-15 and positron tomography. *Brain* 104: 752-778.
37. Heiss, W.D., Herholz, K., Pawlik, G., Wagner, R., and Wienhard, K. (1986). Positron emission tomography in neuropsychology. *Neuropsychologia* 24: 141-149.
38. Haxby, J.V., Grady, C.L., Duara, R., Schlageter, N., Berg, G., and Rapoport, S.I. (1986). Neocortical metabolic abnormalities precede nonmemory cognitive defects in early Alzheimer's type dementia. *Arch. Neurol.* 43: 882-885.
39. Rapoport, S.I., Horwirz, B., Haxby, J.V., and Grady, C.L. (1986). Alzheimer's disease: Metabolic uncoupling of associative brain regions. *Can. J. Neurol. Sci.* 13: (4 Suppl): 540-545.
40. Roth, M., Tomlinson, B.E., and Blessed, G. (1966). Correlation between scores for dementia and counts of 'senile plaques' in cerebral grey matter of elderly subjects. *Nature* 209: 109-110.
41. Cutler, N.R., Haxby, J.V., Duara, R., et al. (1985). Clinical history, brain metabolism and neuropsychological function in Alzheimer's disease. *Ann. Neurol.* 18: 298-309.
42. McGeer, P.L., McGeer, E.G., Kamo, H., and Wong, K. (1986). Positron emission tomography and the possible origins of cytopathology of Alzheimer's disease. *Prog. Neuropsychopharmacol. Biol. Psychiatry* 10: 501-518.
43. Farkas, T., Ferris, S.H., Wolf, A.P., DeLeon, M.J., et al. (1982). 18-F-2-deoxy-2-fluoro-d-glucose as a tracer in the positron tomographic study of senile demential. *Am. J. Psychiatry* 139: 352-353.
44. Frackowiak, R.S.J., Pozzilli, C., Legg, N.J., et al. (1981). Regional cerebral oxygen supply and utilization in dementia: A clinical and psychological study with oxygen-15 and positron tomography. *Brain* 104: 753-778.
45. Foster, N.L., Chase, T.N., Mansi, L., et al. (1984). Cortical abnormalities in Alzheimer's disease. *Ann. Neurol.* 16: 649-654.
46. McGeer, P.L., Kamo, H., Harrop, R., et al. (1986). Positron emission tomography in patients with clinically diagnosed Alzheimer's disease. *Can. Med. Assoc. J.* 134: 597-607.
47. Cutler, N.R., Haxby, J.V., Duara, R., et al. (1985). Brain metabolism as measured with positron emission tomography: Serial assessment in a patient with familial Alzheimer's disease. *Neurology* 35: 1556-1561.
48. Cutler, N.R., Heston, L.L., Davies, P., Haxby, J.V., and Schapiro, M.B. (1985). Alzheimer's disease and Down syndrome: New insights. *Ann. Intern. Med.* 103: 566-578.

49. Cutler, N.R. (1985). Alzheimer's disease and Down's syndrome: New insights. *Ann. Intern. Med.* 103: 566-578.
50. Cutler, N.R., Duara, R., Grady, C.L., Haxby, J.L., Kessler, R., and Rapoport, S.I. (1984). Brain metabolism and neuropsychology in Alzheimer's dementia (abstr.). *Neurology* 34 (Suppl 1): 101.
51. Cutler, N.R., and Schapiro, M.B. (1984). Brain metabolism as measured with positron emission tomography: Alzheimer's disease and Down syndrome. *Clin. Neuropharmacol.* 7 (Suppl 1): S177-S178.
52. Duara, R., Grady, C., Haxby, J., et al. (1986). Positron emission tomography in Alzheimer's disease. *Neurology* 36: 879-887.
53. McGeer, E.G., McGeer, P.L., Kamo, H., Tago, H., and Harrop, R. (1986). Cortical metabolism, acetylcholinesterase staining and pathological changes in Alzheimer's disease. *Can. J. Neurol. Sci.* 13 (4 Suppl): 511-516.
54. Haxby, J.V., and Rapoport, S.I. (1986). Abnormalities of regional brain metabolism in Alzheimer's disease and their relation to functional impairment. *Prog. Neuropsychopharmacol. Biol. Psychiatry* 10: 427-438.
55. Foster, N.L., Chase, T.N., Fedio, P., Patronas, N.J., Brooks, R.A., and DiChiro, G. (1983). Alzheimer's disease: Focal changes shown by positron emission tomography. *Neurology* 33: 961-965.
56. Foster, N.L., Chase, T.N., Patronas, N.J., Gillespie, M.M., and Fedio, P. (1986). Cerebral mapping of apraxia in Alzheimer's disease by positron emission tomography. *Ann. Neurol.* 19: 139-143.
57. Rapoport, S.I. (1986). Positron emission tomography in normal aging and Alzheimer's disease. *Gerontology* 32 (Suppl 1): 6-13.
58. Wagner, H.N. Jr. (1986). Quantitative imaging of neuroreceptors in the living human brain. *Semin. Nucl. Med.* 16: 51-62.
59. Tamminga, C.A., Foster, N.L., Fedio, P., Bird, E.D., and Chase, T.N. (1987). Alzheimer's disease: Low cerebral somatostatin levels correlate with impaired cognitive function and cortical metabolism. *Neurology* 37: 161-165.
60. Holman, B.L., Gibson, R.E., Hill, T.C., et al. (1985). Muscarinic acetylcholine receptors in Alzheimer's disease. In vivo imaging with iodine-123-labeled 3-quinuclidinyl-4-iodobenzolate and emission tomography. *JAMA* 254: 3063-3066.
61. Miatto, O., Gonzalez, R.G., Buonanno, F., and Growdon, J.H. (1986). In vitro 31-P NMR spectroscopy detects altered phospholipid metabolism in Alzheimer's disease. *Can. J. Neurol. Sci.* 13 (suppl): 535-539.
62. Inoue, Y., Wagner, J.R., Wong, D.F., et al. (1985). Atlas of dopamine receptor images (PET) of the human brain. *J. Comput. Assist. Tomogr.* 9: 129-140.
63. Hersovitch, P., Gado, M., Minton, M.A., and Raichle, M.E. (1984). The necessity for correcting for cerebral atrophy in global positron emission tomography measurements (monogr). *Neural. Sci.* 11: 93-97.
64. Herscovitch, P., Auchus, A.P., Gado, M., Chi, D., and Raichle, M.E. (1986). Correction of positron emission tomography data for cerebral atrophy. *J. Cereb. Blood Flow Metab.* 6: 120-124.
65. Hoffman, E.J., Huang, S.C., and Phelps, M.E. (1979). Quantitation in positron emission computed tomography. 1. Effect of object size. *J. Comput. Assist. Tomogr.* 3: 299-308.

66. Mazziotta, J.C., Phelps, M.E., Plummer, D., and Kuhl, D.E. (1981). Quantitation in positron emission computed tomography. 5. Physical-anatomical effects. *J. Comput. Assist. Tomogr.* 5. 734-743.
67. Benson, D.F., Kuhl, D.E., Hawkins, R.A., Phelps, M.E., Cummings, J.L., and Tsai, S.Y. (1983). The fluorodeoxyglucose 18-F scan in Alzheimer's disease and multi-infarct dementia. *Arch. Neurol.* 40: 711-713.
68. Ginsberg, M.D., Yoshii, F., Vibulsresth, S., Chang, J.Y., Duara, R., and Barker, W.W. (1986). Task-specific somatosensory activation of cerebral metabolism in man. *Neurology* 36 (Suppl 1): 281.
69. Besson, J.A.O., Corrigan, F.M., Foreman, E.I., Eastwood, L.M., Smith, F.W., and Ashcroft, G.W. (1985). Nuclear magnetic resonance (NMR). *Br. J. Psychiatry* 146: 31-35.
70. Erkinjuntti, T., Sipponen, J.T., Iivananien, M., Ketonen, L., Sulkava, R., and Sepponen, R.E. (1984). Cerebral NMR and CT imaging in dementia. *J. Comput. Assist. Tomogr.* 8(4): 614-618.
71. Yamaguchi, F., Meyer, J.S., Yamamoto, M., Sakai, F., and Show, T. (1980). Noninvasive regional cerebral flow measurements in dementia. *Arch. Neurol.* 37: 410-418.
72. Felder, R.C., and Parker, J.A. (1985). Principles of nuclear magnetic resonance imaging. *Med. Instrum.* 19: 248-255.
73. Mansfield, P., and Morris, P.G. (1982). *NMR Imaging in Biomedicine.* New York, Academic Press.
74. Edalman, R.R., and Brady, T. 91985). Clinical applications of magnetic resonance imaging. *Med. Instrument.* 19: 257-260.
75. Johnson, K.A., Davis, K.R., Buonanno, F.S., Brady, T.J., Rosen, J., and Growdon, J.H. (1987). Comparison of magnetic resonance and roentgen ray computed tomography in dementia. *Arch. Neurol.* 44: 1075-1080.
76. Yamanashi, W.S., Wheatley, K.K., Lester, P.D., and Anderson, D.W. (1984). Technical artifacts in magnetic resonance imaging. *Physiol. Chem. Phys.* 16: 237-250.
77. Friedland, R.P., Budinger, T.F., Brant-Zawadzki, M.B., and Jaqust, W. (1984). The diagnosis of Alzheimer type dementia. *JAMA* 252: 2748-2752.
78. Brady, W.G., Waluch, V., and Brant-Zawadzki, M. (1984). Patchy preventicular white matter lesions in the elderly: A common observation during NMR imaging. *Noninvas. Med. Imaging* 1: 35-41.
79. Bottomley, P.A., Foster, T.H., Argersinger, R.E., and Pfeifer, L.M. (1984). A review of normal tissue hydrogen NMR relaxation times and relaxation mechanisms from 1-100 MHz: Dependence on tissue, type NMR frequency, temperature species, excision and age. *Med. Phys.* 11: 425-448.
80. Anderson, D.W., Yamanashi, W.S., Ross-Duggan, J.D., Lester, P.D., Harns, S.E., Chan, W.K., Suss, R.A., and Shenoy, R. (1986). Pixel intensity and contrast values as functions of relaxation times and pulse intervals in several commercial MR images. Society of Magnetic Resonance Imaging 4th Annual Meeting, Philadelphia, Pennsylvania, March 1-5.
81. Slichter, C.P. (1963). *Principles of Magnetic Resonance.* New York, Harper & Row.

82. Carrington, A., and McLachlan, A.D. (1967). *Introduction to Magnetic Resonance.* New York, Harper & Row.
83. Gadian, D.G. (1982). *Nuclear Magnetic Resonance and its Application to Living Systems.* Oxford, Clarendon Press.
84. Bottomley, P.A. (1985). Towards clinical 31P spectroscopic imaging. Society of Magnetic Resonance Imaging 4th Annual Meeting, London, August 19-23. Abstract 1: 125-126.
85. Gyulai, L., Schnall, M., Leigh, J., Chance, B., and McLaughlin, A. (1985). Simultaneous determination of lactate and phosphocreatine in the cat brain. 4th Annual Meeting of the Society of Magnetic Resonance in Medicine, London, August 11-23.
86. Besson, J.A.O., Corrigan, F.M., Foreman, E.I., Ashcroft, G.W., Eastwood, L.M., and Smith, F.W. (1983). Differentiating senile dementia of Alzheimer type and multi-infarct dementia by proton NMR imaging. *Lancet* 2: 789.
87. Pettegrew, J.W., Withers, G., Panchalingam, K., and Post, J.F.M. (1987). P nuclear magnetic resonance (NMR) spectroscopy of brain in aging and Alzheimer's disease. *J. Neural. Transm.* 24: 261-268.
88. Greon, J.P., Arnold, D.A., Balerianx, D., and denHollander, J.A. (1986). 31P MR localized spectroscopy of the human brain *in situ* at 1.5 Tesla. 5th Annual Meeting of the Society of Magnetic Resonance, Montreal, Quebec, August 19-22. Abstract 3: 1083-1084.
89. Goodin, D.S. (1986). Event-related (endogenous) potentials. In: *Electrodiagnosis in Clinical Neurology*, 2nd ed, M.J. Aminoff (Ed.) New York, Churchill Livingstone, pp. 575-595.
90. Sadun, A.A., Borchert, M., DeVita, E., Hinton, D.R., and Bassi, C.J. (1987). Assessment of visual impairment in patients with Alzheimer's disease. *Am. J. Ophthalmol.* 104: 113-120.
91. Grimes, A.M., Grady, C.L., and Pijus, A. (1986). Auditory evoked potentials in patients with dementia of the Alzheimer type. *Ear Hearing* 8 (3): 157-161.
92. Atsumi, K., Katila, T., Kotani, M., Williamson, S.J., and Ueno, S. (1987). Tokyo Denki University Press. New method for the study of spontaneous brain activity. In: Biomagnetism 1987, Proceedings of the 6th International Conference on Biomagnetism.

20

Evidence for Altered Neuronal Binding of [^{3}H] Nitrendipine in Dimentia

ROBERT A. COLVIN, RICHARD G. WILLIAMS, DONALD T. EAGLE, RICHARD A. ALLEN, JOSEPH A. OIBO, and IBOK IBOK / *Oral Roberts University, School of Medicine, Tulsa, Oklahoma*

GARY D. MINER / *Familial Alzheimer's Disease Research Foundation, Tulsa, Oklahoma*

Alzheimer's disease (AD) is a degenerative disorder of the human central nervous system characterized by progressive impairment of memory and intellectual function beginning in middle to late adult life (1). No treatment that is effective in preventing or arresting the neurodegenerative process of AD has yet been discovered. Three major areas of AD research can be identified: (a) experiments leading to a complete understanding of the pathomechanism underlying AD, (b) development of a test that can screen and detect patients who are entirely asymptomatic but who will develop the disease later, and (c) once the disease is detected, a method of stopping its progression. For those individuals who already have the disease, a rehabilitative treatment must be found.

The major morphological changes that occur in AD brains include, but are not limited to cortical atrophy and loss of neurons, and formation of neurofibrillary tangles and senile plaques. Although the extent of these changes varies, they occur in all cases of AD (1). It is now thought that senile plaque formation is the result of increased amyloid deposition in the brain (amyloidosis). The clinical symptoms of dementia are the result of the loss of neurons and neuronal function. However, the relationship between neuronal death and senile plaque formation is not well understood. A central unanswered question in AD research is whether amyloidosis is the primary event leading to neuronal disease and death or is an epiphenomenon occurring in association with neuronal death and damage.

To understand more completely the pathomechanism of AD we have chosen to investigate the potential role that calcium may play in the disease process. Recent evidence suggests that AD may be a systemic disease of altered calcium metabolism

(3-10), with the most prominent pathological changes seen in the central nervous system. Studies have shown that the total and intracellular calcium content of cultured skin fibroblasts from Alzheimer's donors is increased compared to age-matched controls (5). Furthermore, microprobe analysis has shown that only aluminum and calcium levels in the brain are consistently increased in relationship to the lesions associated with AD (11).

These findings have led us to investigate cellular mechanisms that control calcium homeostasis and that may be altered in AD. One of the most important pathways for the entry of calcium into the cell, particularly in neurons, is the voltage-sensitive calcium channel of the plasma membrane (17). This channel protein is characterized in receptor binding studies by a high-affinity binding site for 1,4-dihydropyridine calcium antagonists (12). In the present studies we have determined the binding characteristics of the radiolabeled 1,4-dihydropyridine $[^3H]$nitrenpidine in the brains of control, AD, and patients with non-Alzheimer's dementia.

MATERIALS AND METHODS

Sections from the frontal cortex and temporal cortex/hippocampus region of human brains were obtained from the National Neurological Research Bank (NNRB) in Los Angeles. The sections were classified into the following three categories: those from nondemented control patients, those from patients who had a non-Alzheimer's dementia, and those from patients with AD. The control and non-Alzheimer's dementia brains were age-matched with the Alzheimer's brains. Table 1 lists the mean age at death and autolysis times for the brain samples used in this study. Frozen brain sections (−80°C) were thawed and the

Table 1 Average Age and Autolysis Times for Brain Samples Used in this Study (Values are mean ± standard deviation)

	N	Age (yrs)	Autolysis Time (hr)
Control			
Frontal cortex	5	67.2 ± 6.1	17.6 ± 6.4
Temporal/hippocampus	7	71.6 ± 9.2	16.0 ± 6.2
Alzheimer's disease			
Frontal cortex	6	75.8 ± 5.4	16.4 ± 7.3
Temporal/hippocampus	7	75.1 ± 5.3	15.8 ± 6.9
Non-Alzheimer's Dementia			
Frontal cortex	4	75.8 ± 9.7	8.75 ± 4.0
Temporal/hippocampus	4	75.8 ± 9.7	8.75 ± 4.0

tissue was rapidly dissected in an ice bath. Homogenization of the tissue was performed in 20 volumes of a buffer containing 0.32 M sucrose and 10 mM HEPES at pH 7.4, using the Brinkman Polytron homogenizer at a setting of 4 (10 sec, repeated three to four times). The homogenate was then centrifuged at 1000 × g for 10 min. The resulting supernatant fluid was removed and centrifuged at 17,000 × g for 20 min. The pellet (containing membrane fragments) was recovered and resuspended in a "brain buffer" containing 132 mM NaCl, 5mM KCl, 1.3 mM $MgCl_2$, 1.2 mM $CaCl_2$, 10 mM glucose, and 25 mM tris-HCl with a pH of 7.4. Membrane preparations were stored at −80°C until used for a binding assay.

Binding assays were performed in tubes containing a total of 0.2 mg in 5 ml brain buffer, together with increasing concentrations of [^{3}H]nitrendipine (0.1-1.0 nM). Nonspecific binding was defined as the amount of binding obtained in the presence of 1.0 μM nonradioactive nimodipine. The samples were incubated for 90 min at 37°C. Binding reactions were terminated by rapid filtration on the Brandel M-24RP cell harvester filtration system; the filters were rinsed twice with 5 ml of a 50 mM tris-HCl buffer (pH 7.4). Radioactivity trapped on filters was determined by liquid scintillation spectrophotometry. Computer-generated linear least-squares analysis of Scatchard plots of bound [^{3}H]nitrendipine vs. bound/free were obtained to determine the maximal number of binding sites (B_{max}) as well as the equilibrium dissociation constant (K_d) for the ligand.

RESULTS

Table 2 shows cumulative data obtained from Scatchard analysis of saturation isotherms of [^{3}H]nitrendipine binding. The fact that Scatchard plots were linear strongly suggests that [^{3}H]nitrendipine bound to a single class of binding sites in control, AD, and non-Alzheimer's dementia brains. The frontal cortex and temporal/hippocampal regions of control human brain had very similar binding characteristics. The K_d obtained for both regions was 0.642 ± 0.191 and 0.686 ± 0.181 nM, respectively, while the B_{max} was estimated to be 0.133 ± 0.287 and 0.141 ± 0.0217 pmol/mg, respectively (see Table 2). The results obtained in the present study for control brains are very similar to previous data obtained from fresh or autopsy human brain tissues (12-14).

Both AD and non-Alzheimer's dementia brains showed no significant changes in the apparent K_d and B_{max} determined in both the frontal cortex and temporal/hippocampal brain regions (see Table 2). These data suggest that most probably neither the density of calcium channels nor the affinity of the 1,4-dihydropyridine binding site is affected by AD or non-Alzheimer's dementia.

DISCUSSION AND CONCLUSIONS

The present findings demonstrate no change in the apparent K_d and B_{max} estimated for [^{3}H]nitrendipine binding to brain calcium channels in both AD and

TABLE 2 Kinetic Constants Determined for Brain Samples Used in This Study (Values are mean ± standard deviation)

	N	K_d (nM)	B_{max} (pmol/mg)
Control			
Frontal cortex	5	0.642 ± 0.212	0.133 ± 0.0287
Temporal/hippocampus	7	0.686 ± 0.181	0.141 ± 0.0217
Alzheimer's Disease			
Frontal cortex	6	0.672 ± 0.300	0.134 ± 0.0360
Temporal/hippocampus	7	0.939 ± 0.572	0.123 ± 0.0375
Non-Alzheimer's Dementia			
Frontal cortex	4	0.810 ± 0.166	0.124 ± 0.0243
Temporal/hippocampus	4	0.804 ± 0.210	0.134 ± 0.0377

non-Alzheimer's dementia. One previous study (15) has shown reduced affinity of [^{3}H] nitrendipine and reduced sensitivity to calcium (calcium normally enhances binding of [^{3}H]-nitrendipine [16]) of cortical membranes of aging rats. Although the reduction in [^{3}H] nitrendipine binding affinity may be a phenomenon of aging in human brain as well, the present findings indicate that if this reduction does occur, it occurs to the same degree in control, AD, and non-Alzheimer's dementia.

Although the functional nature of the 1,4-dihydropyridine binding site and the voltage-sensitive calcium channel (12,17) is still unclear, it is interesting to speculate that altered calcium transport across the plasma membrane may exist in dementia as a result of altered calcium channel function. Derangements in calcium transport of this sort could result in alterations in neurotransmitter storage and release, nerve impulse conduction, assembly and maintenance of neurofilaments, protein phosphorylation, and could conceivably lead to cell death in severe cases. It is also interesting to speculate on a possible link between calcium and aluminum. Calcium and aluminum bind to similar proteins (e.g., both bind to calmodulin [18]). It is probable that changes in calcium metabolism would subsequently alter the way the cell handles aluminum, perhaps allowing aluminum to accumulate in the cytoplasm or key organelles, leading to derangements in cell function, neurofibrillary tangle and senile plaque formation, and eventual cell death.

Preliminary therapeutic trials using nimodipine have been attempted in AD with limited success. In light of the present study, one can conclude that the beneficial effect obtained with dihydropyridine calcium antagonists may result from its indirect actions of this drug. Although in this study we failed to identify a site of derangement in neuronal cell metabolism, it is important to note the limitations of this study. The dihydropyridine binding site is an allosteric site on the channel protein. It is now recognized that the calcium channel is a subunit structure and that this structure is required for its normal functioning (19). It is therefore possible that despite the dihydropyridine binding site being kinetically the same, channel function could be severely affected by AD and dementia in general. More extensive studies of neuronal calcium metabolism will be required before any conclusions can be made.

REFERENCES

1. Katzman, R. (1986). Alzheimer's disease. *N. Engl. J. Med.* 314: 964-973.
2. Peterson, C., Ratan, R.R., Shelanski, M.L., and Goldman, J.E. (1988). Altered response of fibroblasts from aged and Alzheimer donors to drugs that elevate cytosolic free calcium. *Neurobiol. Aging* 9: 261-266.
3. Peterson, C., Gibson, G.E., and Blass, J.P. (1986). Altered calcium uptake in cultured skin fibroblasts from patients with Alzheimer's disease. *N. Engl. J. Med.* 312: 1063-1065.
4. Deary, I.J., and Hendrickson, A.E. (1986). Calcium and Alzheimer's disease. *Lancet* 1: 1219.
5. Peterson, C., and Goldman, J.E. (1986). Alterations in calcium content and biochemical processes in cultured skin fibroblasts from aged and Alzheimer donors. *Proc. Natl. Acad. Sci. USA* 83: 2758-2762.
6. Gibson, G.E., and Peterson, C. (1986). Considerations of neurotransmitters and calcium metabolism in therapeutic design. In: *Treatment Development Strategies for Alzheimer's and Parkinson's Disease*, Crook, T., Bartus, R., Ferris, S., Gershon, S. (Eds.). Madison CT, Mark Powley Associates, pp. 499-517.
7. Blass, J., Baker, A., Balin, A., Barclay, L., Gibson, G., Peterson, C., and Sims, N. (1986). Biological markers for Alzheimer's disease. In: *Alzheimer's and Parkinson's: Strategies for Research and Development*, A. Fisher, I. Hanin, and C. Lachman (Eds.). New York, Plenum, pp. 299-308.
8. West, R.D. (1985). Aluminosilicates and Alzheimer's disease. *Lancet* 2: 682.
9. Crapper-McLachlan, D.R., Wong, L., Bergeron, C., and Bambridge, K.G. (1987). Calmodulin and calbindin D_{28k} in Alzheimer disease. *Alzheimers Dis. Assoc. Disord.* 1: 171-179.
10. Zubenko, G.S., Wusylko, M., Cohen, B.M., Boller, F., Teply, I. (1987). Family study of platelet membrane fluidity in Alzheimer's disease. *Science* 238: 539-542.
11. Perl, D.P. (1986). The aluminum hypothesis of Alzheimer's disease: A personal view based on microprobe analysis. *Neurobiol. Aging* 7: 550-552.
12. Janis, R.A., Silver, P.J., and Triggle, D.J. (1987). Drug action and cellular calcium regulation. *Adv. Drug Res.* 16: 309-591.
13. Hanada, S., and Tanaka, C. (1985). Regional distribution of [^{3}H]-nitrendipine binding in human brain. *Neurosci. Lett.* 58: 375-380.

14. Quirion, R., Lal, S., Olivier, A., Robitaille, Y., Vassavannar, N.P., Ford, R. M., and Stratford, J.G. (1988). Calcium channel binding sites in human brain. *Proc. N.Y. Acad. Sci.* 522: 203-206.
15. Giovoni, S., Rivs, R.A., Battaini, F., Fianchi, A., and Trabucchi, M. (1985). Age-related reduced affinity in [^{3}H]-nitrendipine labeling of brain voltage-dependent calcium channels. *Brain Res.* 333: 374-377.
16. Luchowski, E.M., Yousif, F., Triggle, D.J., Maurer, S.C., Sarmiento, J.G., and Janis, R.A. (1984). Effects of metal cations and calmodulin antagonists of [^{3}H]-nitrendipine binding in smooth and cardiac muscle. *J. Pharmacol. Exp. Ther.* 230: 607-613.
17. Miller, R.J. (1987). Multiple calcium channels and neuronal function. *Science* 235: 46-52.
18. Seigle, N., and Haug, A. (1983). Aluminum interactions with calmodulin; evidence for altered structure and function from optical and enzymatic studies. *Biochim. Biophys. Acta* 744: 36-45.
19. Ellis, S.B., Williams, M.E., Ways, N.R., Brenner, R., Sharp, A.H., Leung, A. T., Campbell, K.P., McKenna, E., Koch, W.J., Hui, A., Schwartz, A., and Harpold, M.M. (1988). Sequence and expression of mRNAs encoding the α_1 and α_2 subunits of a DHP-sensitive calcium channel. *Science* 241: 1661-1664.

21

The IMAGE Project: A Multimatrix Model for the Study of Alzheimer's Disease

DENIS GAUVREAU / *Institut National de la Recherche Scientifique, Pointe-Claire, Canada*

MARC DE BRAEKELEER / *Université du Québec, Chicoutimi, Quebec, Canada*

RÉMI BOUCHARD / *Hôpital de l'Enfant-Jésus, Quebec, Canada*

SERGE GAUTHIER / *McGill University, Montreal, Canada*

JEAN MATHIEU, CAMIL BOILY, and ANDRÉE CHOLETTE / *Hôpital de Chicoutimi, Chicoutimi, Quebec, Canada*

YVES ROBITAILLE / *McGill University, Montreal, Canada*

PATRICK BOUCHARD / *Hôpital de Jonquière, Jonquière, Canada*

NORMAND BOUCHARD / *Hôpital de la Baie, La Baie, Canada*

LUCIE-PAULE DOYON / *Hôpital de Roberval, Roberval, Canada*

MAURIL GAUDREAULT / *Hôpital de Chicoutimi, Chicoutimi, Quebec, Canada*

ANDRÉ OUELLET / *Hôpital de Dolbeau, Dolbeau, Canada*

MARC DUMONT / *Hôpital d'Alma, Alma, Canada*

PAUL KISHKA and CLAUDE FOURNIER / *Sanatorium Bégin, Lac Etchemin, Canada*

JOSEPHINE NALBANTOGLU, GINETTE LACOSTE-ROYAL, and DENYSE GAUTRIN / *Institut National de la Recherche Scientifique, Pointe-Claire, Canada*

SORANA FRODA / *Université du Québec à Montréal, Montreal, Canada*

GÉRARD BOUCHARD / *Université du Québec, Chicoutimi, Quebec, Canada*

INTRODUCTION

From clinical and socioeconomic standpoints alone, Alzheimer's disease (AD) and senile dementias of the Alzheimer's type rate among the currently most prominent public health problems, which can only get worse in the next decades (1-3). It is interesting, however, that the interpretation of data already gathered on putative risk factors for this particular class of neurodegenerative disorders remains perplexing, although its collection is still sketchy. The fact that establishing a population-based registry of reliable cases is difficult, especially from an operational point of view, no doubt accounts to a large extent for the current lack of major comprehensive epidemiological studies on AD. Designing and satisfactorily analyzing case-control studies have also posed considerable technical demands. Hence, researchers' results cannot be considered entirely conclusive, since progress and potential solutions to the advancement of knowledge on AD have been limited by practical and methodological issues (4).

We knew very well that only a small proportion of patients with AD live in nursing homes and hospitals in any specific area. It is therefore extremely hazardous (not to say impossible) to determine with reasonable statistical precision this proportion of cases; it usually varies according to the institutional caretaking resources available in the area and the socioeconomic status of its population. In those institutions, it may be relatively easy to identify presumptive cases if one wishes, for example, to screen specifically for AD, but a registry built in such a manner will evidently only provide part of the true Alzheimer's disease picture in any selected area. Notwithstanding the quality of medical archives in the hospitals, the cause of death has been seldom labeled, until recently, as senile dementia itself, or even by any other term "historically" associated with senility. Thus, retrospective investigations do not lead to the discovery of a significant number of reliable cases; moreover, this problem is made noticeably worse by the scarcity of pathological data obtained through autopsy to corroborate clinical inclusion criteria.

Tracking down all (or most of) the AD cases residing in the community can be carried out by means of a careful supervision of the physicians in any field of study. The task, however, calls for a solid network of collaborators and key informants, backed up by an effective clerical organization. Furthermore, since the first diagnostic impressions collected in the private office by the general practitioner must be followed up by a rigorous neurological consultation, as well as periodic checkups, the concept of a truly comprehensive and prospective survey constitutes a formidable enterprise. By all accounts, such an initiative remains a particularly onerous challenge. It has therefore not been met so far with great enthusiasm by epidemiologists and clinicians seeking to unveil the mystery of AD. In countries lacking public systems of health care and social welfare, such an initiative can simply not be envisaged on a reasonably high scale.

The fact that the important methodological issues relating to case definition have been tackled in a much more comprehensive fashion in the last few years provides a further incentive to reconsider seriously the project of a population-based study of AD.

Indeed, some major efforts have been investigated in trying to surmount the inherent diagnostic difficulties met by research teams working to establish registries of AD cases. Mainly because a great deal of work has gone into defining more clearly the clinical characteristics of patients with senile dementia of the Alzheimer's type, and also into specifying explicitly the neurological and pathological diagnostic protocols, we have better survey tools. Therefore, we can reasonably expect to obtain through those diagnostic instruments further valuable information on the development of the disease (5,6). These criteria remain principally exclusionary, and they obviously lack (as of yet) standardization. Furthermore, they do not really describe specific markers for the disease. Despite the fact that these criteria still must be tested in different longitudinal studies and need to be evaluated in the context of a pathological follow-up, they have constituted the premise for reconsidering seriously the possibility of a population-based study.

RATIONALE UNDERLYING THE ESTABLISHMENT OF A REGISTRY OF CASES FOR COHORT STUDIES OF GENERAL POPULATION SAMPLES

Although the data gathered by different scientists have not provided any definite answers to the causes of AD (7), the information collected thus far points to unequivocal questions that must be addressed directly in defining the qualities of the research model for the study of this disease. Considered together, the caveats listed below would appear to limit the choice of a research model to the population-based study as the approach most likely to provide valuable clues to our understanding of AD.

First, the definition of AD is a particularly difficult hurdle in interpreting the literature available on this subject; currently, its diagnosis is founded on the equation between specific clinical and neuropathological criteria. It is interesting that researchers seem to have operated until recently on the basic assumption that AD is identifiable, either clinically or neuropathologically, and that it represents a distinct phenomenon. Currently, AD can probably best be described as a "syndrome," but its clinical and pathological features, and their associations over time, need to be more carefully examined on their own merits (8). The lack of a "gold standard" for the identification of AD through longitudinal studies with appropriate comparison groups and neuropathological follow-up, as well as of standardized multifaceted clinical assessment procedures, has severely impeded our understanding of this disease. Alzheimer's disease should be best understood from a diagnostic perspective in order to direct research questions in a much more specific fashion in the field or in the laboratory. Uneasiness in interpreting the epidemiological data so far collected essentially springs from the inherent circularity in the criteria used to define the AD diagnosis. This circularity arises mainly from the fact that a clinical diagnosis requires neuropathological confirmation, while a neuropathological diagnosis requires clinical confirmation. This peculiar situation is borne out by findings showing that brain changes by definition considered characteristic of AD may also appear in the brains of nondemented elderly individuals (9). Indeed, one cannot assume that neuropathological changes constitute per se the only "gold standard" for the disease. Thus, the lack of truly specific neuropathological and clinical markers for the "Alzheimer syndrome" still remains a stumbling block, shrouding somewhat the identification and the reliability of cases at either level. It constitutes a serious caveat in designing experiments (and in interpreting the scientific and medical literature of the past, before the introduction of the more stringent National Institute of Neurological and Communicative Disorders and Stroke-Alzheimer's Disease and Related Diseases Association [NINCDS-ADRDA] criteria). Different studies would appear to suggest that AD could comprise subtypes that may, in fact, represent different diseases (10). Heterogeneity seems to characterize AD as we have come to know (and define) it. This rather "uncertain" situation calls for a prospective design, with the possibility for retrospective analyses, to allow reclassification of cases (and perhaps redefinition of the disease and its subtypes).

Second, the variability in the age of onset of the so-called types I and II AD wold seem to indicate that the question of "expression" is also paramount in setting the criteria for a research model (11,12). The realization that the time window for this disease to manifest itself is large would further suggest that some of the aging phenomena that may act to modulate the clinical and neuropathological expression of AD are very important, and should be accounted for in any study. Hence, any model should attempt, in the ideal circumstances, to cover the whole period or time span of the "at risk period" of AD.

Third, the paradox between, on the one hand, the fact that familial cases of AD would seem to point to a strong genetic causative factor and, on the other hand, that discordance for AD has been observed in many twin sets, suggests that there are many causative factors in this disease (13,14). Since it seems that the environmental features can simply not be ignored in the experimental design, one should also attempt to cover the particular risk factors likely to be influenced by spatial or geographic characteristics.

Fourth, the lack of any significant linkage between the disease trait and the genes apparently implicated in the production of AD lesions would seem to indicate that there may be many missing biochemical links between the true causative factors and what constitutes the most obvious and observable expression of the disease (15,16). That "causative gap" may extend outside the brain, which is considered the site of the disease. To reconstruct the metabolic or physiological steps that lead to what we currently use as diagnostic criteria in neuropathology, one should try to correct for this lack of a systemic history of the disease. A longitudinal approach over a large field provides one way (albeit incomplete) to compensate for this particular obstacle, notably by allowing us to investigate the medical histories of large families (17).

We believe that these four caveats (among the most important ones that can be considered) call for a somewhat different frame of mind in approaching the study of AD. By definition, a comprehensive research model should provide for observations on the milieu within which the disease develops. AD lesions are "normal" features of the aging of the brain; an amplification of the usual phenomena underlying their appearance seems to characterize this disease. If, as proposed, AD is truly a multifactorial condition, with a complex polygenic basis, a simple telescopic research approach can only provide fragmentary information on its cause(s) and its clinical types. With the data already obtained mostly in a "disciplinary fashion" (which translates into a collection of elements that one does not know how to fit into the overall puzzle), we possess few clues as to which physiological or cellular systems might be involved in the development of the disease (17,18). Furthermore, the lessons provided by recent knowledge about "expression" of Duchenne muscular dystrophy clearly demonstrate that what one might consider a "straightforward" single-gene disease seems to be much more complex (19-21). If AD is more than just a "one-factor disease," we believe that as wide an investigative angle as possible should be used in the study of the disease. This would increase the chances of assembling as large a set of clues and help solve its riddle. A population-based study appears best suited to meet these different criteria for the definition of the research model.

A SHORT INTRODUCTION TO THE IMAGE PROJECT

A registry of AD cases is currently being established over the whole area of Saguenay-Lac-Saint-Jean in the Province of Quebec (Canada) (Fig. 1). The IMAGE* Project has now been in progress since late 1985 and is founded on a network of specialists, collaborators, and key informants in the field of study. It has progressively grown into a population-based study. The IMAGE registry is unique of its kind and its strength lies in the ability of its investigators to access a computerized database of all the parish records, currently dating back to 1842. This research is conducted in collaboration with the SOREP Consortium at the University of Quebec at Chicoutimi (SOREP–Centre Interuniversitaire de Recherches sur les Populations–is a triuniversity consortium in human genetics, involving

*IMAGE is a French acronym for "Investigations de la maladie d'Alzheimer: Génétique et épidémiologie," which translates into "Studies on Alzheimer's disease: Genetics and Epidemiology."

Laval University (Quebec), McGill University (Montreal), and University of Quebec at Chicoutimi). Through its ability to reconstruct family pedigrees rapidly and automatically, this special facility offers an opportunity to study in detail the demographic and genetic evolution of the SLSJ community.

The project has been set up to investigate the development of AD in the area using a multidisciplinary approach. The research structure of IMAGE is planned to include eight specific research matrices: (a) the clinicopathological data collected on patients; (b) the population genetics within the field of study, including measurements of genealogical indices of the AD population; (c) epidemiological data on patients; (d) the sociogeographical distribution of patients over the study area; (e) the study of caretaking and case management issues in the field; (f) environmental and toxicological data from the territory investigated; (g) the molecular genetics underlying AD; and (h) the physiocellular analysis of gene products affecting the expression of the disease condition.

THE IMAGE CONCEPT: A MULTIMATRIX MODEL FOR THE STUDY OF ALZHEIMER'S DISEASE

The absence of an adequate animal or experimental model probably remains the single most important obstacle in investigating thoroughly the cause(s) of AD (22). Only a comprehensive approach could provide the best chances of understanding its causes. Hence, a case registry was established over the whole area of SLSJ to create an extended research laboratory. It should be possible to combine analytical techniques in epidemiology, biostatistics, population genetics, as well as in cellular and molecular biology, from a series of measurements all based on a single population. The search for an alternative experimental model to integrate multidisciplinary data is the basic premise that led to the establishment of the IMAGE Project.

The project can be defined as a set of disciplinary projects or research matrices that the IMAGE scientists wish to analyze in a continuum. Through the integration of its multifaceted data into one large Alzheimer's disease picture, IMAGE can be conceived of as a holistic model, providing an opportunity to overlap any number of, or a combination of results from, its disciplinary matrices. We believe that the IMAGE Project will probably lead to creative feedforward or feedback inferences between the different matrices, and that their synergic effects will suggest constructive relationships between the research planes. Above all, the IMAGE Project appears to possess a registry that is eminently suited for investigating the relationships between, and the relative importance of, genetic and environmental factors suspected to interact in the development of AD.

FIELD OF STUDY

The targeted field for the IMAGE Project is the area of Saguenay-Lac-Saint-Jean (SLSJ) in the Province of Quebec, a term that describes all the territory situated

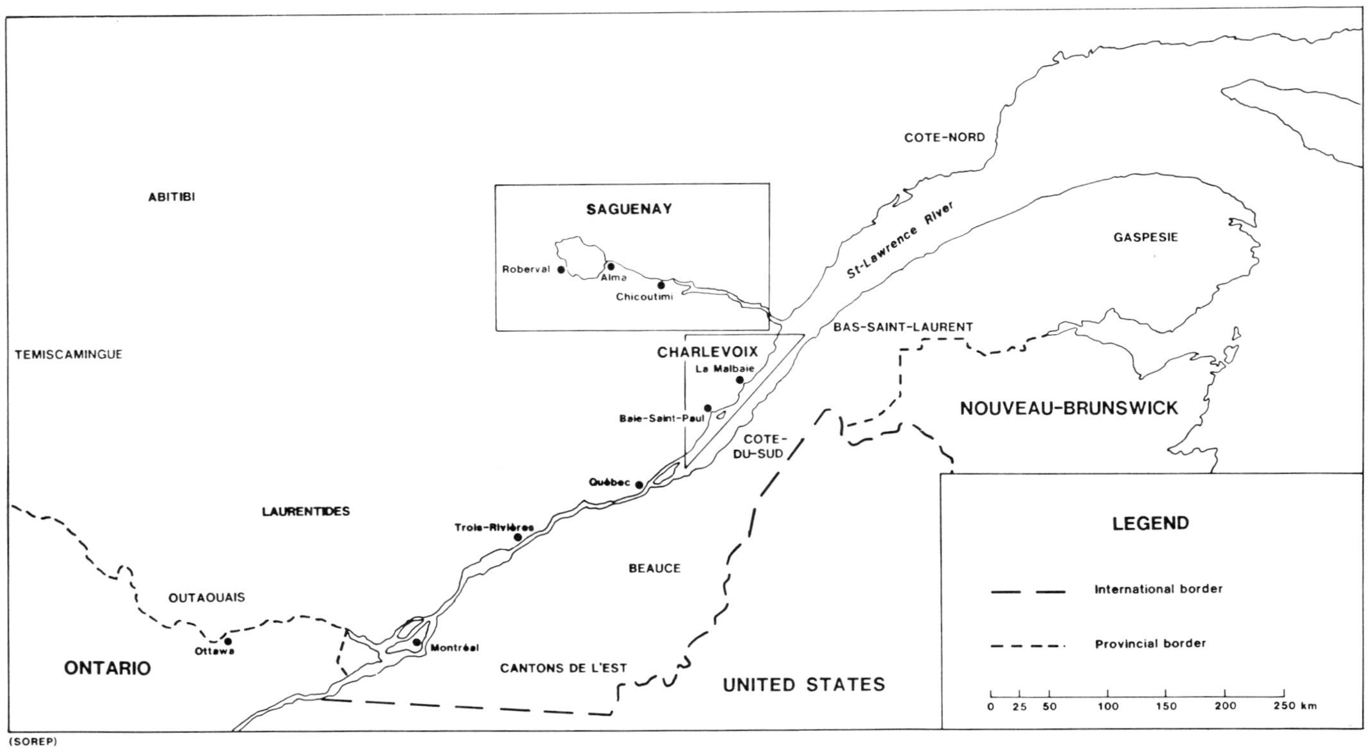

FIGURE 1 The Saguenay-Lac-Saint-Jean territory, selected as field of study for the IMAGE Project. SLSJ is located north of the city of Quebec; it covers an area of approximately 22,500 Km^2, with a population of approximately 290,000 persons.

between the longitudes of 70° and 75°, and between latitudes 48° and 49° north (Fig. 1). The SLSJ area, the center of which is located at some 200 Km north of the city of Quebec, covers approximately 225 Km from east to west and about 100 from north to south. Figure 1 defines clearly the borders of that area, which embraces all the villages and towns included between Petit-Saguenay in the east portion and St-Thomas-Didyme in the west portion, and between Notre-Dame-de-Lorette in the northern portion and Lac des Commissaires in the southern portion. From an administrative standpoint, the SLSJ (as defined in this project) does not correspond exactly to the administrative zone no. 2 of the Ministry of Health and Social Services of the Province of Quebec, which also contains the territory of the cities of Chibougamau and Chapais (located northwest of SLSJ). Situated as they are, halfway between SLSJ and the Abitibi area, their history and resources bring them closer to the latter region. On the other hand, our definition of SLSJ corresponds exactly to the three municipal counties of Chicoutimi, Lac-Saint-Jean-East, and Lac-Saint-Jean-West (also called Roberval). These three counties also coincide with those defined by Statistics Canada in the national population census. It is interesting to underline a characteristic historical feature of SLSJ: its relative isolation from the rest of the Province of Quebec. Indeed, until the end of the 19th century, access was extremely difficult because of very bad roads. The only other means of communications was the river Saguenay, the waters of which are navigable up to the city of Chicoutimi. However, the river was frozen 4-5 months per year, which, until the construction of railways, meant that the area was separated from the rest of Quebec from early December to the end of April. This relative isolation obviously had a direct bearing on the composition of the gene pool found in SLSJ nowadays. The current total population of the area of this study is approximately 290,000.

ORIGINAL FEATURES OF SLSJ AS A FIELD OF STUDY

As stated above, the strength of the IMAGE registry of AD cases is the possibility for its investigators to access a computerized data base of all the parish records. Currently, the SOREP data base provides 145 years of vital data of the field of study, but soon it will be extended into the pool of the Charlevoix area just south of SLSJ (Fig. 1). It is estimated that 70-80% of the gene pool of SLSJ comes from Charlevoix, which means that IMAGE could work back to the 17th century ancestors of its patients. This data base includes information on place and date of birth, place and date of death, as well as on residential and professional itineraries throughout the life of its constituents. On average, any citizen who spent his or her life in SLSJ is recorded 10 times in the data base.

A computerized data base of the geographical and socioeconomic characteristics of the SLSJ (based on the information obtained from Statistics Canada through periodic censuses) also provides a tool for street-by-street analysis of the spatial distribution of cases. It was established by the ECOBES group at the College of Jonquière during their studies of Steinert's disease, but it is equally applicable to AD subjects.

The area also offers very special opportunities to investigate the relative influence of environmental factors in the causes of AD. SLSJ is divided in two distinct regions, with a clearly delimited agricultural section (around the lake), and a concentrated industrial area (along the axis of the cities of Jonquière-Chicoutimi-La Baie). The two sections correspond roughly to rural and urban concentrations, with small villages and medium-size cities, respectively. The territorial limits can be labeled as "reasonable" from the point of view of managing the data, traveling within the field of study, and air transport from the cities of Montreal or Quebec. Geographically, SLSJ allows for adequate management of a network of collaborators and key informants, as well as for frequent contacts with the various hospitals, nursing homes, and medical specialists. There is also in the area a major hospital center equipped with modern neurological instruments and biochemical laboratories. A regional constituent of the University of Quebec network (where IMAGE headquarters in the field have been established) links computer facilities between the laboratories in Montreal (INRS-Santé is also a constituent of the University of Quebec network) and the IMAGE agents and officials in the area.

Most interesting, particularly from a toxicological point of view, is a major aluminum-producing plant, established in the early part of this century (1926). This offers a rather unique chance to test the hypothesis that aluminum is a causative agent of AD.

Above all, IMAGE provides an opportunity for geneticists to locate three generations of living AD cases. The average number of children in that area, between 1880 and 1940, was 10 per family, which is among the highest recorded so far in the world. In fact, IMAGE deals with very large families in successive generations, which generate the best odds of locating simultaneously a proband with affected children, as well as uncles or aunts also affected (i.e., cases of AD in different generations, who are all alive). We believe that this feature of the IMAGE field may turn out to be especially important with regard to the study of the causes of AD, particularly in investigating a polygenic hypothesis.

Since AD appears to develop due to a multifactorial matrix of factors (with some gene dosage possibly operating on the expression of these factors), large numbers of cases in nuclear families may not be sufficient to provide the tight linkage one usually seeks to spot the one causal gene. In fact, it seems more likely that tight linkage to establish the identity of these different genetic factors will require large (or perhaps even very large) clusters of related families or extended families. Furthermore, because AD probably results from a combination of genetic and environmental factors, understanding the genetic-environmental interaction is best afforded by the study of large numbers of blood relatives who live far away.

NEUROLOGICAL DIAGNOSTIC PROCEDURE FOR SCREENING AD CASES

The identification of putative cases across the IMAGE network constitutes the first step in the overall procedure for screening AD cases in the field of study and for subsequently corroborating the AD diagnosis. The Reisberg Global Deterioration Scale is used in an undiscriminating fashion by the key informants in the field to locate patients with memory impairments (23), without regard, at that point in the procedure, to the exact nature of the medical problem. The cases identified at this stage are labeled putative cases.

The two following stages in the diagnostic flow chart of a putative case are based on the elements of the diagnostic scale of exclusion and inclusion criteria (DSEIC) adapted for this study from McKhann et al. (5). Hence, the approach is aimed at identifying specific clinical and neuropathological features. In the first step, the medical files and history of a putative case are reevaluated in a critical fashion with data already available to establish the presumptive character of the preliminary diagnosis of AD. This review is founded on the identification of so-called absolute exclusion criteria in the biological and clinical evaluation of the putative cases. The DSEIC, which follows the distinctive elements of the NINCDS-ADRDA scale, is used in a retrospective fashion at this stage to eliminate from the group of putative cases those whose symptoms are of a different origin, with explicitly documented relevant data (multi-infarcts, long history of alcoholism or primary affective disorders, etc.). All patients identified by this preselection step constitute the group of presumptive cases.

We define as absolute exclusion criteria any of the other pathological conditions from the class of diseases that specifically cause some of the different neuropsychological changes also characteristic of AD. Since we know that some diseases clearly mimic AD clinically, but that they are nonetheless of a distinctly different origin, the identification of one of these diseases is sufficient to exclude any clear, unconfounding diagnosis of AD. Thus, these diseases constitute absolute exclusion criteria, according to the definition given by the DSEIC: any hard evidence of the presence of one of these diseases in the medical history leads to the rejection of the case from the groups of putative cases. A list of these absolute exclusion criteria is given in Table 1.

On the other hand, certain other diseases can also hinder or confuse the establishment of a clinical diagnosis of AD, because we know that they might have caused some of the neuropsychological changes also characteristic of AD. The identification of such diseases in the medical history of the patient, even one likely to have AD, raises some doubt as to the primary cause of the dementia.

These diseases constitute relative exclusion criteria according to the definition given by the DSEIC. The term relative signifies that any evidence of the presence of these diseases has to be appraised in a critical fashion, since it does not neces-

TABLE 1 Absolute and Relative Exclusion Criteria in Establishing the Diagnosis of Alzheimer Disease

Absolute exclusion criteria
Creutzfeldt-Jakob disease
Huntington's disease
Progressive subnuclear palsy
Chronic infections of the nervous system
Multi-infarct dementia
Brain tumors
Subdural hematoma
Multiple sclerosis
Schizophrenia
Uncontrolled severe arterial hypertension
Advanced insulin-dependent diabetes
Relative exclusion criteria
Parkinson's disease
Communicative hydrocephalus
Posttraumatic encephalopathy
Epilepsy-convulsions
Affective and manic-depressive disorders
Alcoholism
Hallucinogen or drug intoxication
Cancers
Systematic disorders
Asymptomatic vitamin B_{12} deficiency
Asymptomatic folic acid deficiency

Based on ref. 5.

sarily mean that the patient is automatically rejected from the group of presumptive cases. In fact, the rejection of a case depends on the severity of one or more than one of the different relative exclusion criteria, and of their clinical importance in the evaluation of the causes of the neuropsychological changes. If the cause of these changes is simply indeterminate or seems to be one or more of those diseases classified as relative exclusion criteria, the patient can be rejected from the group of presumptive cases at the next stage in the diagnostic flow chart. A list of the diseases classified as so-called relative exclusion criteria is given in Table 1.

Thus, the clinical investigation proceeds in two distinctive phases. In the first, the preliminary review of data on putative cases seeks to exclude from the diagnostic flow chart patients with diseases defined as absolute exclusion criteria. The patients not rejected are then referred to a neurologist for an exhaustive evaluation. At this phase, the neurologist seeks to corroborate or invalidate the presumptive diagnosis of AD; this investigation is founded on the criteria laid down by the NINCDS-ADRDA scale.

If they have not been rejected by new evidence of an absolute exclusion criterion, the cases are then classified into two distinctive categories: possible cases and probable cases. The former group is made up of the patients who present evidence of one or more confounding diseases with the dementia of the Alzheimer type, that is, diseases known as relative exclusion criteria. However, the cause of dementia for those patients is very likely Alzheimer's disease, and not one or another of those diseases identified as relative exclusion criteria. In these instances, the patient presents with a clinical history that is not totally clear. Since doubt exists as to the true origin of the dementia, the neurologist would rather reserve his or her diagnosis for another evaluation (or until definite corroboration is obtained through the neuropathological investigation).

The group of probable cases is constituted of patients whose neuropsychological changes correspond in all ways to that of a characteristic Alzheimer's disease pattern, with no evidence of relative or absolute exclusion criteria upon thorough neurological investigation. This group is formed of cases who in all likelihood (and barring neuropathological proof to the contrary) have Alzheimer disease. A possible case can be reclassified as a probable case, when his or her clinical history accentuates the neurological changes typical of AD, while also minimizing the importance of a relative exclusion criterion identified earlier.

THE IMAGE NETWORK OPERATION IN SAGUENAY-LAC-SAINT-JEAN AREA

Key Informants

Collaborators in the institutions providing health or social services across the SLSJ area are defined as key informants. They have been selected individually; they usually hold a supervising or coordinating role for the staff who come into contact with AD patients. IMAGE has recruited key informants in the so-called categories and units of screening: likely contact sites of AD cases throughout the field of study. They have been trained in reporting procedures, and a routine mode of communication has been set up to keep the key informants in contact with the IMAGE network. Official IMAGE forms are used to up-date the registry. Managing agents also maintain personal contact with the key informants by telephone and site visits. Key informants are asked to report any client or patient who has already been labeled as a possible, probable, or definite case of AD; and who shows confusion and memory impairments or related behavior, as defined by the criteria laid down in Reisberg's Global Deterioration Scale for a period spanning at least 6 months. Related behaviors include wandering or getting lost in a familiar environment, requiring to be dressed or fed without obvious physical disability to account for it, and being unable to avoid simple dangers without supervision. Positive manifestation of AD neuropsychological changes described above lead to the identification of a putative case of AD. The case finding is aimed at all cases residing in the targeted geographic area selected as field of study. The sites of contact, or so-called categories and units of screening, have been thoroughly documented to extend the screening to capture all the prevalent cases of AD in the area (see Fig. 2 for a diagram of the funnel structure of the network of IMAGE key informants in the field).

The source of cases for the study is determined by the total number of persons affected by any form of dementia or senility who are reported to IMAGE by means of its network of key informants in the different units of screening across the field. Although the efforts of the group are directed particularly towards those cases born in the area of SLSJ, without regard to their age at onset of the disease, all cases located throughout the network who were born outside the area are also entered into the registry. On the other hand, cases born in SLSJ who are diagnosed outside the area and who are identified to IMAGE officials also become part of the registry.

Medical Officers

Their task is described below in the section on the geographical spheres of screening in SLSJ.

Managing Agents

The managing agents operate within the field from the headquarters in Chicoutimi (Centre-IMAGE). They act mainly as permanent resources for the network and assist field key informants in finding and screening the cases across the SLSJ. They also work on family pedigrees that are automatically reconstructed from the SOREP registry for all the presumptive, probable, possible, and definite cases reported by the clinical core. The family pedigrees serve as a tool in the field to reconstruct the family medical history, in order to investigate heredity as a risk factor. All pedigrees collected are also used for the genetic linkage study to choose informative families in which to seek a DNA marker linked to AD.

Nursing Homes

The head of nursing services in the nursing homes acts as key informant in each nursing home participating in the IMAGE network.

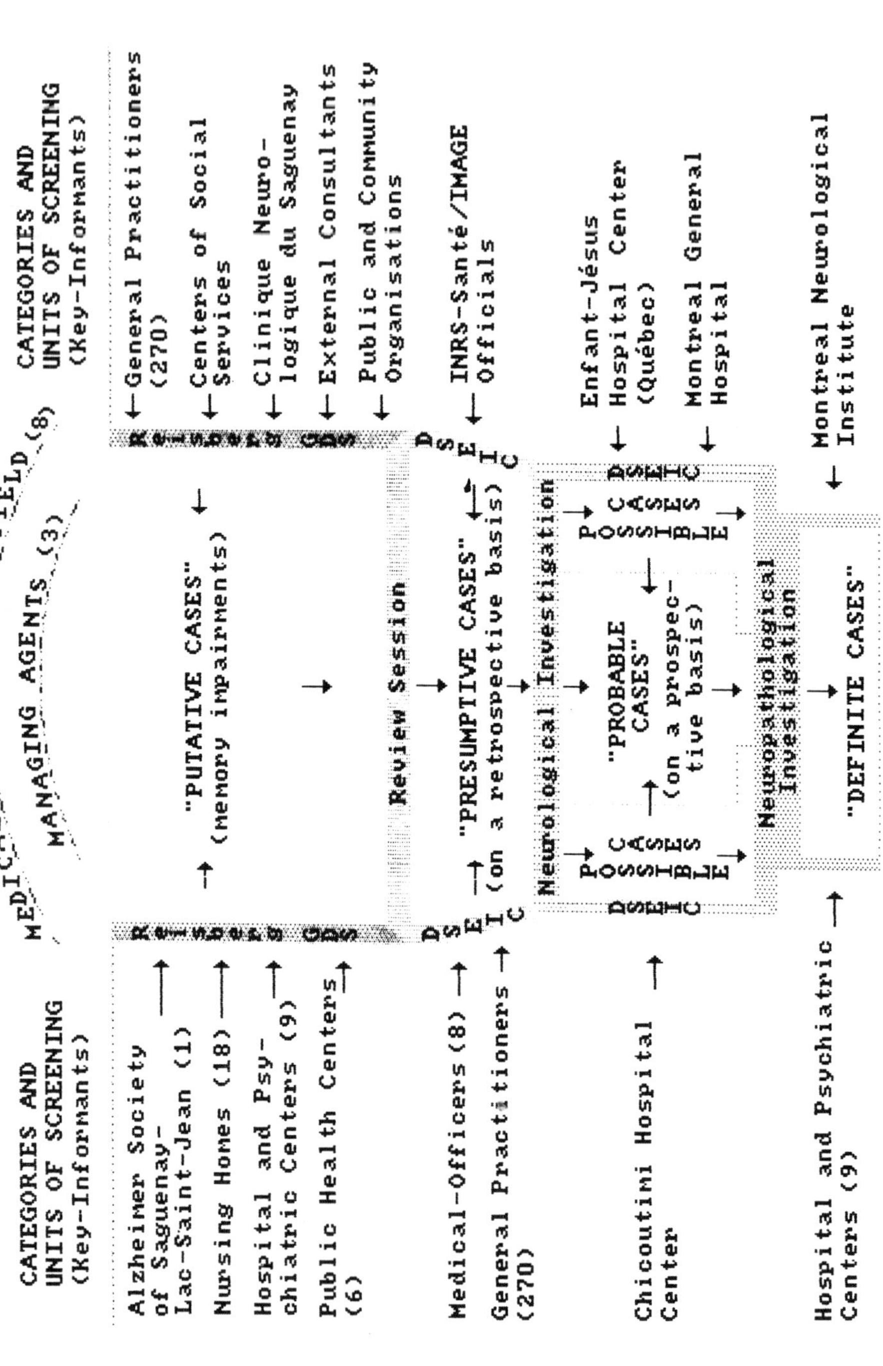
MEDICAL-OFFICERS IN THE FIELD (8)
MANAGING AGENTS (3)
CATEGORIES AND UNITS OF SCREENING (Key-Informants)
Alzheimer Society of Saguenay-Lac-Saint-Jean (1)
Nursing Homes (18)
Hospital and Psychiatric Centers (9)
Public Health Centers (6)
Medical-Officers (8)
General Practitioners (270)
Chicoutimi Hospital Center
Hospital and Psychiatric Centers (9)
Reisberg GDS
"PUTATIVE CASES" (memory impairments)
Review Session
"PRESUMPTIVE CASES" (on a retrospective basis)
DSEIC
Neurological Investigation
POSSIBLE CASES
"PROBABLE CASES" (on a prospective basis)
Neuropathological Investigation
"DEFINITE CASES"
CATEGORIES AND UNITS OF SCREENING (Key-Informants)
General Practitioners (270)
Centers of Social Services
Clinique Neurologique du Saguenay
External Consultants
Public and Community Organisations
INRS-Santé/IMAGE Officials
Enfant-Jésus Hospital Center (Québec)
Montreal General Hospital
Montreal Neurological Institute

Société Alzheimer de Sagamie

The local Alzheimer Society (which is the chapter covering the entire SLSJ area) has an office in Alma. It provides help in organizing support groups. The Society also publicizes the IMAGE Project through its brochure and strongly encourages the families of presumptive cases to get in touch directly with the project officials in Chicoutimi.

Departments of Public Health

The Departments of Public Health (DPH) are research units associated with the large hospitals, whose task and objectives pertain directly to public health problems in the area. Two DPH are found in the SLSJ: one in Roberval and one in Chicoutimi. The DPH occasionally refer administrative information or give advice on general matters regarding field operations.

Center of Social Services

The direction of social services in the field of study is divided in two sections, social workers in the Saguenay area and in the Lac-Saint-Jean area. The social workers provide mainly home help and counseling services across the field; they occasionally supervise the social services in some community agencies, and they may also be in public and private day care centers or senior citizens centers. They encounter putative cases in their routine activities.

Hospital and Psychiatric Centers

Heads of nursing services in the SLSJ hospitals and psychiatric centers have assisted and continue to help managing agents in locating AD cases in their institutions on a retrospective and prospective bases.

FIGURE 2 Funnel structure of the IMAGE key informants in the SLSJ for screening putative cases of Alzheimer disease and for the corroboration of an AD diagnosis. Screening is divided into four distinct steps that correspond to establishing the character of the putative, presumptive, possible or probable, and definitive diagnoses of AD. On the basis of the criteria defined in Reisberg's global deterioration scale (GDS), key informants in the network signal patients with memory impairments to IMAGE officials; cases are then directed according to the procedure described in the chart for screening putative cases and for corroboration of an AD diagnosis. Case segregation is based on the elements prescribed by the diagnostic scale of exclusion and inclusion criteria adapted from McKhann et al. (5). DSEIC, Diagnostic scale of exclusion and inclusion criteria.

SLSJ Physicians

Physicians in the field of study are gathered once a year in subgroups corresponding to those of the six geographical spheres of screening. A meeting is then organized by the medical officer of the sphere to deliver copies of the Cartable-IMAGE with the form for the identification of a putative case. Managing agents also call them individually every 4 months to enquire about new cases and remind them of the existence of Alzheimer computed tomographic (CT) scan clinics at the Hospital of Chicoutimi.

District Medical Examiner

The district medical examiners have been informed of the IMAGE Project in detail and are met with on a regular basis. They are aware of the procedure for autopsy and of the identity of key informants involved in helping with this procedure and transporting brains to Chicoutimi.

Public and Community Organizations

Since the targeted population of IMAGE is found almost exclusively in a specific age segment of the population, a certain number of organizations devoted to their needs have been identified as possible sources of key informants for the IMAGE Project. These include the Fédération de l'Age d'Or du Québec of SLSJ, which is the principal organization of senior citizens in the province (established as a general federation of the social clubs of senior citizens), and the Catholic Church.

Geographical Spheres of Screening

For the IMAGE Project, the field of study of SLSJ has been divided in six geographical spheres of screening. Each sphere of screening is supervised by a medical officer. His or her task consists of overlooking the activities of the network, and making sure that the rules and procedures of screening for cases within the framework of the IMAGE Project are followed in the different units of screening of his or her own geographical sphere of screening. The field research objectives of the medical officers in their own community also include providing assistance in completing the medical and genealogical (if necessary) histories of possible, probable, and definite cases and their families. They contribute their influence to make public opinion sensitive to the subject of research on Alzheimer's disease, as well as encouraging the general practitioners in their respective geographical sphere of screening to refer presumptive cases for neurological consultation.

Categories and Units of Screening

With a view to reassembling under selective classes all prospective sources of putative cases, and cataloguing them in distinctly representative groups (which differ from one another only in their mode of caretaking and/or type of intervention), we have established categories and units of screening (CUS). A category of screening represents a group of public or private institutions dispensing similar health services to the community. As illustrated in Figure 2, different categories of screening are involved in the IMAGE search for putative cases in SLSJ. These include the regional Alzheimer Society, the 18 nursing homes, the 9 psychiatric and hospital centers, the local centers for public health, the general practitioners, the 2 Departments of Public Health servicing the area, the Regional Council for Health and Social Services, the neurological clinic of SLSJ, and a certain number of public and community organizations. Each institution within a category represents a distinct unit of screening (e.g., a specific nursing home or a particular hospital). Identification codes have been introduced to facilitate computer management of the network and to ensure the follow-up of key infornants' activities in locating putative cases across the different units of screening in the field.

Forms and Lists for Field Operations

The term form designates any document necessary to collect data in the field of study. The forms used in the procedure for screening putative cases and for the corroboration of an AD diagnosis have a rigid structure. The key informants in the field have samples of the specific forms they require at their level of operation so that they can transmit relevant information on the cases directly to the IMAGE registry. All the collaborators in the field have an IMAGE official ring binder (Cartable-IMAGE) that gives all the details necessary to communicate rapidly with project officials.

The term list is used to designate all the matrices produced when the field activities are updated. Each line of the matrix corresponds to one particular case; every column corresponds to a bit of information collected within the IMAGE framework. The lists allow for efficient and coherent management of the IMAGE registry, since they provide the information required to plan the subsequent steps to corroborate a diagnosis of AD.

Procedure for Screening Putative Cases and for the Corroboration of an AD Diagnosis

Across the different categories and specific units of screening, prospective screening of putative cases is based on Reisberg's global deterioration scale (GDS). As mentioned above, key informants in the network will identify any person who presents symptoms that fit the description of the characteristic stages as defined by the GDS. In the beginning, managing agents also helped out the collaborators in the field with the retrospective screening of putative cases. All the cases with senile or presenile dementia were identified on the basis of the diagnostic codes enumerated in Table 2. As illustrated in Figure 3, the identification of a putative case is initially supervised by the administrative loop formed by the IMAGE officials in Chicoutimi, the different key informants in the categories and units of screening, and the medical officers in the six geographical spheres of screening. Reporting a putative case to the project, whether by means of a key informant in the field, or by a systematic search in the medical records of living patients in the hospitals and nursing homes, constitutes the first step in the classification of cases in the overall procedure for screening AD cases and for the corroboration of an AD diagnosis. The form for the identification of a putative case (item 1 in the flow diagram of Fig. 3) is used at this step; the name of the case is then entered into the IMAGE registry. If the family of a putative case has not been directly in touch with the IMAGE officials, the key informant in the field informs the family of the existence of our research group, and takes that opportunity to make them aware of our scientific objectives. A verbal authorization is then obtained from the family of a putative case to allow our managing agents to communicate with them (item 0 in the flow chart of Fig. 3). The IMAGE managing agents then meet the family of the putative case to explain in summary what the aims of the study are, and in what way the patient and family will be involved in the work if they agree to participate.

The information collected during that meeting (as well as at all subsequent meetings) is recorded on the form for the family information service (item 3 in

---

FIGURE 3 Stepwise flow chart of the operations in the field for screening putative cases and for the corroboration of an AD diagnosis. C.U.S., Categories and units of screening; M.O., Medical officers. 0. Introduction to IMAGE and verbal authorization for screening. 1. Form for the identification of a putative case. 2. Family information service. 3. Form for the family information service. 4. Forms for the authorization to consult medical records, for autopsy, and for a blood sample. 5a. Form for the diagnostic scale of exclusion and inclusion criteria (retrospective). 5b. Form for the diagnostic scale of exclusion and inclusion criteria (prospective). 6. Form for the DSEIC completed. 7. List of putative cases for the review session of medical records. 8. Form for the results of the review session of medical records. 9. Form for the neurological clinics. 10. Form for the results of the neurological consultation. 11. Check list of possible and probable cases for the neuropathological investigation. 12. Form for the results of the neuropsychological investigation. 13. Form for the results of the neuropathological investigation. 14. Form for the transfer of a case: A. Label BEWARE-AUTOPSY; B. Notice of death; C. Catalogue of the managing agent: a. Check list of the IMAGE registry; b. Check list of resources for the family information service; c. Check list of DSEIC to be completed; d. Check list of clinical and laboratory investigations; e. Check list of presumptive cases for the neurological consultation; f. Check list of cases transferred; D. Catalogue of the medical officer (Catalogue of the managing agent subdivided by geographical sphere of screening); E. Catalogue of the pathologist: a. List of names of the living cases; b. Check list of family resources for living cases.

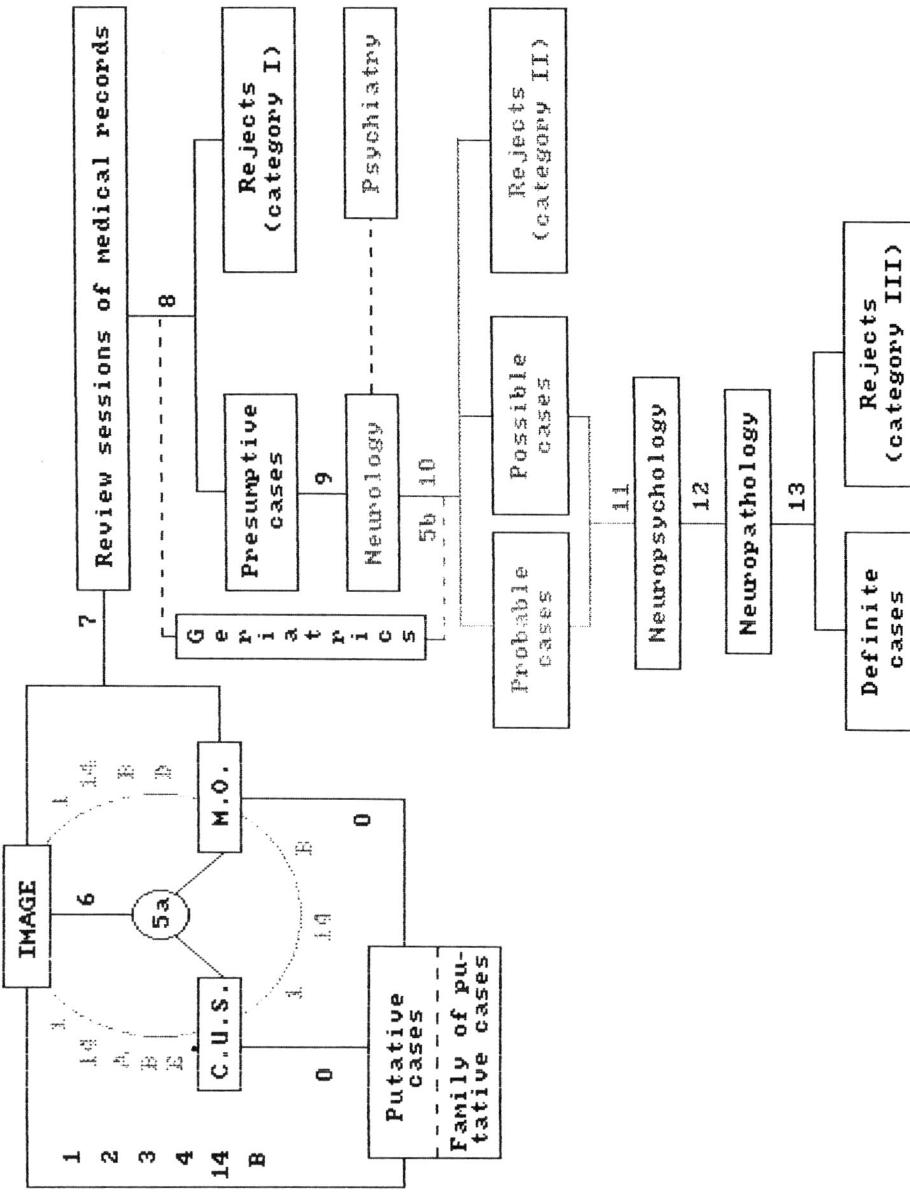
IMAGE
C.U.S.
M.O.
5a
6
0
Putative cases
Family of putative cases
1
2
3
4
14
B
7
Review sessions of medical records
8
Presumptive cases
Rejects (category I)
9
Neurology
Psychiatry
Geriatrics
5b
10
Probable cases
Possible cases
Rejects (category II)
11
Neuropsychology
12
Neuropathology
13
Definite cases
Rejects (category III)

TABLE 2 Diagnostic Codes Used for the Retrospective Screening of Putative Cases of Alzheimer's Disease

Number 290	Senile and presenile organic psychotic conditions
290.0	Senile dementia, simple type
290.1	Presenile dementia
290.2	Senile dementia, depressed or paranoid type
290.3	Senile dementia with acute confusional state
290.4	Arteriosclerotic dementia
290.8	Other
290.9	Unspecified
Number 294	Other organic psychotic conditions (chronic)
294.0	Karsakov's psychosis or syndrome (nonalcoholic)
294.1	Dementia in conditions classified elsewhere
294.8	Other
294.9	Unspecified
Number 310	Specific nonpsychotic mental disorders following organic brain damage
310.0	Frontal lobe syndrome
310.1	Cognitive or personality change of other type
310.2	Postconcussional syndrome
310.8	Other
310.9	Unspecified
Number 331	Other cerebral degenerations
331.0	Alzheimer's disease
331.1	Pick's disease
331.2	Senile degeneration of brain
331.3	Communicating hydrocephalus
331.4	Obstructive hydrocephalus
331.5	Jakob-Creutzfeldt disease
331.6	Progressive multifocal leukoencephalopathy
331.7	Cerebral degeneration in other diseases classified elsewhere
331.8	Other
331.9	Unspecified
Number 437	Cerebrovascular disease, other, and ill-defined
437.0	Cerebral atherosclerosis
437.1	Other generalized ischemic cerebrovascular disease
437.2	Hypertensive encephalopathy
437.3	Cerebral aneurysm, nonruptured
437.4	Cerebral arteritis
437.5	Moyamoya disease
437.6	Nonpyogenic thrombosis of intracranial venous sinus
437.8	Other
437.9	Nonspecified
Number 440	Arteriosclerosis
440.9	Arteriosclerosis (senile)

Codes synonymous or similar to the general expression of dementia-senility and used to screen on a retrospective basis the patients labeled with conditions akin to dementia of the Alzheimer type.

the flow chart of Fig. 3). On that occasion, and if necessary, the managing agents will also fill in the forms for the authorization to consult medical records, the form for the authorization for autopsy, and the form for the authorization for a blood sample (item 4 in the flow chart of Fig. 3). The managing agents will then proceed to the unit of screening to complete the diagnostic scale of exclusion and inclusion criteria (on a retrospective basis) with the data available in the medical records of the putative case. At that step in the procedure (item 5a in the flow chart of Fig. 3), the managing agent fills in on a retrospective basis a form for the DSEIC for each case, collecting the information already recorded in the patient's medical history. This work is signaled to the IMAGE registry by way of the form for the DSEIC completed (item 6 in the flow chart of Fig. 3), as well as the form for the DSEIC (on a retrospective basis) itself.

On the basis of the exclusion and inclusion criteria defined for this study, all the putative cases for whom a form for the DSEIC (on a retrospective basis) has been completed are reevaluated one by one during the review session of medical records. A list of putative cases for the review session of medical records is regularly prepared. This session is directed by a geriatrician. The selection of presumptive cases represents the second step in the procedure for screening Alzheimer cases and for the corroboration of an AD diagnosis. The review session of a putative case is designed to entice the IMAGE officials to gather as much information as possible from the family physician and the nurses (if the case arises) in order to evaluate the evidence of obvious exclusion criteria. As mentioned above, the search for absolute exclusion criteria in the clinical evaluation of the case represents the objective of the review sessions. When there is clear evidence or a strong suspicion of the presence of an absolute exclusion criterion, the case is automatically classified as reject-category I. In the contrary situation, the case proceeds to the level of presumptiveness, which means that upon preliminary examination of the case by a general practitioner and after review of the medical history, there does not appear to be any other obvious disease likely to have caused the neuropsychological changes observed in the patient. Observations and comments gathered at this step are entered into the IMAGE registry by means of the form for the results of the review session of the medical records (item 8 in the flow chart of Fig. 3).

The neurological consultation represents the third step in the overall procedure for screening Alzheimer's disease cases and for the corroboration of an AD diagnosis. In stating the importance of a neurological consultation, the IMAGE Project encourages the families of presumptive cases to ask their family physician to refer the case to a neurologist in the field. At that step, all the exclusion and inclusion criteria prescribed by the diagnostic scale developed for the study are reviewed one by one by the neurologist. At regular intervals, IMAGE organizes Alzheimer CT scan clinics at the Hospital of Chicoutimi with the battery of compulsory neurological exams, in order to reduce the number of patients in the IMAGE diagnostic funnel. The form for the neurological clinics is used to plan these special sessions (item 9 in the flow chart of Fig. 3). The form for the results of the neurological consultation (item 10 in the flow chart of Fig. 3) and the form for the DSEIC (on a prospective basis) (item 5b in the flow chart of Fig. 3) are used to transmit the results of the neurological exams to the IMAGE registry. At this step, the cases may be classified as rejects-category II, if an absolute exclusion criterion has been identified by the neurologist; alternatively, they will be classified as possible or probable cases. The group of probable cases is constituted of patients whose neuropsychological changes correspond in all likelihood to those characteristic of AD, with a medical history that shows no evidence of relative or absolute exclusion criteria. The group of possible cases is constituted of patients presenting one or more confounding disease(s) in the medical history, identified by these relative or absolute exclusion criteria. The neuropsychological changes experienced by these patients, however, seem nonetheless to be caused by Alzheimer's disease (item 12 in the flow chart of Fig. 3).

The IMAGE registry produces a check list of possible and probable cases for the neuropathological investigation, that is, a global list of cases that the pathologists of the area are likely to get as patients for autopsy within the framework of IMAGE. This list is regularly updated for the pathologists (item 11 in the flow chart of Fig. 3).

The different units of screening can also report to the IMAGE registry patients' changes in location by means of the form for the transfer of a case (item 14 in the flow chart of Fig. 3).

The labels Beware-Autopsy appended to the active file of a case (item A in the flow chart of Fig. 3) are there to remind medical authorities and nurses in the institutions collaborating with the IMAGE Project that the person identified has been selected within the framework of a research project for a neuropathological study and that autopsy is required for full corroboration of a diagnosis of Alzheimer's disease. A list of telephone numbers to be dialed as death is nearing or at death itself are given on the label Beware-Autopsy in order for the notice of decease to be given to IMAGE officials, to allow for prompt autopsy procedures to be set in motion, and for the biological specimens to be collected as quickly as possible (item B in the flow chart of Fig. 3).

The neuropathological investigation constitutes the fourth and last step in the procedure for screening Alzheimer cases and for the corroboration of an AD diagnosis. At this step, a case may be identified as reject-category III, when the criteria of the neuropathological scale have not been met, or as a definite case if the counts of senile plaques and neurofibrillary tangles correspond to the criteria used for the study (24-29). The results collected by the neuropathologist are transmitted to the IMAGE registry by means of the form for the results of the neuropathological investigation (item 13 in the flow chart of Fig. 3).

In the field of study, the IMAGE officials are assisted by managing agents; their task consists in monitoring step by step the progression of cases along the four stages of the diagnostic procedure and ensuring collection of data. To assist them in their functions, they are equipped with the catalogue of the managing agents, which represents the logbook of the project in the field of study. It is made up of the following lists: check list of the IMAGE registry; check list of resources for the family information service; check list of DSEIC to be completed; check list of clinical and laboratory investigations; check list of presumptive cases for the neurological consultation; and check list of cases transferred.

The check list of the IMAGE registry provides a detailed account of the state of the operations in the field of study, recording the stage reached by the case in the procedure for the corroboration of an AD diagnosis. The object of this list is to help project officials to follow the evolution of the IMAGE file of every single case identified, along all the stages prescribed by the general diagnostic funnel. The list provides information for the identification of cases, the nature of the category and unit of screening through which the case was first referred to IMAGE, the resources in the family of a case who have been contacted through the family information service, the location and identification of the current medical records, as well as a series of details pertinent to collecting data in the field and to managing the IMAGE registry (retrospective DSEIC completed, results of the neurological consultation, prospective DSEIC completed, authorizations for autopsy and to take a blood sample, death records, availability of other biological specimens, results of the neuropathological investigation, as well as the diagnostic impression on a prospective or retrospective basis).

The check list of resources for the family information service gives the names, addresses, and telephone numbers of resources identified for every case (e.g., spouse, child, sibling). This information is obviously needed by the IMAGE official to communicate with the family of a case. Meetings are organized with family members to explain the objectives of our medical and scientific research program, and to discuss authorizations to consult medical records, to perform autopsy, and to take a blood sample. The form for the family information service is used by the managing agent to report on the discussions and exchanges with the family resources identified for each case.

The check list of DSEIC to be completed is a nominative list of putative cases for whom no general retrospective information has been obtained yet. The form for the DSEIC (on a retrospective basis) is used to gather data already present in the medical records.

The check list of clinical and laboratory investigations gives the results of the neurological consultation for each case. The exams prescribed by the DSEIC are aimed at excluding confounding diseases that, while mimicking Alzheimer's disease's neuropsychological changes, are of a totally different nature and origin.

The check list of presumptive cases for the neurologic consultation is a nominative list of presumptive cases for whom a neurological consultation has been requested. This list is used as a planning tool for the Alzheimer CT scan clinics organized at the Hospital of Chicoutimi.

The check list of cases transferred is a nominative list of the cases that have been transferred from the unit of screening in which they were last residing to a new location. The list identifies the new unit of screening of the case who has just been transferred, the dates of entry and exit, as well as its new location. The list is designed to help ensure geographical supervision of the cases within the IMAGE network.

The catalogue of the medical officer is identical to that of the managing agent, except that it only provides the information on the cases of one particular geographical sphere of screening, that is, that of each medical officer. The catalogue of the pathologist contains a check list of the names of probable and possible cases expected to be referred for autopsy and neuropathological investigation, as well as the check list of resources for the family information services of the living cases.

THE CORES FOR MEDICAL INVESTIGATIONS: PROTOCOLS FOR TRIALS

The clinical core consists of four components: the neurological, neuropsychological, geriatric, and neuropathological investigations. The protocol for neurological trials is based on the diagnostic scale of inclusion and exclusion criteria developed for IMAGE and adapted from McKhann et al. (5). The Hospital of Chicoutimi provides the resources for the neurological consultations (CT scan, biochemical laboratories, etc). IMAGE Alzheimer CT scan clinics are organized on a regular basic (generally every 4-5 weeks) at the Hospital of Chicoutimi for the overflow of presumptive cases identified in the network. The protocol for neuropsychological trials is adapted from the tools developed by the American Consortium to establish registries of AD cases. The neuropathological scale of the IMAGE Project is based on the criteria established by Ball (30). The Hospital of Chicoutimi also provides the resources for the neuropathological investigations (laboratories, microscope, freezers etc.) as part of their involvement and collaboration in the project. By special arrangement with the public security of Chicoutimi, police agents have taken charge of all transportation of brains collected within the framework of the IMAGE Project in SLSJ, following the instructions laid down by IMAGE officials.

ETHICS

Screening for putative cases of AD within the framework of the IMAGE Project is carried out following the articles prescribed by the laws on the protection of individual rights and privacy of the Province of Quebec. Our procedures have also been approved by the Quebec Commission of Access to Information.

Key informants in the network, often keepers of medical records, will take the initiative of informing the families of presumptive cases of the objectives of the research group. Generally, a verbal authorization for IMAGE officials to communicate with the family members is obtained on the occasion of a visit by the latter at the nursing home or the hospital where the case is residing, or by telephone. In the early stages of the disease, when the case is still living in the community, the authorization is obtained on the occasion of the first visits to the physician's office, or again from the case him- or herself. Upon meeting the presumptive case or members of the family of a presumptive case, the managing agents provide detailed information about the project. They also give the following guarantees: the patient does not have to undergo invasive tests or treatments, or to be subjected to any direct form of participation into the project, if he or his surrogates are unwilling to do so; only the neurologists, physicians, and other research personnel duly authorized on oath by the direction of the IMAGE project have access to medical records, for all medical, scientific, and statistical analyses; no public mention of the conclusions of the clinical investigations of a particular case will be made during or after the study; the strictest confidentiality is assured in dealing with the information obtained on the case.

All the collaborators have to sign an internal document that serves as a guarantee of confidentiality for the family of a case. This document bears the signatures of the director of IMAGE, as well as that of the collaborator, and it stipulates that the signatories undertake to respect the anonymity of cases and the confidentiality of all data collected within the framework of IMAGE.

The request to participate in IMAGE, as it is presented to the family of a presumptive case or the case him- or herself, is in keeping with the ethical rules and dispositions in force in scientific and medical projects of this type. It explains clearly the requirements and particular nature of an eventual participation; it does not lead to the disclosure of information that may cause moral harm to the patient or family; the strictest confidentiality is guaranteed in data manipulation; the patients, or their families, are entirely free to accept or refuse participation in IMAGE; all the information collected on a case within IMAGE can be consulted by the patient or family. The patients or families who refused to participate in the study are generally not solicited twice. All the names of cases are transcribed in alphanumerical codes in the IMAGE registry. Codification of names ensures that confidentiality and anonymity of data are preserved during handling of the registry. All questionnaires, forms, and lists containing data are stored under key in private IMAGE filing cabinets. The guide to the internal rules of IMAGE Project governing the confidentiality of the data collected within the registry and in the field is available upon request.

PRELIMINARY RESULTS OBTAINED ON THE IMAGE REGISTRY

Parental Age and Birth Order

Parental age (more particularly maternal age), as well as birth order, are well-known risk factors in Down's syndrome (31,32). These findings led a number of researchers to investigate a possible relationship between AD and parental age or birth order (33-40). Although no paternal effect was found, analyses of the maternal age and birth order showed conflicting results. In view of the ease with which we can select a variety of control groups out of the SOREP registry, IMAGE has undertaken to determine whether parental age and birth order were risk factors in a population of 133 clinically diagnosed Alzheimer's disease patients from the SLSJ. The cases had been classified as definite, probable, or possible AD patients on the basis of the criteria described above. A method devised by Haldane and Smith (41) was used in order to decide whether, in our 133 subships, AD cases tended to be born later. The Haldane-Smith test is based on the sum of the birth ranks of all affected members in all sibships. Hence, this test uses only the affected sibships and no controls. In case there is no information on some sibs, the method proposes to eliminate these "unspecified" members. For the present analysis, the deceased sibs and those younger than 40 years of age were considered "unspecified" since their disease status remained unknown.

Maternal age was known in 120 cases and paternal age in 122 cases. The mean parental age for the normal sibs of the Alzheimer patients was calculated using the SOREP population registry. Parental age at the time of birth of the spouses of AD patients was also determined. Six control groups were created using the SOREP registry. Controls 1-2-3 were matched by the date of marriage of the parents of the Alzheimer patients (± 5 days), their socioeconomic status as defined by the father's profession, the residence of parents, and the birth rank of the AD patients. Controls 4-5-6 were randomly selected births matched by sex and year of birth of the Alzheimer's disease patients, as well as by the socioeconomic status of the parents. The statistical analysis was performed using the Student's paired t test, two-tailed.

The Haldane-Smith test was applied for testing "no birth order effect" against a "born later" alternative. No significant result was found (test statistic = −3.075, $p > 0.99$). Table 3 shows the parental age at time of birth for Alzheimer's disease patients, normal siblings, spouses, and controls. Both maternal and paternal mean ages at the time of birth of the Alzheimer's disease patients were found to be significantly lower than the ages at the time of birth of the normal siblings (respectively, $F = 2.64$, $p < 0.001$ and $F = 2.25$, $p = 0.001$). No significant difference was found between parental age at the time of birth of the Alzheimer's disease patients and their spouses, or any of the six control groups ($p < 0.10$).

In a previous report, Larsson et al. (34) found that 199 of 408 patients with senile dementia belonged to the first half of the birth series and the remaining 209 the second half of the birth series. Using the method devised by Carothers et al. (42), Whalley et al. (35) did not find any significant birth order effect. Amaducci et al. (39) found a borderline significant relationship between a high birth rank and AD. White et al. (40) showed that the average birth order of 126 autopsy-proven Alzheimer s disease patients was significantly less than the average

TABLE 3 Parental Age at Time of Birth for Alzheimer's Disease Patients, Normal Siblings, Spouses, and Controls

	Mother's age (years)		Father's age (years)	
	Mean	S.D.	Mean	S.D.
Alzheimer's disease patients	29.4	6.7	32.6	7.5
Normal siblings	31.5[a]	4.1	34.9[a]	5.0
Spouses	29.5	6.1	33.4	6.7
Control 1	29.7	4.2	33.3	4.7
Control 2	30.1	4.3	33.5	4.3
Control 3	29.2	4.3	33.4	5.6
Control 4	30.2	4.5	33.2	7.0
Control 5	30.0	4.2	32.5	5.1
Control 6	29.1	5.7	32.2	6.8

[a]$p < 0.05$.

birth order of the controls selected among the births recorded in Anoka County (Minnesota). However, the average birth order for the Alzheimer's disease patients was not significantly different from the expected average computed assuming random distribution of the AD cases throughout the sibship.

Our results did not show any evidence of a relationship between a high birth order and AD. In fact, it was noted that testing "no birth order effect" against an "early-born" alternative would have given highly significant results ($p < 0.001$). White et al. (40) suggested that their result was probably due to the control families being larger than the AD families. However, the present analysis was based only on the affected sibships and, therefore, there is no possible bias due to the choice of the control families. An "early-born" effect may sometimes be explained by the lack of ascertainment of younger cases (secondary cases) who have not yet developed the disease or been screened. The use of the Haldane-Smith method, which allows one to eliminate the very young sibling in the computing (less than 40 years old), has helped to circumvent this problem.

A younger maternal age at the time of birth of the Alzheimer's disease patients as compared to that of the normal siblings (29.4 versus 31.5 years) was found in our preliminary studies. The direction of this difference is opposite to what would be expected if there was a maternal age effect in AD. The difference in the mean maternal age at the time of birth of the Alzheimer's disease patients compared with that of the spouses and controls was not statistically significant. Similar results have already been reported by Heyman et al. (37) in comparing maternal age at the time of birth of 36 clinically diagnosed AD patients with their spouses, and by Corkin et al. (38) in comparing the maternal age at the time of birth of 37 clinically diagnosed AD patients with the age at birth of 34 controls of comparable age and socioeconomic status. A similar conclusion was reached by English and Cohen (38), who compared 64 clinically diagnosed AD patients with their spouses and spouses of 87 patients with Parkinson's disease. White et al. (40) did not find any significant difference in maternal age at the time of birth of 112 AD patients (most of them autopsy proven), their normal siblings, and 200 randomly selected briths in Anoka County (Minnesota). Cohen et al. (36) found an association between maternal age and AD, but their controls were not matched on factors such as socioeconomic status. Amaducci et al. (39) found a maternal age effect for AD but their controls were not matched on characteristics of AD patients.

A younger paternal age at the time of birth of the Alzheimer's disease patients as compared to that of the normal siblings (32.6 versus 34.9 years) was also found in our prelininary studies. The mean age of fathers at the time of birth of AD cases was not significantly different from the mean age for the spouses or the controls. Such findings have already been reported by several workers (36,37, 39,40).

Whalley et al. (35) compared 69 autopsy-proven AD cases with 207 unrelated controls matched for year of birth, sex, and paternal occupation. They found a significant increase in maternal and paternal ages for the AD cases. However, they did not find any significant parental age effect when using the method of Carothers et al. (42), which estimates a relative risk as a function of parental age and birth order and, therefore, uses the siblings as controls.

In conclusion, we believe that the controversial results described in the literature may be a consequence of control selection. The studies that used the siblings or the spouses as controls or matched the controls on socioeconomic status did not show any parental age or birth order effects for Alzheimer's disease. Our results, which are based on six different control groups, are in agreement with these conclusions.

Season of Birth

A second series of measurements was undertaken to study seasonality of birth in the Alzheimer's disease patients from the IMAGE registry. The sample of cases consisted of 55 men born between 1893 and 1930, and 70 women born between 1898 and 1932. Only five cases were known to be of the familial type. It should be mentioned, however, that family medical history had not been established on a systematic basis at the time of these measurements. The age of onset was known for 78 cases. Eight control groups were defined to carry out the analyses. The first group of controls consisted of the patients' spouses; unfortunately the information was available for only 69 cases. The second group represented the cumulative month of the 118,202 births registered between 1891 and 1930 in SLSJ. The third group was obtained by pooling 3 samples of 125 persons matched on the year of marriage of parents, their residence, as well as the father's occupation and parity. The fourth group was matched on the year of parents' marriage, their residence, the father's occupation, the sex of the case, and his or her order in family of married sibs (to control for infantile mortality); this group consisted of 125 controls and their spouses. Four other control groups of randomly selected individuals matched on sex and year of birth who survived at least until the age of 40 were also constituted (control groups 5-8).

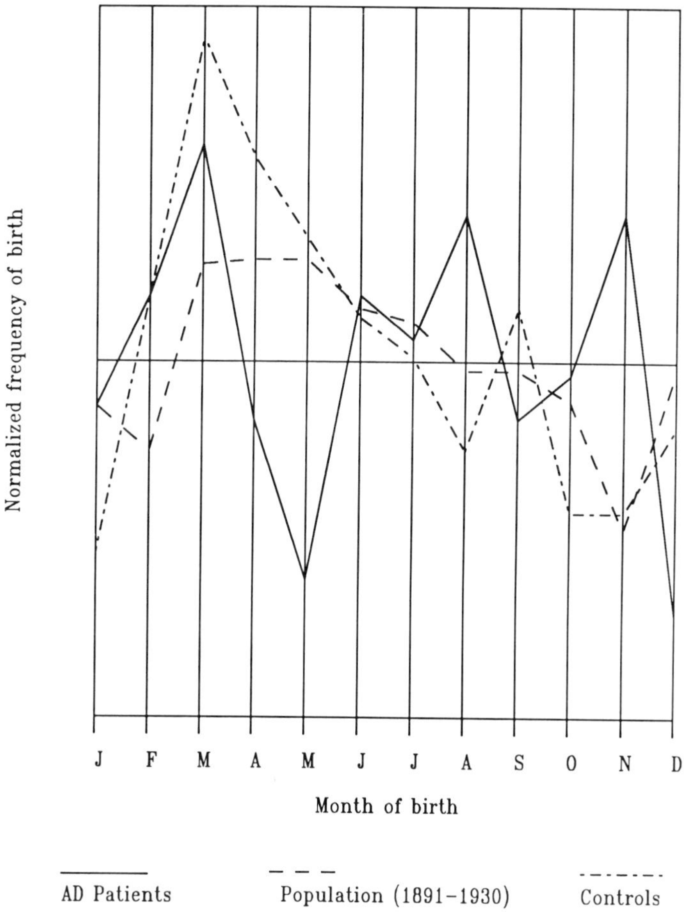

FIGURE 4 Monthly birth distribution in Alzheimer's disease patients and in control groups.

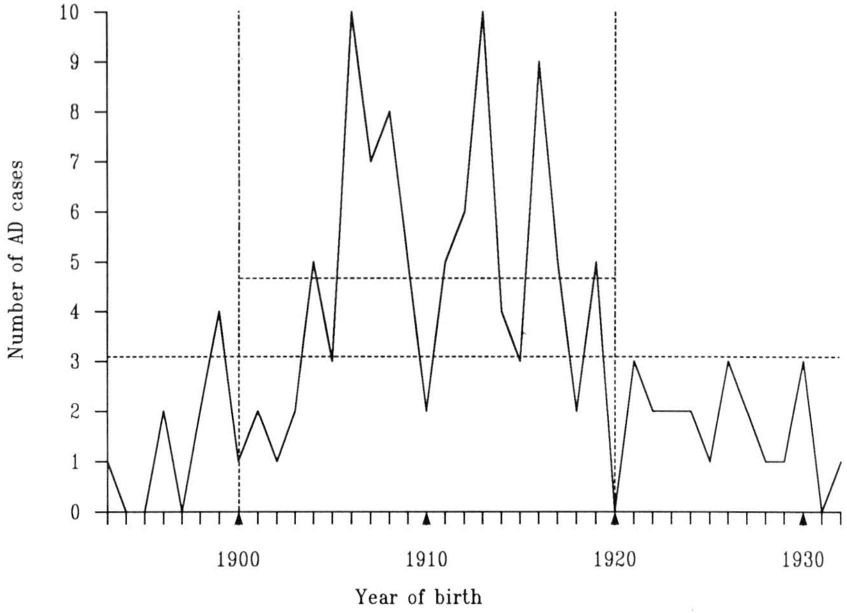

FIGURE 5 Yearly birth distribution of patients with Alzheimer's disease.

The distributions of months of birth were analyzed by the test of goodness-of-fit of sample marginal distribution to the relative length of month using a small chi-square test (43-45). Figure 4 shows the monthly birth distribution for the Alzheimer's disease patients, the general population between 1891 and 1930, and the third control group (as defined above). A statistically significant difference was found between Alzheimer's disease patients and the general population between 1891 and 1930. A significant difference was also found between Alzheimer's disease patients and the third control group and between Alzheimer's disease patients and the fourth control group, whereas this was not observed between the Alzheimer's disease patients and their spouses, or between the Alzheimer's disease patients and control groups 5-8.

Yearly Birth Distribution

Figure 5 shows the yearly birth distribution of the 125 Alzheimer's disease patients. Most of the cases were found to be born between 1900 and 1920. Since the project was started in 1985, most of the patients born before 1900 have died, whereas most of those born after 1920 and who may develop AD have not been diagnosed yet. The distribution was found to be highly uneven with a 2- or 3-year cycle (peaks in 1904, 1906-1908, 1911-1913, 1916, and 1919). We are now studying on a yearbasis the distribution of mortality of all individuals born between 1891 and 1930, as well as the yearly distribution of stillbirth and infant mortality.

Although it may still be too early to draw conclusions from the yearly birth distribution, with an alternation of peaks and depressions and a periodicity of 2-3 years, different working hypotheses can be generated. These preliminary results would appear to suggest that genetic factors or exposures occurring during the gestation period could play an important role in the causes of AD. Hence, one could hypothesize that a modification of the genome by viral DNA might take place during intrauterine life, and that gene function would then be more easily disrupted in a later period of life if promoted by some other environmental agent(s). This model applies perhaps more readily to the sporadic form of the disease. On the other hand, one could also hypothesize that through viral infection or some exposure to an environmental toxin during intrauterine life, an important phenomenon of cell depletion takes place in specific areas, not interfering at that time, however, with the development of the brain. As a result of aging, the number of cells in the particular locus of the viral scar would go below that of the threshold number of cells required to preserve normal cerebral functions.

Horner has used Sartwell's incubation period model as a tool to approach the question of the relative importance of genetic and environmental factors in AD (46). Sartwell has demonstrated that the incubation period for infectious disease fits a log normal distribution; therefore, if genetic factors are predominant in the development of a disease, age at disease onset is considered the end of the incubation period. Horner's preliminary analysis of four series of AD cases has established that age at onset consistently follows a log normal distribution. Despite a number of inherent limitations in the method, this finding would support the hypothesis of a genetic cause, but may also suggest that the search for environmental risk factors should focus on the prenatal life of the cases. The fact that Alzheimer's disease is widespread throughout any given population might find its explanation in a very common cause, that is, a ubiquitous causal factor (e.g., measles, or another common virus, for example).

CONCLUSION

Research on AD has so far been largely compartmentalized within specialities, such as neurology, neurochemistry, neuropsychology, epidemiology, and radiology. The major challenge of AD research in the future will be to seek means of merging the substantive findings across specialities. Ideally, this challenge can best be met by collecting all the data on the same subjects, since using a common rigorous set of both diagnostic criteria and disciplinary measurements across various studies hardly seems realistic and feasible; controls would be extremely costly. Indeed, exhaustive multidisciplinary comparisons that were to be trusted would require a replication of either of its cross-sectional or case-control studies, in the various sets of cases investigated separately. In this context, the IMAGE Project has opted for the multidisciplinary approach and seeks to establish a registry of AD cases on a general population, since we believe that any serious investigative effort to cover the widest range of risk factors should aim at surveying a targeted field in the most exhaustive fashion. This should be done with a view to screening as systematically as possible for all living AD cases in the entire population selected for the study and evaluating them for a relatively long period of time.

Sample sizes have typically been too small to identify the differential patterns unique to AD. Since AD is a progressively deteriorating condition with enormous individual variations in expression, it seems essential to evaluate large samples of individuals who meet the diagnostic criteria. In doing so, we can anticipate being able to determine whether common clinical features are consistent across the individuals, while remaining distinct from both normal aging and other dementing conditions. In order to characterize AD at both the neuropathological and clinical levels, it is imperative to make comparisons among individuals with diagnoses of AD, diagnoses of dementias of other causes, as well as normals. A majority of studies investigating the distinct characteristics of AD have focused on the differences between the latter and normals, while studies comparing AD with other dementias were conducted on small samples. Differentiating between AD and other forms of dementia remains to be done using various batteries of clinical and neuropsychological measurements. True statistically significant results, which may provide the basis for a clear distinction between subtypes and for developing specific markers for AD, will probably only be obtained from large samples.

The IMAGE research design is based on prospective and longitudinal screening of one population. Until recently, the majority of studies on AD were retrospective cross-sectional designs, with a typical lack of control over inclusion and exclusion criteria for diagnostic decisions. In our case, as well as with a limited number of experiments across the world, only after specifically defined criteria have been documented are individuals entered into the study and evaluated at specific intervals over the course of their disease.

While providing the experimental set to develop an operational model for establishing a population-based registry of cases of AD over a large geographical area, IMAGE will permit an evaluation of the reliability of diagnostic procedures, since the criteria for diagnostic decisions have been developed beforehand and are applied similarly to all cases in the study. Through this project, is should be possible to gather sufficient data to create a pool of longitudinal information to examine the interrelationships between scores of the clinical, neuropsychological, and neuropathological measures, to determine which particular measures identify the differences among the dementias, and particularly between the subtypes of senile dementia of the Alzheimer's type (SDAT).

Most importantly, IMAGE should provide the elements to establish the basis for a comprehensive research model that allows decompartmentalization of research specialities and integration of multidisciplinary data on the same subjects within one registry.

ACKNOWLEDGMENTS

This study was supported by research grants from the Medical Research Council of Canada, the Fonds de la Réchérche en Santé du Québec, La Fondation Jean-Louis Lévesque, the Alzheimer Society of Canada, and La Fédération de l'Age d'Or du Québec.

The authors are grateful to Dr. Ken Morgan (Department of Epidemiology and Biostatistics, McGill University, Montreal) for performing the statistical analyses. They also wish to thank Mrs. Muriel Grenon and Lisette Tremblay and Messrs. Hugues Tétreault and Jocelyn Martel for assistance in the field operations, as well as Mrs. Hélène Faucher for typing the manuscript.

REFERENCES

1. Ineichen, B. (1987). Measuring the rising tide: How many dementia cases will there be by 2001? *Br. J. Psychiatry* 150: 193-200.
2. Weiler, P.G. (1987). The public health impact of Alzheimer's disease. *Am. J. Public Health* 77: 1157-1158.
3. Hay, J.W., and Ernst, R.L. (1987). The economic costs of Alzheimer's disease. *Am. J. Public Health* 77: 1169-1175.
4. Henderson, A.S. (1986). The epidemiology of Alzheimer's disease. *Br. Med. Bull.* 42: 3-10.
5. McKhann, G., Drachman, D., Folstein, M., et al. (1984). Clinical diagnosis of Alzheimer's disease: Report of the NINCDS-ADRDA work group under the auspices of Department of Health and Human Services Task Force on Alzheimer's disease. *Neurology* 34: 939-944.
6. Wade, J.P.H., Mirsen, T.R., Hachinski, V.C., Fisman, M., Lau, C., and Merskey, H. (1987). The clinical diagnosis of Alzheimer's disease. *Arch. Neurol.* 44: 24-29.
7. Katzman, R. (1987). Alzheimer's disease: Advances and opportunities. *J. Am. Geriatr. Soc.* 35: 69-73.
8. Tierney, M.C., Reid, D.W., Zorzitto, M.L., Snow, W.G., Fisher, R.H., Campbell-Taylor, I., and Lewis, A. (1986). The differential diagnosis of Alzheimer's disease: Conceptual and methodological issues. *Can. J. Neurol. Sci.* 13: 424-426.
9. Traber, J., and Gispen, W.H. (1985). In: *Senile Dementia of the Alzheimer Type.* Berlin, Springer Verlag.
10. Kay, D.W.K. (1987). Heterogeneity in Alzheimer's disease: Epidemiological and family studies. *Trends Neurosci.* 10: 194-195.

11. Mayeux, R., Stern, Y., and Spanton, S. (1985). Heterogeneity in dementia of the Alzheimer type: Evidence of subgroups. *Neurology* 35: 453-461.
12. Berg, L. (1985). Does Alzheimer's disease represent an exaggeration of normal aging? *Arch. Neurol.* 42: 737-739.
13. Nee, L.E., Eldridge, R., Sunderland, T., Thomas, C.B., Katz, D., Thompson, K.E., Weingartner, H., Weiss, H., Julian, C., and Cohen, R. (1987). Dementia of the Alzheimer type: Clinical and family study of 22 twin pairs. *Neurology* 37: 359-363.
14. Mozar, H.N., Bal, D.G., and Howard, J.T. (1987). Perspectives on the etiology of Alzheimer's disease. *JAMA* 257: 1503-1507.
15. Broeckhoven, C.V., Genthe, A.M., Vandenberghe, A., Horsthemke, B., Backhovens, H., Raeymaekers, P., Hul, W.V., Wehnert, A., Gheuens, J., Cras, P., Bruyland, M., Martin, J.J., Slabaum, M., Multhaup, G., Masters, C.L., Beyreuther, K., Gurling, H.M.D., Mullan, M.J., Holland, A., Barton, A., Irving, N., Williamson, R., Richards, S.J., and Hardy, J.A. (1987). Failure of familial Alzheimer's disease to segregate with the A4-amyloid gene in several European families. *Nature* 329: 153-155.
16. Tanzi, R.E., St. George-Hyslop, P.H., Haines, J.L., Polinsky, R.J., Nee, L., Foncin, J.-F., Neve, R.L., McClatchey, A.I., Conneally, P.M., and Gusella, J.F. (1987). The genetic defect in familial Alzheimer's disease is not tightly linked to the amyloid β-protein gene. *Nature* 329: 156-157.
17. Brody, J.A. (1982). An epidemiologist views senile dementia–facts and fragments. *Am. J. Epidemiol.* 115: 155-162.
18. Schoenberg, B.S. (1986). Epidemiology of Alzheimer's disease and other dementing illnesses. *J. Chron. Dis.* 39: 1095-1104.
19. Worton, R.G. (1987). Molecular analysis of Duchenne and Becker muscular dystrophy. *Bio Essays* 7: 57-62.
20. Monaco, A.P., and Kunkel, L.M. (1987). A giant locus for the Duchenne and Becker muscular dystrophy gene. *TIG* 3: 33-37.
21. Robertson, M. (1987). Muscular dystrophy: Mapping the disease phenotype. *Nature* 327: 372-373.
22. Cork, L.C., Kitt, C.A., Struble, R.G., Griffin, J.W., and Price, D.L. (1987). Animal models of degenerative neurological disease. In: *Animal Models: Assessing the Scope of their Use in Biomedical Research.* New York, Alan R. Liss, Inc., pp. 241-269.
23. Reisberg, B. (1983). Clinical diagnosis and differential diagnosis of Alzheimer's disease and related disorders. In: *Alzheimer's Disease: The Standard Reference.* New York, Free Press, pp. 173-187.
24. Yamamoto, T., and Hirano, A. (1986). A comparative study of modified Bielschowsky, Bodian and thioflavine S stains on Alzheimer's neurofibrillary tangles. *Neuropathol. Appl. Neurobiol.* 12: 3-9.
25. Ball, M.J. (1977). Neuronal loss, neurofibrillary tangles and granulovacuolar degeneration in the hippocampus with aging and dementia. *Acta Neuropathol.* 37: 111-118.
26. Ball, M.J. (1978). Topographic distribution of neurofibrillary tangles and granulovacuolar degeneration in hippocampal cortex of aging and demented patients: A quantitative study. *Acta Neuropathol.* 42: 73-80.

27. Rogers, J., and Morrison, J.H. (1985). Quantitative morphology and regional and lacunar distributions of senile plaques in Alzheimer's disease. *J. Neurol.* 5: 2801-2808.
28. Hedreen, J.C., Struble, R.G., Whitehouse, P.J., and Price, D.L. (1984). Topography of the magnocellular basal forebrain system in human brain. *J. Neuropathol. Exp. Neurol.* 43: 1-21.
29. Abercrombie, M. (1946). Estimation of nuclear population from microtome sections. *Anat. Rec.* 94: 239-247.
30. M. Ball, Personal communication.
31. Penrose, L.S. (1933). The relative effects of paternal and maternal age in mongolism. *J. Genet.* 27: 219-233.
32. Erickson, J.D. (1978). Down's syndrome, paternal age, maternal age and birth order. *Ann. Hum. Genet.* 41: 289-293.
33. Stene, J., and Stene, E. (1977). Statistical methods for detecting a moderate paternal age effect on the incidence of a disorder when a maternal one is present. *Ann. Hum. Genet.* 40: 343-347.
34. Larsson, T., Sjogren, T., and Jacobson, G. (1963). Senile dementia, clinical, sociomedical and genetic study. *Acta Psychiatr. Scand.* 39: 190-191.
35. Whalley, L.J., Carothers, A.D., Collyer, S., et al. (1982). A study of familial factors in Alzheimer's disease. *Br. J. Psychiatry* 140: 249-256.
36. Cohen, D., Eisdorfer, C., and Leverenz, J. (1982). Alzheimer's disease and maternal age. *J. Am. Geriatr. Soc.* 30: 656-659.
37. Heyman, A., Wilkinson, W.E., Hurwitz, B.J., et al. (1983). Alzheimer's disease, genetic aspects and associated clinical disorders. *Ann. Neurol.* 14: 507-515.
38. Corkin, S., Growdon, J.H., and Rasmussen, S.L. (1983). Parental age as a risk factor in Alzheimer's disease. *Ann. Neurol.* 13: 674-676.
39. English, D., and Cohen, D. (1985). A case-control study of maternal age in Alzheimer's disease. *J. Am. Geriatr. Soc.* 33: 167-169.
40. Amaducci, L.A., Fratiglioni, L., Rocca, W.A., et al. (1986). Risk factors for clinically diagnosed Alzheimer's disease, a case-control study of an Italian population. *Neurology* 36: 922-931.
41. White, J.A., McGue, M., and Heston, L.L. (1986). Fertility and parental age in Alzheimer's disease. *J. Gerontol.* 41: 40-43.
42. Haldane, J.B.S., and Smith, C.A.B. (1947). A simple exact test for birth-order effect. *Ann. Eugen.* 14: 117-124.
43. Carothers, A.D., Collyer, S., De Mey, R., et al. (1978). Parental age and birth order in the etiology of some sex chromosome aneuploidies. *Ann. Hum. Genet.* 41: 277-287.
44. Smith, C.A.B. (1952). A test for heterogeneity of proportions. *Ann. Eugen.* 16: 16-25.
45. Smith, C.A.B. (1953). A simplified heterogeneity test. *Ann. Eugen.* 17: 35-36.
46. Smith, C.A.B. (1986). Chi-squared tests with small numbers. *Ann. Hum. Genet.* 50: 163-167.
47. Horner, R.D. (1987). Age at onset of Alzheimer's disease: Clue to the relative importance of etiologic factors? *Am. J. Epidemiol.* 126: 409-414.

Part IV
Overview and Directions for the Future

22

New Challenges in Alzheimer's Disease and Dementia Research

Z. S. KHACHATURIAN / *National Institute on Aging, National Institutes of Health, Bethesda, Maryland*

Speculations concerning the aging brain and systematic studies of age-related changes in the nervous system have a long history. However, only during the last decade have neuroscientists begun to investigate seriously a broad spectrum of topics in the neurobiology of aging. These range from basic molecular to clinical issues, and from the physical chemistry of membrane transport mechanisms to the neuropsychiatric assessment of the aging brain. Not long ago, little was known about "senility," and Alzheimer's disease (AD) was considered a hopeless affliction of the aged. Now we know that chemical and physical changes in the brain can account for some of the memory deficits in AD and benign forgetfulness of the aged. The remarkable pace of scientific progress in this area of research increases the likelihood that some forms of dementia may be treatable by pharmacological agents.

During the past few years, it has been clearly established that the hallmark of AD is a serious defect in the cholinergic system. This finding has stimulated considerable scientific activity aimed at identifying the exact nature of this neurochemical defect and finding a pharmacological means of ameliorating the disease. This type of research has been driven by the assumption that the neurochemical deficits in AD result primarily from biochemical abnormalities in the synthesis or release of acetylcholine. It is assumed that the affected neurons would function normally if these biochemical abnormalities could be corrected. This, the search for treatment has focused on pharmacological manipulations aimed at increasing the supply of the substrate necessary for the synthesis of the neurotransmitter, increasing the amount of the neurotransmitter released, prolonging the availability of the neurotransmitter at the synaptic junction by blocking its breakdown, using neurotransmitter agonists, manipulating the sensitivity of receptors at the postsynaptic membrane, and attempting to manipulate the metabolic activity within the neuron.

Despite some promising initial results in the treatment of AD with agents such as choline, lecithin, and physostigmine, the effort to manipulate cholinergic pharmacology has not produced any consistent or long-lasting treatments for AD. Several possible explanations could account for this lack of success:

1. It is unlikely that AD results from a deficit in a single neurotransmitter system. There is mounting evidence that the pathophysiology of this disease involves multiple neurotransmitter systems and neuropeptides.
2. The observed neurochemical changes or deficits in AD might be epiphenomena associated with or a consequence of cell death. In patients with AD, cell death occurs in specific regions of the brain, particularly in areas richly innervated with cholinergic cells.
3. The neurochemical deficits might be a consequence of other changes within the cell, such as abnormal oxidative or glucose metabolism.

At present it is not known why certain types of neurons are at risk for cell death in AD and whether such cell death can be averted by pharmacological means. There are several working hypotheses concerning the possible mechanisms of cell death. One of the most active areas of study focuses on the chemistry of neurofibrillary tangles. Paired helical filaments make up the neurofibrillary tangles within nerve cells that are the classic pathological markers of AD. It is now known that these filaments are composed of proteins with unusual solubility characteristics derived either by a cross-linking reaction or by the formation of beta-pleated proteins. These insoluble protein masses may form a physical blockage that interferes with axoplasmic transport mechanisms, thus leading to cell death. It is essential that future research focus on the biochemistry and physical chemistry of such proteins and on the enzymology of beta-pleated proteins and cross-linking reactions.

Another important area of study concerns the role of neuromodulators and neurotrophic factors affecting the functioning and viability of cells. There is some evidence that the function and viability of the nerve cell might be compromised when there is no chemical feedback or lack of neurotrophic factor from a target cell. The role of neuropeptides such as somatostatin and the mechanisms by which they modulate neuronal activity are not well understood. Whether such neuromodulators also serve as trophic factors is not known. The chemistry of neuromodulators and the neurotrophic factors is an area that needs greater emphasis.

Recent findings that a pharmacological agent such as methyl phenyl tetrahydropyridine (MPTP) might interact with enzymes in the body and produce neurotoxins for specific types of cells (e.g., substantia nigra), and thus might be involved in a neurodegenerative disorder, has given further credence to the possibility that similar sequences of events might be involved in AD. We need to know more about environmental toxins and infectious viral agents that have been associated with cell death. The chemistry of how such agents interfere with cell functioning is still not well understood.

There is some evidence that in AD, at least in some regions of the brain, there are reductions in glucose utilization. These findings stem from positron emission tomographic (PET) imaging studies as well as biochemical studies on pyruvate dehydrogenase complex (PDHC) using biopsy material. There is a great need to learn more about the biochemistry of metabolism within the cytosol, especially oxidative metabolism and glucose utilization. It is important to have a better understanding of changes in such metabolic pathways associated with aging and disease states. Disruptions in such metabolic activity might be an important factor in cell death. Also, we do not know why there appears to be selective vulnerability; the role of genetic factors in such selectivity is an area requiring greater study.

Another essential cluster of studies that are needed concerns membrane biophysics and how age-related membrane changes influence transport and homeostasis of essential ions such as calcium. There is some evidence that aging, as well as certain diseases, causes changes in the transport mechanisms that regulate cytosol-free calcium concentration. We need to learn more about the biophysics of ion channels, pumps, and transport systems associated with cell and organelle membranes.

The types of studies discussed above are extremely important because they provide a crucial beginning for piecing together the AD puzzle. It is now possible to formulate testable hypotheses that can provide a common framework for interrelating a number of the discrete results discussed here. For example, in study after study we are seeing the importance of calcium levels within the cell in terms of cell-to-cell communication and even the viability of the cell itself. Many of the AD-related changes in the brain point to the possibility that the underlying cellular pathological change is associated with a disruption in the delicately balanced homeostatic system of transporting calcium across the cell membrane. Such a disruption of the system could be a consequence of changes in the transport mechanism of the blood-brain-barrier; pathological changes associated with walls of the brain microvasculature (e.g., amyloid deposition, severe hypoxia, ischemia, or hypoglycemia); exposure to a neurotoxin; pathogenic, or infectious agents; other insults; or aging. Further study should allow us to develop integrated theories of aging and better understand the biological mechanism of diseases such as AD.

An important issue associated with AD is that of accurate diagnosis. There are as yet no specific studies identifying the frequency and cause of reversible cognitive impairments in the elderly, but it is estimated that up to 20% of persons aged 65 and over who have been labeled as "demented" have reversible brain disorders that require evaluation and treatment. Misdiagnosis is extremely costly and a tragic waste when it leads to long-term institutionalization. There is clearly an urgent need to continue the quest for scientific knowledge about diagnosis and treatment possibilities for dementia and the biological mechanisms of aging and of such dementing disorders as AD. In 1983, the National Institute on Aging, in collaboration with the American Association of Retired Persons, sponsored a research planning workshop on the Diagnosis of Alzheimer's Disease. This workshop identified some crucial scientific opportunities for further research on diagnosis. This meeting has begun to bear fruit.

The first finding concerns a protein present in nerve cells involved in the formation of the two types of brain lesions (neuritic plaques and neurofibrillary tangles) that are the hallmark of AD. The significance of this finding is that this abnormal protein is unique to the brains of AD patients. It is not found in normal brain and it is found only in very specific regions of the AD brain that have significant cell loss. This is a crucial finding because it provides the medical scientist with a potential clear diagnosis of this disease. It also opens the door for finding out the mechanism by which the abnormal lesions develop in the brain of AD patients.

The second important discovery concerns another protein called "tau" in the normal nerve cell, but shown to be the major component of paired helical filaments (the neurofibrillary tangles), which are the abnormal protein associated with AD. Tau is known to promote the assembly of microtubules (ingredient parts inside of a nerve cell) that are involved in the transport of biological molecules between the nerve body and its terminals. The significance of finding that a normal protein, such as tau, is associated with a major lesion in AD raises the possibility that, in selected nerve cells in this disease, certain chemical modifications of tau might occur that will allow the nerve cell to form tangles. This finding now will allow scientists another avenue to explore the exact mechanism by which this lesion is caused in AD.

To advance research on the diagnosis of AD there is a need for longitudinal studies. Long-term studies based on standardized procedures and careful controls would allow pooling and comparison of data from all disciplines involved in the study and treatment of AD. Such studies could be classified into two broad categories: studies collecting detailed information on individuals who already have AD and studies involving general aged populations to collect information on premorbid events and conditions of those who might show the disease. This approach should include efforts to establish and link centers in a network for the care and study of AD patients; to establish a central resource for data and a processing center accessible to all investigators in the network; and to establish standard guidelines and procedures for psychological testing, neuropsychiatric protocols, neuroimaging, autopsy, storage and handling of brain tissue, data storage and handling, computer programs, measurements, and nomenclature.

The major difficulty in diagnosing AD involves the definition of the disease itself and its varied and subtle manifestations. Alzheimer's disease requires a combined clinical-pathological diagnosis. The relationships among neuropsychological, neuroradiological, and neuropathological indices of the disease are not well understood. The patient who appears to be borderline on the basis of near-normal neuropsychological test scores might show brain atrophy in neuroradiological examinations. Neuropathological study may show little or no changes in postmortem examinations of the brain of a patient whose dementia had fulfilled all psychological-behavioral requirements for the disease during life. An additional problem is that of clinically differentiating AD from diseases such as multi-infarct dementia, severe depression, nutritional deficiencies, or Pick's disease that may mimic or coexist with it. A continuing effort to define the disease precisely must remain the basis of all research in the field.

There seems to be a genetic component in AD, but external toxic or infectious processes probably also play a significant role. The role of environmental factors is, therefore, another central research theme that needs to be emphasized. Schizophrenia, which also has been shown to have a genetic component, is a useful model for elucidating possible mechanisms for AD. As may be the case with schizophrenia, a susceptibility to AD may be genetically transmitted, but a particular still unknown environmental factor (or factors) must be present for the disease to appear. The wide range of symptoms and pathological lesions seen in AD suggests that it is a complex of related diseases involving more than one gene and more than one precipitating environmental factor in each case. A concerted interdisciplinary effort to investigate all likely environmental possibilities will be necessary, not only to establish firmly the natural history of the disease and its causes but also to identify risk factors and warn those who, through family case registries, have been found to be susceptible.

The process of normal aging is relatively poorly understood. There are no consistent, established determinants of "normal" cognitive impairment and memory loss with advancing years, nor are the neurological, neurochemical, and neurophysiological changes or the gross and fine anatomical changes that accompany normal aging understood well enough to provide a firm base for determining "abnormal" changes. Until we achieve a better understanding of the normal aging process, the diagnosis of AD will continue to be a difficult and sometimes inaccurate combined clinicopathological process.

Because no clinical feature of AD is unique to the disease, differentiating it from other similar disorders is difficult. Other diseases that can be confused with AD include Pick's disease, multi-infarct dementia and other forms of cerebrovascular disease, hydrocephalus, nutritional deficiencies, amyotrophic lateral sclerosis and multiple sclerosis, and dementias resulting from tumors and brain injury. The co-occurrence of many diseases with AD adds to the difficulty of diagnosis. Carefully sorting out the presence of overlapping diseases is important to allow for effective diagnosis and treatment.

Although effective treatment for AD is not yet available, there are useful therapies for various diseases that produce the symptoms of dementia. The danger exists that appropriate therapy that might bring relief, even cure, may be withheld from some patients if they are misdiagnosed. For example, the aged patient with dementia produced by severe depression might be helped by antidepressant drug treatment. Developing methods of firmly differentiating AD from other nervous system diseases should be a high priority of research on diagnosis.

Pedigree studies investigating the familial-genetic aspects of AD should be initiated. Familial studies will help to predict persons who are at risk for the disease. Current observations indicate that individuals with close family members who have, or have had, the disease are more likely to develop it than those with no cases of AD in their families. Genetic parameters of the disease need to be confirmed; a broad cooperative program of centralized record-keeping and pooling of familial records, from worldwide as well as American sources, would speed this process.

One way of encouraging pedigree studies is the establishment of family registries that would maintain records on well-characterized, well-confirmed AD cases. The registries would provide the means to study the natural history of AD and foster the collection of extensive longitudinal neuropsychological data of cognitive function in individuals who might be at risk. These registries would also aid in the scrupulous tracing of pedigrees necessary in establishing cell lines for genetic research.

Research conducted in isolated communities or groups may be especially useful in studying the familial incidence of AD. More studies are needed to establish a familial incidence. To be truly representative, these studies must go beyond clinics and nursing homes and reach into the community.

The dimensions of the health problems posed by age-related changes in the central nervous system are vast. Basic research into the neurobiology of aging as the route to resolving these problems has been demonstrably successful in advancing knowledge of the human brain and providing the first real insights into some of the more baffling neurological disorders. The treatment of Parkinson's disease patients with L-dopa to replace the loss of a vital brain chemical, dopamine, and the discovery of the enkephalins and endorphins—the brain's own "opiate" drugs—are important examples.

These advances have come about because of a critical combination of talent and technology in neuroscience. It is now possible to obtain a detailed picture of what happens at the molecular level of a nerve cell as well as a clearer idea of how large clusters of nerve cells and systems operate in elaborating complex human behaviors. Enthusiasm in the field of neuroscience is running high, and researchers are optimistic about the future of brain research. In several areas of investigation, convergent approaches are focusing on key issues of neurobiology. In order to move toward the fundamental goal of preventing nervous system disorders, developing effective treatments for those presently affected, and ensuring the rapid transfer of research advances to clinical applications, it is essential to capitalize on this new momentum in neuroscience. Progress in biological science needs good ideas, appropriate biological models, and the necessary technology: the methods and tools to make the observations fruitful. The neurosciences can now command all three of these elements. There has never been a lack of good ideas or experimental models, but only in the past 20 or 30 years have there been significant gains in technological progress. These achievements in technology are expected to continue making a substantial difference in the rate of advancement of knowledge in neuroscience.

In summary, the systematic study of AD began only within the last decade, despite the fact that the disease was first described nearly three-quarters of a century ago. In this brief period of time, our knowledge of this disease has advanced from nearly total ignorance to a level where it is possible to begin testing possible treatments, and formulating viable hypotheses to explain its causes. These achievements in technology are expected to continue making a substantial difference in the rate of advancement of knowledge in neuroscience.

23

Legal Perspectives in Alzheimer's Disease

ANTHONY B. SANDOE / *Suffolk University Law School, Boston, Massachusetts*

INTRODUCTION

In the initial stages of Alzheimer's disease (AD), patients experience a gradually diminishing capacity to manage their personal and business affairs. As their disability becomes more acute, patients require increasing degrees of assistance. Accordingly, patients' property interests and their assets and sources of income must be identified and located and decisions made regarding the objectives of their management and who will have the authority to make such decisions due to the patient's diminishing capacity.

As the disease progresses, further and more difficult issues emerge. Patients experience a gradually diminishing capacity to care for themselves physically as well as financially. As this disability grows more acute, patients require increasing degrees of assistance. Considerations must now transcend mere management of property interests to focus upon matters of personal care. Accordingly, the nature and type of care required at each successive stage of the deterioration must be ascertained and decisions made with respect to the objectives of patient care as well as the issue of who will have the authority to make such decisions on behalf of the patient.

Overshadowing all of these considerations of patient and property management are issues of patients' ultimate medical prognosis. At some point during this progressively degenerative process, a medical diagnosis will be made. At this time, it becomes clear that a patient's normal life expectancy will in most cases be shortened, sometimes significantly. Whenever this occurs, attention must then also focus upon the inevitability of a patient's complete mental and physical decline, his or her death, and issues of property and personal management.

Accordingly, consideration must be given to such traditional estate planning issues as whether there is a will or other estate planning instruments established for the transfer of the patient's property interests upon death. Moreover, consideration should also be given to some other unique yet more immediate financial planning issues, such as whether there are sufficient financial resources available to pay for the degree of extended custodial care that may eventually be required; whether there will be sufficient financial resources remaining to care for the patient's spouse and other dependents; and whether, indeed, there will be any assets to transfer upon the patient's death at all. In all of these matters, decisions must be made with respect to the adequacy of such an estate and financial plan to accomplish the objectives of both patients and patients' families during the rest of a patient's life and after their death, together with desirable modifications.

Clearly, Alzheimer's patients and their families have a variety of legal concerns. These concerns arrange themselves into four principal topics for consideration: (a) management of patients' property interests during their lifetime; (b) personal care of the patient; (c) conservation and preservation of property interests for the benefit of the patient and of patient's dependents (financial planning); and (d) transfer of property interests upon the patient's death (estate planning). This chapter reviews some of the more important considerations in each of these areas. With the exception of patients' physical care, these matters are, to a considerable extent, property-oriented.

MANAGEMENT OF PROPERTY INTERESTS

During the early stages of Alzheimer's disease, frequently before it is diagnosed, the disease seems to manifest itself through small lapses of memory and capacity too minute to notice. As the disease progresses, however, and memory problems increase, it becomes gradually more difficult for patients to perform once routine daily tasks. Yet a patient can still manage to disguise the problem and cope with daily management matters with slight behavioral modifications. Significant problems and issues, however, may emerge when memory loss and diminished capacity begin to intrude more seriously into the management of an individual's business and personal financial affairs. At this stage of the disease a person may begin to forget appointments, and fail to meet important deadlines. Significant amounts of cash may be misplaced, deposits and withdrawals forgotten, and a checking account inadvertantly overdrawn. Insurance policies may be allowed to lapse, investments may be allowed to mature untended, recurring bills and other obligations may be neglected. Clearly, such lapses of memory are now becoming more than the occasional, inadvertent oversights that everyone experiences, to their embarrassment, at one time or another. These lapses are becoming chronic and, therefore, of a much more serious nature. Because of such mistakes such as these, undiagnosed patients have lost personal possessions of monetary and sentimental value, significant amounts of cash and other property, their credit standing, and, even worse, their jobs.

As the frequency and severity of these mental lapses and the seriousness of their consequences increase, it eventually becomes apparent that the deteriorating mental condition has placed personal financial affairs at considerable risk and that appropriate measures must immediately be taken to remedy the situation. Depending upon the extent of the deterioration, it may be sufficient, initially for someone merely to assist the patient. Eventually, however, it will become necessary for someone to assume complete control.

While no two individuals or family situations are identical, the patient will in all probability have an interest in a variety of assets. Such assets might typically include real estate, such as a family home or condominium, and perhaps some investment property; securities, such as stocks, bonds, and notes of publicly traded companies and governmental units; cash and cash equivalents, such as demand and term deposit accounts and fund investments; life insurance policies issued on the pattient's life and perhaps on others'; business interests, such as a family or other closely held business; and tangible personal property, such as art, antiques, precious metals, a coin or stamp collection held for investment or heuristic value, as well as an automobile, furniture, furnishings, and other household possessions held principally for use and consumption.

Complementing these assets may be sources of income requiring similar attention. These might include entitlement income such as Social Security or Veterans Administration, retirement income, such as a pension plan or an individual retirement account, and beneficiary income such as some form of insurance, annuity, or trust.

An individual's property interests may certainly be far more extensive and perhaps far more sophisticated and complex. Yet most individuals will have an aggregate of interests as described above. The nature of these interests will be affected by the manner in which title is held: individually or together with others either as joint tenants or as tenants in common.

Beyond the task of locating these assets and sources of income, which may prove to be a formidable challenge because of the behavior modifications incidental to AD, there are several important and interrelated considerations of property management: What are the immediate and longer-term objectives of management? What form will that management take? Who will assume the necessary control?

Of most immediate concern, clearly, is the physical security of the property. Accordingly, the manager should take possession and assume control of all of the patient's property to preserve and protect its integrity. Attention may then be turned to matters of their daily management: the maintenance of real and personal property, the collection of income, and the payments of recurring obligations. Thereafter, consideration may be given to more long-range matters such as investment management. The propriety of a patient's present investments require review both in the context of present objectives and in relation to constantly changing market conditions. Moreover, the prospects of long-term institutional care at extraordinary expense might well require a complete reassessment of the investment objectives of the patient as well as of the entire family.

A variety of legal management forms are available that may be utilized for the care, maintenance, and preservation of such property interests during the remainder of the patient's life. Those most frequently considered for this purpose are discussed below.

Guardianship/Conservatorship

A guardian or a conservator, referred to as a committee in some states, is a person(s) or institution(s) appointed by the court to have jurisdiction over such matters, and who is judicially charged with the duty of caring for the property and/or the person of someone adjudged incapable. This form of management is traditionally used when a person lacks required capacity, and is imposed upon the incompetant person by judicial decree, a characteristic that distinguishes them from the other available forms that might be selected if the patient is competent to select them. While the terminology and the precise form vary somewhat among the various states, a formal court proceeding is generally required and the appointment is based upon a factual finding that a requisite degree of capacity is absent. Most states differentiate among degrees of mental capacity. Such distinctions may determine the degree of care authorized or ordered. Many states, for example, differentiate between a person's capacity to care for their assets and their capacity to care for themselves. It is possible, therefore, for a court to appoint an individual or an institution to manage the financial affairs of the person while the person retains the capacity and freedom to make decisions with respect to their physical needs. In some states, therefore, a conservator will be vested with limited authority for the care of the incompetant and will have custody of assets only and not the person. A guardian, on the other hand, will have custody of both the assets and the person, and will be charged with the complete responsibility of making decisions for that person. Accordingly, this form may be used exclusively for asset management and, under appropriate circumstances, may also be used for management of the patient's person, which will be considered in the following section.

Powers of Attorney

A power of attorney is merely an agency agreement wherein the patient appoints another as an agent to transact a variety of matters on the patient's behalf for some period of time. Depending upon the nature of these matters, the patient may also give the agent possession of certain property for whatever purposes are desired. Although the creation of such a relationship requires no formal transfer of title and no court authority, it does require a requisite degree of mental capacity. The design of these agreements may be exceedingly simple or highly sophisticated, particularly when combined with other forms. As an asset management vehicle, the power permits the agent to conduct, within designated limits, all of the patient's financial affairs for the patient's lifetime, even in some states after the patient becomes incompetent, the so-called "durable power."

Intervivos Trusts

A trust created during the lifetime of the patient (intervivos) is an agreement by which a patient formally transfers property to a trustee who agrees to hold and manage the property pursuant to the terms of the agreement on behalf of the patient and perhaps for others for some particular period of time. As with agency agreements, the creation of this relationship requires no court authority. It does, however, require a requisite degree of mental capacity. In its simplest form, the trust can be compared to the power of attorney. As a legal concept, however, it is more complex and capable of far greater sophistication. It can accomplish an almost limitless array of objectives, far beyond the capacity of the power of attorney, durable or otherwise. As an asset management instrument, the trust permits the trustee to manage all of the assets transferred for the patient's life. Unlike conservatorships, guardianships, and powers of attorney, however, the life of the trust may be designed to extend beyond the life of the patient, thereby providing an instrument through which the trustee may continue to manage the patient's assets for the benefit of those who survive, which presents significant estate and financial planning advantages.

Joint Tenancies

Joint tenancies are merely forms of joint ownership established when one individual places funds in a deposit type account or purchases other types of assets such as securities or real property in his name and that of another person. This form of transfer technically requires a requisite degree of mental capacity. Depending upon the creator's intent, such joint tenancies may have survivorship attributes, thereby entitling the surviving joint tenant to the entire balance or asset upon the death of the cotenant. As an asset management instrument (albeit an extremely simple one) the joint arrangement permits the joint tenant to manage these assets until the patient's death. Because of their simplicity and ease of creation, forms of joint ownership, with and without rights of survivorship, are a frequently sought and commonly utilized form of management. They require neither court action nor the services of an attorney. However, due to their inherent limitations and cumbersome nature, as a practical matter their use is effectively limited to certain types of assets.

Transfers with a Retained Interest

Such an arrangement involves the transfer of an asset, such as a house or securities, by the patient to another while reserving to the patient certain legal rights to enjoy that property, such as the right to reside or to receive income, for some period of time, most commonly, for the rest of the patient's life. During that period, the responsibilities of management and the burdens of ownership may be shifted by contract to the transferee while the transferor retains the benefits of ownership. Inherently cumbersome, this form is often passed over.

Outright and Complete Transfers

As its name implies, this arrangement involves the transfer of an asset by the patient to another. Unlike the previous form, this transfer involves no retained legal rights, perhaps only moral ones. Ownership as a legal matter, and accordingly management, is irrevocably transferred, and the right to any continued use by the transferor/patient is at the discretion of the transferee. Accordingly, this transaction involves a complete loss of legal control by the patient, which presents obvious problems and no little amount of anxiety. Yet, as a management vehicle, this transfer does successfully shift management responsibilities to another and can be an effective device provided the transferee thereafter honors the moral obligation to permit whatever use of the property is envisioned.

Private Annuities

This arrangement typically involves the transfer of income-producing assets such as cash and securities by the patient to another, pursuant to an agreement providing that the transferee will pay an annuity to the patient for some particular period of time, most commonly for the rest of the patient's life. During this period, management responsibilities are shifted to the transferee, as with the retained interest.

While a person's circumstances, objectives, assets, and income are clearly important factors in the selection of the appropriate form, they are by no means the only considerations. The mental capacity of the patient may well be the most significant factor. As mentioned, the law recognizes different degrees of mental capacity. An individual may, for example, be perfectly competent to execute a simple will, and yet lack the capacity to enter into a complex contract. The standards for the determination of such degrees of capacity vary somewhat among the states, but because some degree of competency is a necessary prerequisite to the application of many of these management forms, the patient's relative mental capacity at the time of analysis will be a critical and sometimes determinative factor in their selection. Moreover, while the objectives of the management, the nature of the assets, and the capacity of the patient may help determine, and, in certain circumstances, dictate, the choice of management form, the form or forms themselves may help determine the identity of the manager. Although a clear and probably desirable choice of manager will often be one or more family members, the management form together with the relative sophistication of the assets and of the management objectives may prompt a search outside of the family for a professional or corporate manager. In certain circumstances a bank, trust company, lawyer, accountant, or financial advisor, serving alone or together with a family member, may be a desirable alternative.

MANAGEMENT OF THE PATIENT

As AD progresses and the attendant mental deterioration increases, patients experience gradually increasing difficulties in making appropriate decisions and judgements regarding their own personal physical care. Initially, for example, clothing selected may be inappropriate for the season and personal hygiene may begin to deteriorate. Such difficulties, though embarrassing, may be easily remedied with varying degrees of daily assistance from a family member or a visiting professional as the situation requires.

As the deterioration progresses, the lapses and forgetfulness may become more threatening. Range burners may be left unattended. The distinction between red and green traffic lights may not be as clear as fellow motorists would prefer. Worse, the patient may wander from home, become confused, and hopelessly lost. It may become physically dangerous for the patient to live alone or to function without some form of supervision. Moreover, the patient's irrational behavior, previously confined to relatively harmless matters, may now begin to manifest itself in a far more serious and dangerous manner: in a refusal, for instance, to relinquish the automobile keys when driving has become a hazard; in a refusal to seek appropriate medical assistance and treatment when such is required; and in a refusal to consider alternative living arrangements when the current living accommodations are no longer appropriate.

As the severity of these matters mount, the patient's potential to be of harm to himself or others becomes increasingly apparent. Moreover, the potential of legal liability both to the patient and to the patient's family becomes a source of significant concern. Appropriate measures must therefore be taken immediately to remedy the situation. Depending upon the extent of the deterioration, it may be sufficient initially for someone merely to assist the patient during the day. Eventually, however, it will become necessary for someone to provide constant supervision. As with property management, there are several important and interrelated considerations of personal (or more appropriately "personnel") management: What are the immediate and longer-term objectives of management? What form will that management take? Who will assume the necessary control?

Of immediate concern is the physical security of the patient. The initial objective will be to provide a "safe environment" within which the patient may live. Thereafter, attention may focus upon providing the type of care required at each successive stage of the deterioration.

When it is time for such critical decisions to be made concerning a patient's physical care and management, it would be preferable if the patient were both willing and able to make them. Given the progressively degenerative nature of the disease, however, it is unlikely that he or she will be mentally competent either to make such decisions personally or to designate another to make them in his or her stead. Moreover, even during the earlier stages of the disease not all patients are cooperative and agreeable to necessary treatment and practical living arrangements. Eventually, someone will have to make those decisions on behalf of the patient without their advice and consent. In the absence of personal decision-making, there are generally three sources of decision making authority: judicial determination, personal grant, and de facto management.

Judicial Determination: Guardianship

When patients can no longer make appropriate decisions concerning their physical care, it may be necessary to seek that authority from the courts in the form of the previously considered guardianship. In the case of AD, diagnosis may have been made sufficiently early to enable the family to institute a conservatorship to manage property interests. Early in the course of the disease, while still possessed of sufficient mental capacity, patients themselves could personally institute such a proceeding. By the time the AD patient is unable physically to care for himself, however, the conservatorship (or whatever the appropriate designation within the particular jurisdiction) is no longer an appropriate legal vehicle. Guardianship is generally the only alternative available in most states for the care and management of the AD patient. If such a conservatorship was established earlier in the course of the disease as a form of asset management, such form may readily by "upgraded" to a guardianship (or whatever the appropriate designation) by judicial decree when the requisite degree of mental deterioration has been reached and custody and control of the patient are then at issue. Accordingly, the guardian will have physical custody of both the assets and the person, and will be charged with the complete responsibility of making decisions with respect to that person, much as a parent acts on behalf of a minor child. While guardians often are authorized to make routine decisions regarding medical care, sometimes physicians, medical care institutions, and the courts require special authorization to administer certain medication in nonemergency situations and to withhold the giving of extraordinary medical care.

Personal Grant: Power of Attorney

If AD is diagnosed while the patient still possesses the requisite mental capacity to make decisions regarding property and personal care, the patient may empower another individual to make these decisions on his or her behalf at such time as he or she becomes incapable, through the use of the previously considered special form of agency known as the durable power of attorney. Such a power may accordingly become an informal alternative to the formality of the judicially determined guardianship. Customarily, powers of attorney, both traditional and durable, have been used for property management and for financial and estate planning. Such powers, however, have been used far less frequently for management of the principal's person. Though principals may specifically designate their conservators or guardians in their powers of attorney, such designations are nonetheless generally accorded the judicial status of nominations (mere expressions of intent and preference), which must be judicially confirmed. Unless there is good and sufficient reason not to appoint the nominee and thereby honor the request of the patient, such as, for example, a conflict of interest, such nominations routinely receive judicial confirmation. There is, however, an increasing awareness nationwide of the need for medical powers to be included within the scope of agency powers. In recognition of this, one enlightened jurisdiction recently legislated a durable power specifically for health care. Such an agent is now empowered to make health care decisions for the patient including the power to give or withhold medical treatment, as would a court-appointed guardian. Unfortunately, this form is not available in all states. Given the pressing need for such an alternative, however, it is anticipated that such a form may soon become more widely available.

De Facto Management

Guardianships and durable powers may not always prove to be absolutely necessary for the personal management of the AD patient. Many nursing homes do not require that there be a guardian to authorize the admission of patients or to approve routine care and treatment, although more and more private institutions are requiring it. As a purely practical matter, medical practitioners may accept the judgement of the immediate family with respect to ordinary care and treatment, particularly where there is agreement among family members, and the patient is cooperative. Such acceptance would obviously save the considerable expenditure of time, emotional energy, and financial resources necessary to obtain a judicially appointed guardian.

Sometimes, however, there is no choice but to seek a judicial determination. The AD patient may insist on a course of action that would jeopardize his or her safety and the safety of others, the family members may not be in accord on a particular course of action, or the health provider or physician may simply require authority.

It would perhaps be fair to say that the proliferation of lawsuits in recent years has resulted in a cautionary approach by the medical community with respect to such decisions. Without property authority, it is unlikely that any physician or medical facility will authorize a treatment program that may be subject to question, criticism, and, ultimately litigation.

It would make sense for the family, physician, and health care facility to consult about practices and procedures before seeking the formal guardianship. Foresight and planning among them might alieviate the need for a "legal" alternative, and permit all concerned to seek and successfully use simple, pragmatic, nonlegalistic solutions to the issues of health care and management.

FINANCIAL PLANNING

When AD is finally diagnosed and the patient's prognosis becomes clear—probable long-term residence in a health care facility followed by a premature death—issues of financial and estate planning must be considered.

In any financial and estate planning context there should be two principal components (a) a so-called intervivos estate or financial plan, which involves the creation of an estate, its maintenance and conservation, together with its use to provide support and security for the family, which reflects in a number of significant ways the current popular trend in financial planning; and (b) the traditional estate plan, a so-called postmortem estate plan, which provides for the distribution of the estate thus created, used, and preserved.

The lifetime, or intervivos, financial planning aspect of any AD estate plan should have at least two primary objectives: (a) current property management for the benefit of the patient, previously considered; and (b) future asset conservation and preservation for the needs of the patient, the patient's spouse, and others for whom the patient may be financially responsible, as well as for the benefit of the patient's heirs, considered here.

Given the nature of the disease, however, it is unlikely that in most cases there will be an opportunity for further estate creation. At this point the principal concern should be the preservation and conservation of those assets and sources of income presently available to the patient and family as well as those that may become available.

There are also a variety of traditional postmortem estate planning objectives common in any estate planning context, including the orderly transfer of assets, their subsequent management, minimization of taxes, and the avoidance of costly and time-consuming probate entanglements. All these essentially death-oriented issues are considered in the following section.

In the accomplishment of all of these objectives, both intervivos as well as postmortem, estate planning for the AD patient is not entirely dissimilar to estate planning for anyone else. There are, however, two potentially troublesome issues that set the AD estate plan apart: the probability of long-term custodial care and the patient's loss of mental capacity.

Presently, the expenses of the extended type of custodial care generally required by an advanced Alzheimer's patient are covered neither by Medicare nor by private insurance contracts. Moreover, Medicaid benefits are available only to those who qualify under severely restrictive financial qualification tests permitting minimally available assets and income. Accordingly, the patient and the patient's family, whose personal financial resources are inadequate to afford such costs, are confronted with potential impoverishment. In the absence of proper lifetime estate planning, a healthy spouse could be left with inadequate financial resources for support, dependent children could be deprived of an anticipated education, and subsequent generations could be unintentionally but unavoidably disinherited. In anticipation of such potentially devastating custodial expenses, the financial and estate plan of the Alzheimer's patient with limited personal financial resources should be designed specifically to respond to this potential problem.

The timing of the response to this problem, however, is critical. Unfortunately, by the time the nature and extent of the problem are finally appreciated and the family eventually seeks legal advice, the requisite degree of mental capacity required for many components of a well-designed financial and estate plan may be rapidly diminishing, or may be absent altogether. The estate planner may, therefore, have severely limited options available with which to cope with the inevitable. This loss of capacity and planning options increases the importance of developing a comprehensive plan as early as possible.

Accordingly, when confronted with the probability of extended custodial health care for a member, all families, regardless of the nature and extent of their resources, should develop a financial plan in a timely fashion to preempt the impending crisis and to deal with it as effectively as possible. A logical starting point for such a plan would seem to be to analyze individual requirements and available family resources. Generally, any such analysis would seem to have at least two important components: (a) an analysis of the present and future physical management needs of the patient, together with an estimate of their cost, and (b) an analysis of the family resources, financial and personal, that can be assembled to meet them. Thereafter, depending upon the outcome of the analysis, further consideration should be given to the availability of public resources either to supplement or supersede the family's own resources. However, any consideration of the availability of public financial assistance for whatever level of support might be necessary and must commence with an understanding of Medicaid and Medicare.

Medicare, the federal health insurance program, is designed to assist those who are receiving Social Security retirement benefits as well as those who are receiving Social Security disability benefits. Medicare pays for necessary doctor's services and for necessary inpatient hospital care. Generally, however, coverage is extremely limited thereafter for inpatient skilled nursing home care and for health agency care in a patient's home. It provides no coverage for the kind of total care required by the Alzheimer's patient.

Medicaid, the medical assistance program administered by the various states with federal aid, is designed to assist only those with extremely limited financial resources. While Medicaid pays for a broad range of medical and medically related services, including extended nursing home care, a person must qualify under a variety of tests and special rules to be eligible to receive such assistance.

Generally, to qualify for Medicaid benefits a patient must be both categorically and financially eligible. To be categorically eligible, a patient must be over the age of 65, blind, or disabled as defined by Social Security Administration regulations. To be financially eligible, a patient must qualify under an asset test as well as an income test, both of which establish maximum acceptable levels. Currently, to qualify for Medicaid benefits an individual may not receive income in excess of approximately $450.00 a month, and with certain exceptions, may not own assets in excess of $2000. Certain assets are considered exempt from this asset test such as a home, certain personal property, certain life insurance, and certain assets specifically designated for burial. If a patient's income or assets exceed these minimal levels, the patient must "spend the difference" on medical expenses in order to qualify.

The foregoing is an extremely general overview of the Medicaid framework as it relates to qualification for medical assistance. Within this framework, there is a wide latitude for interpretation. Each state has a different approach to these matters. Depending upon a particular state's attitude toward welfare assistance generally, the public policy of the various jurisdictions span the spectrum from the very liberal to the ultraconservative. The practical application of the laws and regulations promulgated thereunder reflects this diversity. However, given these differences, to qualify for public assistance, within the broad design of the Medicaid program, one must be impoverished or become so.

Fortunately, however, these are not the only alternatives available to the AD family with insufficient resources to support both the patient and family members. With foresight, an understanding of available estate planning opportunities, and timely action, there are other options available. Such a plan might include two measures in particular: (a) the removal of those assets and other resources necessary for support of the patient's spouse and other financial dependents from the pool of resources available for such expenses; and (b) the availability of public financial resources to support the patient's medical and physical care requirements thereafter. The first measure involves restructuring the patient's assets to avoid their eventual depletion. This requires their transfer into other forms of ownership. The second measure involves the qualification of the patient for public medical assistance in a legally permissible manner within the framework of the public welfare laws and regulations. If the family resources fall short, as may well be expected, or even if they marginally exceed projected family needs, it would seem prudent for the family to give serious consideration to the availability of public financial assistance at this time.

This contemplated asset and resource "removal" may be accomplished in a number of different ways. The most obvious and straightforward among them is simple asset transfer. An applicant should consider the advisability of a transfer of both individually owned and jointly held assets to a spouse, child, or other beneficiary. Such a transfer could assume the form of an outright transfer, a transfer with a retained interest, or a transfer in trust depending upon the overall objectives of the transfer. Such assets would, of course, no longer be "available" to meet the patient's personal expenses. Being no longer "available," assets thus transferred would not be counted in determining Medicaid eligibility, subject, however, to certain specific limitations. Medicaid regulations, for example, currently deny eligibility to applicants who transfer assets within a certain period of application, generally 24 months, but only if such transfer is motivated with the intent and purpose of qualifying for medical assistance. But a "properly motivated" or a "timely" transfer would not so disqualify the patient from receiving benefits.

While such transfers may achieve the immediate desired result of removing the patient's property from "harm's way," they are not without their potential problems including, for instance, the psychological impact of transfer upon the patient, and upon his or her admission to a health care facility. Asset transfer, however, is not the only measure available to the family to accomplish such a removal of the patient's assets from "availability." Several other specific measures generally available to the patient and family include severence of jointly owned assets between cotenants, segregation of income between spouses, and purchase of so-called "excempt" assets with "available" income or assets.

Overshadowing all aspects of a comprehensive patient plan is the mental capacity of the Alzheimer's patient, which is usually in a state of continual deterioration throughout the planning process. Virtually all of the planning objectives of the AD patient, intervivos or postmortem, involve a present transfer of property or the present provision for a future transfer, regardless of the extent of the estate.

A certain degree of mental capacity is required for the execution of a valid Last Will and Testament. In the absence of such capacity, the will cannot be effective to provide for property transfer at death. What may not be so widely understood is that a requisite degree of mental capacity, perhaps even higher, is also required for all intervivos transfers, whether outright, in trust, or with a retained interest. If the required degree of capacity is absent at the time of the transfer, a patient will be deemed legally incompetent to effect a transfer and, accordingly, any transfer made by such patient, individually, will lack full legal force and effect. If a patient is to effect immediate property transfers for asset management and preservation purposes, or to provide for their future transfer by will at death, it is critical that such transfers or arrangements be accomplished while sufficient capacity remains.

If, however, Alzheimer's is diagnosed late in the course of the disease, in particular, after the patient has lost the necessary mental capacity to make decisions regarding his or her assets, planning options unfortunately become severely circumscribed. Furthermore, depending upon the relative level of incapacity, the execution of any kind of estate-planning documents, such as a will, may well be beyond the capacity of the patient. The only remaining option in most states may be the establishment of a conservatorship or guardianship to effect such transfers. Once that agent is appointed by the court, any further financial arrangements, such as asset transfer, must be accomplished by the guardian or conservator with the court's advice and consent. While courts generally permit use of the those assets and income not specifically required for the ward's own personal maintenance to be "used" for the "support" of the ward's spouse and other dependents, any "divestiture" of the ward's property for "preservation" purposes, however small, would probably not be approved.

Accordingly, it is these two issues then—the possibilities of extended confinement to a health care facility at potentially exorbitant cost together with the continual mental deterioration of the patient—that lend a rather unique and somewhat difficult perspective to the AD estate plan in particular. Their presence adds an air of critical urgency to the creation of the plan and places an extraordinary premium upon intervivos estate planning considerations in the case of the Alzheimer's patient, perhaps even more so than in any other estate planning context.

ESTATE PLANNING

In addition to the foregoing intervivos financial planning issues, a variety of traditional death-oriented estate planning objectives are normally considered by estate planners. They should be considered by the patient, if the patient is still capable, and by the patient's family. Most commonly, these would include a consideration of the orderly transfer of the patient's assets to whomever the patient wishes to receive them. This is an objective that must consider a variety of personal interests, both of the patient and of the family. Consideration of this objective forces a consideration of the management of assets for those who will receive them in the event that they are unable or unwilling to manage the assets so received. Moreover, there is the usual concern with minimizing taxes: the preservation of the assets against state and federal income and estate taxes and the corresponding concern with avoiding costly and time-consuming probate entanglements.

As previously noted, estate planning for the Alzheimer's disease patient is not entirely dissimilar to estate planning for anyone else. It is, however, the continuing mental deterioration of the patient that lends a unique and difficult perspective to this particular plan. Since the patient's mental capacity may be seriously diminished or altogether absent by the time legal advice is sought, available planning options may be severely limited.

Assuming the presence of a requisite degree of capacity, there are, however, a number of estate planning devices available to the Alzheimer's disease patient and family with which to accomplish the lifetime and postmortem estate planning objectives discussed. For purposes of analysis, these planning devices may be classified into two principal categories based upon the time they become effective for

purposes of transferring property interests: (a) testamentary devices: instruments intended to take effect only upon the patient's death, which transfer no property interests to others until that time; and (b) intervivos devices: instruments intended to take effect immediately, which transfer property interests at that time and/or at the patient's death.

Those testamentary devices most frequently considered for this purpose would, in summary, include those described here.

Wills: Simple and Complex

Technically, there is really only one truly testamentary device: the Last Will and Testament. Simply defined, a will is a person's declaration of intention. While traditionally considered as expressing a plan for property disposition, wills may, in addition, express wishes with respect to other matters as well, such as the nomination of an executor and a guardian for minor children. However simple or extensive the plan, the purpose of the will is to place an obligation upon the executor to carry out the legitimate intentions of the testator under the supervision of the courts. Although the creation of a will requires no court authority, it does, as previously noted, require a certain degree of mental capacity, which in some states may be less than that required for the execution of a contract and other similar matters of personal property management. Not all wills, however, are simple wills designed exclusively for purposes of property transfer at death. Occasionally, the will itself may contain a trust, as a variation on the intervivos trust form. Accordingly, as an alternative to outright distribution to beneficiaries, some or all of property interests passing through the will may be subsequently held in trust for the accomplishment of the testator's objectives.

Intestacy

A consideration of wills as an estate planning device would be incomplete without reference to their statutory counterpart, the intestacy laws. Ownership and use of property is universally subject to certain general rules. A number of these (statutes of descent and distribution) govern distribution of property interests and control in the absence of a conscious distribution plan. They act as an estate planning device by default when a person fails to leave a valid will and they confer the patient's property interests, in certain proportions, upon those individuals specifically preferred by the law. although the actual distribution plans vary in their preferences among the various states, their design applies uniformly to all family situations, regardless of the differences in individual needs, deeds, and abilities.

In contrast to the limited number of testamentary forms—one active (the will) and one passive (the intestate statute)—there are a number of intervivos estate planning forms available to effect a patient's estate planning objectives. Several of these intervivos devices were briefly outlined in the consideration of asset management, since they are effective forms for that purpose as well. Those intervivos devices most frequently considered for this purpose would include the following.

Intervivos Trusts

These fiduciary agreements may be used for asset management when a patient transfers assets to a trustee during his or her lifetime. They may, in addition, be designed to control the disposition of the assets so transferred upon the death of the patient and may be used to achieve a number of the patient's estate-planning objectives. Since the terms of the trust instrument would control the disposition of the assets held therein, rather than the terms of the patient's will, the trust could be considered as an alternative to the will as a device for transferring assets.

Joint Tenancies

These forms of joint ownership may be used for management purposes when a patient transfers assets to a joint account during his or her lifetime. They may, in addition, control the disposition of the asset to the cotenant upon the death of the patient, provided the joint tenancy was created with rights of survivorship. While they may be used to achieve some of the estate-planning objectives of the patient, joint tenancies possess neither the flexibility nor the potential sophistication of the intervivos trust. Nonetheless, they can control the disposition of the particular asset rather than the will, and may be viewed as an alternative to the will as a device for transferring assets.

Deeds of Conveyance

These asset transfers with or without retained interests (legal rights), may be used for management purposes when a patient transfers assets to another during his or her lifetime. These arrangements, however, are primarily asset transfer devices since the deed serves to transfer the asset immediately subject to the interest retained, if any, which generally terminates upon the death of the transferor. As a practical matter, their capacity for asset management is an adjunct to this principal function. While these transfers may achieve some of the estate-planning objectives of the patient, they do not possess either the flexibility or the potential sophistication of the intervivos trust. Nevertheless, the deed controls the disposition of the particular asset—a portion upon delivery of the deed, and the balance upon the death of the transferor—rather than the terms of the will. Again, in this sense the deed of conveyance could be viewed as still another alternative to the will.

Life Insurance Policies

Although frequently overlooked as an estate *planning* device, life insurance often is the key element of an estate plan, which may accomplish some postmortem objectives. In modest estates, proceeds of life insurance frequently make up a significant portion of the estate. In larger estates, proceeds are used to provide necessary funds to prevent unnecessary liquidation of estate assets at a potential loss. Fundamentally, a life insurance policy is a contractual agreement by which a patient transfers assets in the form of periodic premiums during his lifetime to an insurance company that agrees to pay a sum upon the death of the patient to a designated beneficiary, which contract accordingly controls the disposition of the assets.

Retirement Plans: Pension Plans, Profit-Sharing Plans, Corporate Savings Plans, Individual Retirement Plans, Deferred Compensation Plans, Self-Employment Retirement Plans

No survey of estate planning devices would be complete without some reference to retirement plans. Again these are frequently overlooked and not generally considered as an estate-planning device. The income received from a retirement plan together with some form of entitlement income such as Social Security often make up the foundation of most retirement arrangements. Moreover, depending upon the terms of the particular plan and individual circumstances, these plans may be an element of a postmortem estate plan as well. Fundamentally, these various plans are contractual agreements whereby a patient and/or the patient's employer may contribute assets to a retirement plan during the patient's lifetime for management purposes and for subsequent payment to the patient upon retirement. Yet this contract, like life insurance, may control the disposition of unpaid portions to designated beneficiaries upon the patient's death and may effectively transfer assets, thereby achieving some of the postmortem objectives of the patient.

Private Annuities

These contractual agreements may be used for asset management purposes when a patient transfers assets to a transferee during his or her lifetime. Like both insurance policies and retirement plans, private annuities are frequently overlooked as estate-planning devices. Nevertheless, they are, in addition, designed to control the disposition of the assets so transferred upon the death of the patient and may therefore be used to achieve some of the patient's postmortem estate planning objectives. Accordingly, as an asset-transfer device, the private annuity could be considered as yet another alternative to the will.

CONCLUSION

This chapter has considered a few of the more important legal considerations confronting the AD patient and family as they contend with the various issues of patient care and property management. If there is to be an organized approach to these multiple issues and considerations, a comprehensive plan that adequately responds to them is required. The creation of such a comprehensive plan must achieve a number of objectives. This chapter has also sought to outline the more important among these objectives and to suggest a few select measures that might be utilized to achieve them. Finally, it has sought to summarize the various legal forms generally available to implement the suggested measures.

While these various objectives were considered independently in the context of a particular issue of patient care or property management, it should be clear following a consideration of all of the issues that they are highly interdependent. The confluence of all the objectives determines the measures to be taken as well as the legal forms to be used.

Each of the various legal forms considered here possess unique advantages as well as inherent limitations. They vary considerably in terms of flexibility and sophistication. While the various legal forms discussed were likewise considered and analyzed separately, they are by no means mutually exclusive. They are frequently used together as circumstances require. Not all, however, are necessarily appropriate for every patient or family situation. Rather, each patient's particular financial and family circumstance and objectives require careful analysis, and selection of the appropriate measures together with the appropriate legal forms or combination of them by one skilled in their use.

The day when a person's estate consisted solely of real and personal property managed individually and transferred by will has largely disappeared. The nature and types of property interests held by individuals have increased dramatically, as have the measures for their management and transfer. Nowadays, sophisticated asset-management as well as financial and estate planning will utilize a variety of legal devices, both testamentary and intervivos, and an array of strategies to accomplish the various lifetime and postmortem objectives of the owner. When properly integrated, the combination of devices and strategies will frequently overcome the inherent limitations of any one of them and should result in a substantial savings of time, expenses, and taxes, as well as the critical preservation of the assets themselves.

It should also be noted that state laws do vary, sometimes significantly, Moreover, the maze of Medicaid laws, in particular, and the regulations promulgated under them are highly technical and complex, and subject to a broad range of interpretation among the various states. Furthermore, given the senstivity of the areas, it is anticipated that there will be periodic changes in the law, as there have been recently. Accordingly, competent local counsel should be sought to refine the options and perhaps to expand upon them within the permissible context of the current laws and regulations of the particular jurisdiction and to place them appropriately within the perspective of the other concerns of the AD patient and family.

It is perhaps axiomatic to the process of financial and estate planning that the earlier it is begun, the better. Such an admonition is certainly interwoven throughout this summary, implicitly if not explicitly. As perhaps in no other planning context immaginable, the problems and issues presented here dramatically emphasize the critical importance of timing to a comprehensive plan that successfully accomplishes the objectives of the patient and his or her family.

Because of the progressively degenerative nature of the disease, at some point the patient will become incompetent. Since some level of mental capacity is required for the utilization of nearly all of the management and planning options discussed, its loss will significantly reduce the available options. Moreover, since Medicaid regulations require timely action, failure or inability to comply likewise reduces available options. As options decrease so does the flexibility optimally desired to provide creative solutions to difficult asset management, preservation, and transfer problems.

A substantial benefit to be derived from an attorney skilled in management and planning lies not simply in the execution of estate-planning instruments, but in the formulation of a comprehensive design that will respond creatively to the unique requirements of a particular family. Legal counsel should be sought immediately. The advice and the assistance of a capable attorney, however, is only part of the solution. The issues considered here are both complex and frustrating. Because of the diverse nature of the problems and objectives and well as the diversity of local laws, regulations, and practices, families need information and assistance from a wide variety of sources: support groups, medical personnel, social workers, and friends as well as attorneys. Even with such an array of assistance, assuming the responsibility for the care and management of the AD patient is at best a monumental task.

Appendix
Research Bibliography on Familial Alzheimer's Disease

ROBERT MULLAN COOK-DEEGAN / *Georgetown University, Washington, D.C.*

LINDA A. WINTERS-MINER / *Familial Alzheimer's Disease Research Foundation, Tulsa, Oklahoma*

1907

Alzheimer, A. (1907). Uber eine eigenartige Erkrankung der Hirnrinde. *Ges. Psych.* 64: 146-148.

1926

Meggendorfer, F. (1926). Uber die hereditare disposition zur dementia senilis. *Z Neurol. Psychiatry* 101: 387-405.

1929

Flugel, F.E. (1929). Zur diagnostik der Alzheimerschen Krankheit. *Ges. Psych.* 120: 783-787.

1932

Schottky, J. (1932). Uber präsenile Verblödungen. *Ges. Neurol. Psych.* 140: 333-397.

von Braunmuhl, A. (1932). Kolloidchemische Betrachtungsweise seniler and präseniler Gewebsveranderungen. *Ges. Neurol. Psych.* 142: 1-54.

1933

Gillespie, R.D. (1933). Discussion on the mental and physical symptoms of the presenile dementias. *Proc. R. Soc. Med.* 26: 1080-1084.

1934

Lowenberg, K., and Waggoner, R.W. (1934). Familial organic psychosis (Alzheimer's type). *Arch. Neurol. Psychiatry* 31: 737-754.

1939

McMenemey, W.H., Worster-Drought, C., Flind, J., et al. (1939). Familial presenile dementia. *J. Neurol. Psychiatr.* 2: 293-302.

1942

English, W.H. (1942). Alzheimer's disease. *Psychiatry Q.* 16: 98.

1946

Essen-Moller, E. (1946). A family with Alzheimer's disease. *Acta Psychiatr. Neurol. (Scand.)* 21: 233-244.

1947

Luers, T. (1947). Uber die familiäre juvenile Form der Alzheimerschen Krankheit mit neurologischen Herderscheinungen. *Arch. Psychiatr. Nervenkr.* 179: 132-145.

1948

De Risio, C., Ridoldo, P., and Conterio, F. (1948). Il problema dell-creditarieta nella demenza preseniie di Alzheimer. *Boll. Soc. Ital. Biol. Sper.* 24: 188-196.

1951

Arndt, M. (1951). La forma familiar de al enfermedad de Alzheimer. *Neuropsiquiatria* 2: 169-181.

1952

Sjogren, T. (1952). A genetic study of morbus Alzheimer and morbus Pick. *Acta Psychiatrica Neurol. Scand.* (Suppl. 82): 9-63.

1955

Davidson, E.A., and Robertson, E.E. (1955). Alzheimer's disease with acne rosacea in one of identical twins. *J. Neurol. Neurosurg. Psychiatry* 18: 72-77.

1956

Josephy, H. (1956). Discussion note. *J. Neuropathol. Exp. Neurol.* 15: 234-235.

Marchand, L., Leconte, M., and Halpern, B. (1956). Considerations pathogeniques sur les demences atrophiques. *Presse Medi.* 64: 1412-1415.

1957

Frank, H. cited by von Braunmuch, A., in Lubarseh, O., Henke, F., Rossie, R. (Eds). (1957). *Handbuch der Speziellen Pathologischen Anatomie Und Histologie.* Berlin, Springer-Verlag, 500-501.

1959

Wheelan, L. (1959). Familial Alzheimer's disease. *Ann. Hum. Genet.* 23: 300-310.

1960

Zawuski, G. (1960). Zur erblichkeit der Alzheimerschen Krankheit. *Arch. J. Psychiatr. Ges. Neurol.* 201: 123-132.

1961

Lauter, H. (1961). Genealogische Erhebungen in einer Familie mit Alzheimerschen Krankheit. *Arch. Psychiatr. Ges. Neurol.* 202: 126-139.

1962

Friede, R.L., and Magee, K.R. (1962). Alzheimer's disease. *Neurology* 12: 213-222.

1963

Bucci, L. (1963). A familial organic psychosis of Alzheimer type in six kinship of three generations. *Am. J. Psychiatry* 119: 863-866.

Feldman, R.H., Chandler, K.A., Levy, L.L., and Glaser, G.H. (1963). Familial Alzheimer's disease. *Neurology* 13: 811-824.

1965

Constantinidis, J., Garrone, G., Tissot, R., et al. (1965). L'incidence familiale des alterations neurofibrillaires corticales d'Alzheimer. *Psychiatr. Neurol.* 150: 235-247.

1966

Heston, L.L., Lowther, D.L.W., and Leventhal, C.M. (1966). Alzheimer's disease. *Arch. Neurol.* 15: 225-233.

1967

Pratt, R.T.C. (1967). The presenile and senile dementias. In: *The Genetics of Neurological Disorders.* London, Oxford University Press, pp. 69-77.

1970

Jacob, H. (1970). Muscular twitchings in Alzheimer's disease. In: *Alzheimer's Disease*, Wolstenholme, G.E.W. (Eds.) London, Churchill Press, pp. 75-89.
Landy, P.J. (1970). Alzheimer's disease in siblings. *Med. J. Aust.* 1: 832-834.
Nielsen, J. (1970). Chromosomes in senile, presenile and arteriosclerotic dementia. *J. Gerontol.* 25: 312-315.
Pratt, R.T.C. (1970). The genetics of Alzheimer's disease. In: *Alzheimer's Disease*, Wolstenholme, G.E.W. (Ed.) London, Churchill Press, pp. 137-144.

1971

Beighton, P.H., and Lindenberg, R. (1971). Alzheimer's disease in multiple members of a family. *Birth Defects* 7: 232-233.
Clark, D.B. (1971). The clinical approach to neurologic disorders. *Birth Defects* 7: 8.

1972

Hunter, R., Dayan, A.D., and Wilson, J. (1972). Alzheimer's disease in one monozygotic twin. *J. Neurol. Neurosurg. Psychiatry* 35: 707-710.

1973

Bergener, M., and Jungklaass, F.K. (1973). Genetische befunde bei morbus alzheimer und seiner demenz. *Gerontol. Clin.* 12: 71-75.
Mark, J., and Brun, A. (1973). Chromosomal deviations in Alzheimer's disease compared to those in senescence and senile dementia. *Gerontol. Clin.* 15: 253-258.

1976

Homma, A., and Nielsen, J. (1976). Chromosome aneuploidy associated with aging. *Neuropsychobiology* 2: 104-111.

1977

Gaches, J., Supino-Viterbo, V., and Foncin, J.F. (1977). Association de maladies d'Alzheimer et de Creutzfeldt-Jakob. *Acta Neurol. Belg.* 77: 202-212.

Heston, L.L. (1977). Alzhcimer's disease, trisomy 21, and myeloproliferative disorders: Associations suggesting a genetic diathesis. *Science* 196: 322-323.
Heston, L.L., and Mastri, A.R. (1977). The genetics of Alzheimer's disease. Associations with hematologic malignancy and Down's syndrome. *Arch. Gen. Psychiatry* 34: 976-981.
Traub, R., Gajdusek, D.C., and Gibbs, C.J. (1977). Transmissible virus dementia: The relation of transmissible spongiform encephalopathy to Creutzfeldt-Jakob disease. In: *Aging and Dementia*, Kinsbourne, M., and Smith, W.L. (Eds.) New York, Spectrum, pp. 110-114.

1978

Brun, A., Gustafson, L., and Mitelman, F. (1978). Normal chromosome banding pattern in Alzheimer's disease. *Gerontology* 24: 369-373.
Cook, R.H., and Austin, J.H. (1978). Precautions in familial transmissible dementia, including familial Alzheimer's disease. *Arch. Neurol.* 5: 697-698.
Heston, L.L., and White, J. (1978). Pedigrees of 30 families with Alzheimer disease: Associations with defective organization of microfilaments and microtubules. *Behav. Genet.* 8: 315-331.

1979

Cook, R.H., Ward, B.E., and Austin, J.H. (1979). Studies in aging of the brain: IV. Familial Alzheimer disease: Relation to transmissible dementia, aneuploidy, and microtubular defects. *Neurology* 29: 1402-1412.
Masters, C.L., Gajdasek, D.C., Gibbs, C.J., et al. (1979). Familial Creutzfeldt-Jakob disease and other familial dementias: An inquiry into possible modes of transmission of virus-induced familial diseases. In: *Slow Transmissible Diseases of the Nervous System*, Prusiner, S.W., Hadlow, W. (Eds.) New York, Academic Press, pp. 143-191.
Sulkava, R., Rossi, L., and Knuutia, S. (1979). No elevated sister chromatid exchange in Alzheimer's disease. *Acta Neurol. Scand.* 59: 156-159.
Ward, B., Cook, R., Robinson, A., and Austin, J. (1979). Increased aneuploidy in Alzheimer disease. *Am. J. Med. Genet.* 3: 137-144.

1980

Botstein, D., White, R.L., Skolnick, et al. (1980). Construction of a genetic linkage map in man using restriction fragment length polymorphisms. *Am. J. Hum. Genet.* 32: 314-333.
Goudsmit, J., Morrow, C.H., Asher, D.H., et al. (1980). Evidence for and against the transmissibility of Alzheimer's disease. *Neurology* 30: 945-950.
Moreau-Dubois, M.C., Cathala, F., Brown, P., and Gajdusek, D.C. (1980). Application d'un test de fusion cellulaire aux maladies de Creutzfeldt-Jakob et d'Alzheimer. *Rev. Neurol.* 136: 409-409.

Nordenson, I., Adolfsson, R., Beckman, G., Bucht, G., and Winblad, B. (1980). Chromosomal abnormality in dementia of Alzheimer type. *Lancet* 1: 481-482.

Pro, J.D., Smith, C.H., and Sumi, S.M. (1980). Presenile Alzheimer disease: Amyloid plaques in the cerebellum. *Neurology* 30: 820-825.

Selkoe, D.J. (1980). Altered protein composition of isolated human cortical neurons in Alzheimer disease. *Ann. Neurol.* 8: 468-478.

1981

Cook, R.H., Schneck, S.A., and Clark, D.B. (1981). Twins with Alzheimer's disease. *Arch. Neurol.* 38: 300-301.

Folstein, M.F., and Breitner, J.C. (1981). Language disorder predicts familial Alzheimer's disease. *Med. J.* 149: 145-147.

Goudsmit, J., White, B.J., Weitkamp, L.R., Keats, B.J.P., Morrow, C.H., and Gajdusek, D.C. (1981). Familial Alzheimer's disease in two kindreds of the same geographic and ethnic origin: A clinical and genetic study. *J. Neurol. Sci.* 49: 79-89.

Heston, L.L., Mastri, A.R., Anderson, V.E., et al. (1981). Dementia of the Alzheimer type: clinical genetics, natural history and associated conditions. *Arch. Gen. Psychiatry* 38: 1085-1090.

Heston, L.L. (1981). Genetic studies of dementia: With emphasis on Parkinson's disease and Alzheimer's neuropathology. In: *The Epidemiology of Dementia*, Mortimer, J.A., and Schuman, L.M. (Eds.) New York & Oxford, Oxford University Press.

Krucke, W. (1981). Familial Alzheimer's disease with cerebral amyloid angiopathy, senile plaques, and neurofibrillary tangles. *Gerontology* 27: 108-109.

Martin, J.M., Kellet, J.M., and Kahn, J. (1981). Aneuploidy in cultured human lymphocytes: II. A comparison between senescence and dementia. *Age Aging* 10: 24-28.

Masters, C.L., Gajdasek, D.C., and Gibbs, C.J., Jr. (1981). The familial occurrence of Creutzfeldt-Jakob disease and Alzheimer's disease. *Brain* 104: 535-538.

Moreau-Dubois, M.C., Brown, P., Goudsmit, J., Cathala, F., and Gajdusek, D.C. (1981). Biologic distinction between sporadic and familial Alzheimer disease by an in vitro cell fusion test. *Neurology* 31: 323-325.

White, B.J., Crandall, C., Goudsmit, J., Morrow, C., Alling, D., and Tjio, J.-H. (1981). Cytogenetic studies of familial and sporadic Alzheimer disease. *Am. J. Med. Genet.* 10: 77-89.

1982

Harris, R. (1982). Genetics of Alzheimer's disease. *Br. Med. J.* 284: 1065-1066.

Heston, L.L. (1982). Alzheimer's dementia and Down's syndrome: Genetic evidence suggesting an association. *Ann. N.Y. Acad. Sci.* 396: 2938.

Muramoto, O., Nanke, S., Kosaka, R., et al. (1982). Suspected cases of familial Alzheimer's disease: A case report and a study on aneuploids in leucocytes. *Brain Nerve* 34: 71-76.

Staiano-Coico, L., Darzynkiewicz, Z., Melamed, M.R., and Wersler, M. (1982). Changes in DNA content of human blood mononuclear cells with senescence. *Cytometry* 3: 79-83.

Walford, R.L. (1982). Immunologic studies of Down's syndrome and Alzheimer's disease. *Ann. N.Y. Acad. Sci.* 396: 95-106.

Whalley, L.J., Carothers, A.D., Collyer, S., Demey, R., and Frackiewicz, A. (1982). A study of familial factors in Alzheimer's disease. *Br. J. Psychiatry* 140: 249-256.

1983

Chase, G.A., Folstein, M.F., Breitner, J.C.S., Beary, T.H., and Self, S.G. (1983). The use of life tables and survival analysis in testing genetic hypotheses, with an application to Alzheimer's disease. *Am. J. Epidemiol.* 117: 590-597.

Cook-Deegan, R.M., and Austin, J.H. (1983). Implications of normal lymphocyte DNA content in familial Alzheimer disease [letter]. *Am. J. Med. Genet.* 15: 511-513.

Delasnerie-Lauprete, N., Calot, M., Ohayon, E., Foucault, C., Cambon-de-Mouzon, A., Clanet, M., and Cathala, F. (1983). Alzheimer familiar: Étude des marquers HLA. [Familial Alzheimer's disease: A study of HLA markers.] *Biomed. Pharmacother.* 37: 186-188.

Heston, L.L., and White, J.A. (1983). *Dementia: A Practical Guide to Alzheimer's Disease and Related Illnesses.* New York, W.H. Freeman.

Heston, L.L. (1983). Dementia of the Alzheimer's type. In: *Biological Aspects of Alzheimer's Disease.* Cold Spring Harbor, New York, Cold Spring Harbor Laboratory Press, pp. 183-192.

Heyman, A., Wilkinson, W.E., Hurwitz, B.J., et al. (1983). Alzheimer's disease: Genetic aspects and associated clinical disorders. *Ann. Neurol.* 14: 507-515.

Kilpatrick, C., Bruns, R., and Blumbers, F.C. (1983). Identical twins with Alzheimer disease. *J. Neurol. Neurosurg. Psychiatry* 46: 421-425.

Mowshowitz, S.L., Dawson, G.J., and Elizan, T.S. (1983). Antiviral response of fibroblasts from familial Alzheimer's disease and Down's syndrome to human interferonalpha. *J. Neurol. Transm.* 57: 121-126.

Nee, L.E., Polinsky, R.J., Eldridge, R., et al. (1983). A family with histologically confirmed Alzheimer's disease. *Arch. Neurol.* 40: 203-208.

Sargent, M. (1983). NIMH researcher traces Alzheimer's Disease through eight generations in one family. *NIH Record*, Feb. 15, p. 8.

1984

Amano, N., Matsuishi, T., Suzuki, K., Yokoi, S., Saitoh, A., and Yashishita, S. (1984). Ultrastructural study of the neuronal lipofuscin–an autopsy case of familial Alzheimer's disease. *Brain Nerve* 36: 657-663.

Breitner, J.C.S. (1984). Familial nature of Alzheimer's disease. *N. Engl. J. Med.* 311: 1318-1319.

Breitner, J.C.S. (1984). Aphasia/apraxia and familial aggregation in Alzheimer's disease. *Ann. Neurol.* 15: 614-615.

Breitner, J.C.S., and Folstein, M.F. (1984). Familial Alzheimer dementia: A prevalent disorder with specific clinical features. *Psychol. Med.* 14: 63-80.

Heyman, A., Wilkinson, W.E., Stafford, J.A., et al. (1984). Alzheimer's disease: A study of epidemiological aspects. *Ann. Neurol.* 15: 335-341.

Powell, D., and Folstein, M.F. (1984). Pedigree study of familial Alzheimer disease. *Med. J. Neurogenet.* 1: 189-197.

Reisberg, B., DeLeon, M.J., and Ferris, S.H. (1984). Familial nature of Alzheimer's disease? *N. Engl. J. Med.* 311: 1318-1319.

Smith, A., Broe, G.A., and Williamson, M. (1984). Chromosome fragility in Alzheimer's disease. *Clin. Genet.* 25: 416-421.

1985

Azzarelli, B., Muller, J., Ghetti, B., Dyken, M., and Conneally, P.M. (1985). Cerebellar plaques in familial Alzheimer's disease (Gerstmann-Straussler-Scheinker variant-questionable). *Acta Neuropathol.* 65: 235-246.

Boll, T.J. (1985). Developing issues in clinical neuropsychology. *J. Clin. Exp. Neuropsychol.* 7: 473-485.

Chui, H.C., Teng, E.L., Henderson, V.W., et al. (1985). Clinical subtypes of dementia of the Alzheimer type. *Neurology* 35: 1544-1550.

Cutler, N.R., Haxy, J.V., Duara, R., Grady, C.L., Moore, A.M., Parisi, J.E., White, J., Heston, L., Margolin, R.M., and Rapoport, S.I. (1985). Brain metabolism as measured with positron emission tomography—serial assessment in a patient with familial Alzheimer's disease. *Neurology* 35: 1556-1561.

Cutler, N.R., Heston, L.L., Davies, P., Haxy, J.V., and Schapiro, M.B. (1985). NIH Conference, Alzheimer's disease and Down's syndrome: New insights. *Ann. Intern. Med.* 103: 566-578.

Embry, C., and Lippmann, S. (1985). Presumed Alzheimer's disease beginning at different ages in two twins. *J. Am. Geriatr. Soc.* 33: 61-62.

English, D., and Cohen, D. (1985). A case-control study of maternal age in Alzheimer's disease. *J. Am. Geriatr. Soc.* 33: 167.

Foncin, J.F., Salmon, D., Supino-Viterbo, V., Feldman, R.G., Macchi, G., Mariotti, P., Scoppetta, C., Caruso, G., and Bruni, A.C. (1985). Demence présénile d'Alzheimer transmise dans unes famille étendue. *Rev. Neurol.* 141: 194-202.

Heston, L.L. (1985). Ask the doctor: Genetics and dementia of the Alzheimer type. *ADRDA Newsletter* 5: 4.

Knesevich, J.W., Toro, F.R., Morris, J.C., et al. (1985). Aphasia, family history, and the longitudinal course of senile dementia of the Alzheimer type. *Psychiatry Res.* 14: 255-263.

Kosada, K., Arai, H., and Ikeda, K. (1985). Familial presenile dementia with CJD-like lesions, preliminary results. *Clin. Neuropathol.* 4: 149-155.

Li, J.C., and Kaminskas, E. (1985). Deficient repair of DNA lesions in Alzheimer's disease fibroblasts. *Biochem. Biophys. Res. Commun.* 129: 733.

Mayeux, R., Stern, Y., and Spanton, S. (1985). Heterogeneity in dementia of the Alzheimer type: Evidence of subgroups. *Neurology* 35: 453-461.

Schweber, M. (1985). A possible unitary genetic hypothesis for Alzheimer's disease and Down's syndrome. *Ann. N.Y. Acad. Sci.* 450: 223-238.

Sevush, S., and Turkewitz, L.J. (1985). Brain biopsy: Risks, benefits, and indications. *Mt. Sinai J. Med.* 52: 380-383.

1986

Breitner, J.C.S., Folstein, M.F., and Murphy, E.A. (1986). Familial aggregation in Alzheimer dementia. I. A model for the age-dependent expression of an autosomal dominant gene. *J. Psychiatr. Res.* 20: 31-43.

Breitner, J.C.S., Mohs, R.C., Silverman, J.M., and Davis, K.L. (1986). Genetic factors in the etiology of Alzheimer's disease. American College of Neuropsychopharmacology 25th Annual Meeting, Washington DC, December.

Breitner, J.C.S., Murphy, E.A., and Folstein, M.F. (1986). Familial aggregation in Alzheimer dementia. II. Clinical genetic implications of age-dependent onset. *J. Psychiatr. Res.* 20: 45-55.

Heston, L.L., and Morris, M.L. (1986). Family studies of Alzheimer's dementia: Results and prospects. *Can. J. Neurol. Sci.* 13: 432-434.

Kay, D.W.K. (1986). The genetics of Alzheimer's disease. *Br. Med. Bull.* 42: 19-23.

Mayeux, R., Kupsky, W., and Duffy, P. (1986). Familial Alzheimer's disease with spongy change. *Neurology* 36: 272.

Newald, J. (1986). Plans under way for Alzheimer's center in Illinois. *Hospital* 60: 92.

Renvoize, E.B., Minham, R.H.S., Stewart, M., McDonald, R., and Wallace, D.R.D. (1986). Identical twins discordant for presenile dementia of the Alzheimer type. *Br. J. Psychiatry* 149: 509-512.

Robison, S.H., Polinsky, R., Kubic, S., and Bradley, W.G. (1986). DNA-repair in familial Alzheimer's disease. *Neurology* 36: 300.

Seltzer, B., and Sherwin, I. (1986). Fingerprint pattern differences in early- and late-onset primary degenerative dementia. *Arch. Neurol.* 43: 665-668.

Small, G.U., and Matsuyama, S.S. (1986). HLA-A2 as a possible marker for early-onset Alzheimer disease in men. *Neurobiol. Aging* 7: 211-214.

Sobel, E., Davanipour, Z., and Alter, M. (1986). Re: the use of life tables and survival analysis in testing genetic hypotheses, with an application to Alzheimer's disease (letter). *Am. J. Epidemiol.* 124: 341-342.

Spence, M.A., Heyman, A., Harazita, M.L., Sparkes, R.S., and Weinberg, T. (1986). Genetic linkage studies in Alzheimer's disease. *Neurology* 36: 581-584.

Weinreb, H.J. (1986). Dermatoglyphic patterns in Alzheimer's disease. *J. Neurogenet.* 3: 233-246.

Wolozin, B.L., Pruchnick, A., and Dickson, D.W., et al. (1986). A neuronal antigen in the brains of Alzheimer Patients. *Science* 232: 648-650.

1987

Goldgaber, D., Lerman, M.I., McBride, O.W., Saffiotti, U., and Gajdusek, D.C. (1987). Characterization and chromosomal localization of a cDNA encoding brain amyloid of Alzheimer's disease. *Science* 235: 877-880.

Jenkins, E.C., Devine-Gage, E.A., Yao, X.-L., Houck, G.E., Jr., Brown, W.T., Wisniewski, H.M., and Robakis, N.K. (1987). In-situ hybridisation of the β-amyloid protein probe to chromosome 9 in patients with familial Alzheimer's disease. *Lancet* 2: 1155-1156.

Kang, J., Lemaire, H.-G., Unterbeck, A., Salbaum, J.M., Masters, C.L., Grzeschik, K.H., Multhaup, G., Beyreuther, K., and Müller-Hill, B. (1987). The precursor of Alzheimer's disease amyloid A4 protein resembles a cell-surface receptor. *Nature* 325: 733-736.

Kay, D.W.K. (1987). Heterogeneity in Alzheimer's disease: Epidemiological and family studies. *Trends Neurosci.* 10: 194-195.

Luxenberg, J.S., May, C., Haxy, J.V., Grady, C., Moore, A., Berg, G., White, B.J., Robinette, D., and Rapoport, S.I. (1987). Cerebral metabolism, anatomy, and cognition in monozygotic twins discordant for dementia of the Alzheimer type. *J. Neurol.* 50: 333-340.

Nee, L.E., Eldridge, R., Sunderland, T., Thomas, C.B., Katz, D., Thompson, K.E., Weingartner, H., Weis, H., Julian, C., and Cohen, R. (1987). Dementia of the Alzheimer type: Clinical and family study of 22 twin pairs. *Neurology* 37: 359-363.

Podlisny, M.B., Lee, G., and Selkoe, D.J. (1987). Gene dosage of the amyloid precursor protein in Alzheimer's disease. *Science* 238: 669-671.

Robakis, N.K., Wisniewski, H.M., Jenkins, E.C., Devine-Gage, E.A., Houck, G.E., Yao, X.-L., Ramakrishna, N., Wolfe, G., Silverman, W.P., and Brown, W.T. (1987). Chromosome 21q21 sublocalisation of gene encoding beta-amyloid peptide in cerebral vessels and neuritic (senile) plaques of people with Alzheimer disease and Down's syndrome. *Lancet* 1: 384-385.

Schellenberg, G.D., Deeb, S.S., Boehnke, M., Bryant, E.M., Martin, C.M., Lampe, T.H., and Bird, T.D. (1987). Association of an apolipoprotein CII allele with familial dementia of the Alzheimer type. *J. Neurogenet.* 4: 97-108.

Selkoe, D.J., Bell, D.S., Podlisny, M.B., Price, D.L., and Cork, L.C. (1987). Conservation of brain amyloid proteins in aged mammals and humans with Alzheimer's disease. *Science* 235: 873-877.

St. George-Hyslop, P.H., Tanzi, R.E., Polinsky, R.J., Haines, J.L., Nee, L., Watkins, P.C., Myers, R.H., Feldman, R.G., Pollen, D., Drachman, D., Growdon, J., Bruni, A., Foncin, J.-F., Salomin, D., Frommelt, P., Amaducci, L., Sorbi, S., Piacentini, S., Stewart, G.D., Hobbs, W.J., Conneally, P.M., and Gusella, J.F. (1987). The genetic defect causing familial Alzheimer's disease maps on chromosome 21. *Science* 235: 885-890.

St. George-Hyslop, P.H., Tanzi, R.E., Polinsky, R.J., Neve, R.L., Pollen, D., Drachman, D., Growdon, J., Cupples, L.A., Nee, L., Myers, R.H., O'Sullivan, D., Watkins, P.C., Amos, J.A., Deutsch, C.K., Bodfish, J.W., Kinsbourne, M., Feldman, R.G., Bruni, A., Amaducci, L., Foncin, J.-F., and Gusella, J.F. (1987). Absence of duplication of chromosome 21 genes in familial and sporadic Alzheimer's disease. *Science* 238: 664-666.

Tanzi, R.E., Bird, E.D., Latt, S.A., and Neve, R.L. (1987). The amyloid protein gene is not duplicated in brains from patients with Alzheimer's disease. *Science* 238: 666-669.

Tanzi, R.E., St. George-Hyslop, P.H., Haines, J.L., Polinsky, R.J., Nee, L., Foncin, J.-F., Neve, R.L., McClatchey, A.I., Conneally, P.M., and Gusella, J.F. (1987). The genetic defect in familial Alzheimer's disease is not tightly linked to the amyloid β-protein gene. *Nature* 329: 156-157.

Tanzi, R.E., Gusella, J.F., Watkins, P.C., Bruns, G.A.P., St. George-Hyslop, P., Van Keuren, M.L., Patterson, D., Pagan, S., Kurnit, D.M., and Neve, R.L. (1987). Amyloid beta protein gene: cDNA, mRNA distribution, and genetic linkage near the Alzheimer locus. *Science* 235: 880 884.

Van Broeckhoven, C., Genthe, A.M., Vanderberghe, A., Horsthemke, B., Backhovens, H., Raeymaekers, R., Van Hul, W., Wehnert, A., Gheuens, J., Cras, P., Bruyland, M., Martin, J.J., Salbaum, M., Multhaup, G., Masters, C.L., Beyreuther, K., Gurling, H.M.D., Mullan, M.J., Holland, A., Barton, A., Irving, N., Williamson, R., Richards, S.J., and Hardy, J.A. (1987). Failure of familial Alzheimer's disease to segregate with the A4-amyloid gene in several European families. *Nature* 329: 153-155.

1988

Bird, T.D., Lampe, T.H., Nemens, E.J., Miner, G.D., Sumi, S.M., Schellenberg, G.D. (1988). Familial Alzheimer's disease in American descendants of the Volga Germans: Probably Genetic Founder Effect. *Ann. Neurol.* 23: 25-31.

Bird, T.D., Sumi, S.M., Nemens, E.J., Nochlin, D., Schellenberg, G., Lampe, T.H., Sadovnick, A., Chui, H., Miner, G.D., Tinklenberg, J., and Masters, C. (1988). Evidence for phenotypic heterogeneity in Familial Alzheimer's Disease. In: Finch, C.A. and Davies, P. (Editors): *The Molecular Biology of Alzheimer's Disease*, New York: Cold Spring Harbor Laboratory [Box 100, Cold Spring Harbor, New York 11724]. pp. 169-173.

Bird, T.D., Lampe, T., Nemens, E.J., Sumi, S.M., Nochlin, D., Schellenberg, G., Wijaman, E., Miner, G. (1988). Characteristics of familial Alzheimer's disease in nine kindreds of Volga German descent. *Alz. Dis. Assoc. Dis.* 2: 286.

Breitner, J.C.S., Silverman, J.M., Mohs, R.C., and Davis, K.L. (1988). Familial aggregation in Alzheimer's disease: Comparison of risk among relatives of early- and late-onset cases, and among male and female relatives in successive generations. *Neurology* 38: 207-212.

Brown, W.T., Devine-Gage, E.A., Jenkins, E.C., Wu, Y., Harris, M., Yao, X., Rubinstein, R., Kascsak, R., Wisniewski, H., Schellenberg, G., Bird, T.D. (1988). Genetics of familial Alzheimer's disease. *Alz. Dis. Assoc. Dis.* 2: 273.

Furuya, H., Sasaki, H., Goto, I., Wong, C.W., Glenner, G.G., and Sakasi, Y. (1988). Amyloid β-protein gene duplication is not common in Alzheimer's disease: Analysis by polymorphic restriction fragments. *Biochem. Biophys. Res. Commun.* 150: 75-81.

Miner, G.D., and Richter, R.W. (1988). Meeting Report: First International Symposium on Familial Alzheimer's Disease. *Neurobiol. Aging* 9: 415-419.

Murdoch, G.H., Manuelidis, L., Kin, J.H., and Manuelidis, E.E. (1988). β-amyloid gene dosage in Alzheimer's disease. *Nucleic Acids Res.* 16: 357.

Nochlin, D., Sumi, S.M., Snow, A.D., et al. (1988). Familial dementia with unusual "senile" plaques with multiple amyloid cores positive for prion protein. *Neurology* 38 (Suppl. 1): 266.

Pericak-Vance, M.A., Yamanoka, L.H., Haynes, C.S., Speer, M.C., Haines, J.L., Gaskell, P.C., Hung, W.-Y., Clark, C.M., Heyman, A.L., Trofatter, J.A., Eisenmenger, J.P., Gilbert, J.R., Lee, J.E., Alberts, M.J., Conneally, P.M., and Roses, A.D. (1988). Genetic linkage studies in Alzheimer's disease families. *Exper. Neurol.* 102: 271-279.

Schellenberg, G.D., Bird, T.D., Wijsman, E.M., Moore, D.K., Doehnke, M., Bryant, E.M., Lampe, T.H., Nochlin, D., Sumi, S.M., Deeb, S.S., Beyereuther, K., and Martin, G.M. (1988). Absence of chromosome 21q21 markers to familial Alzheimer's disease. *Science* 241: 1507-1510.

Snow, A.D., Nochlin, D., Sumi, S.M., Bird, T.D., Wight, T.N. (1988). Immunolocalization of Heparan Sulfate proteoglycans to primitive plaques and multicore prior positive plaques in familial dementia. *Alz. Dis. Assoc. Dis.* 2: 232.

Tanzi, R.E., Haines, J.L., Watkins, P.C., Stewart, G.D., Wallace, M.R., Hallewell, R., Wong, C., Wexler, N.S., Conneally, P.M., and Gusella, J.F. (1988). Genetic Linkage Map of Human Chromosome 21. *Genomics* 3: 129-136.

Zubenko, G.S., and Ferrell, R.E. (1988). Monozygotic twins concordant for probable Alzheimer's disease and increased platelet membrane fluidity. *Am. J. Med. Genet.* 29: 431-436.

1989

January:

Bird, T.D., Sumi, S.M., Nemens, E.J., Nochlin, D., Schellenberg, G., Lampe, T.H., Sadovnick, A., Chui, H., Miner, G.D., and Tinklenberg, J. (1989). Phenotypic heterogeneity in Familial Alzheimer's Disease: A study of 24 kindreds. *Ann. Neurol.* 25: 12-25.

Index

B

C

D

E

H

I

J

K

L

M

N

O

P

About the Editors

GARY D. MINER is Cofounder and Chief-Executive-Officer of the Familial Alzheimer's Disease Research Foundation in Tulsa, Oklahoma. He also serves as an Affiliate Research Scientist at the Oklahoma Medical Research Foundation; and is working with the University of Oklahoma Health Sciences Center, Oklahoma City, and with institutions in adjacent states to develop a regional Alzheimer's Center. He previously served as Associate Professor of Pharmacology at Oral Roberts University School of Medicine, and Director of the Alzheimer's Disease and Geriatric Disorders Research Laboratory at the City of Faith Medical & Research Center in Tulsa, Oklahoma. Dr. Miner has authored or coauthored numerous articles and abstracts in leading medical journals, and he is a member of the American Association for the Advancement of Science, Behavior Genetics Association, American Geriatrics Society, American Federation for Aging Research, and Society for Sigma Xi. He received the B.S. degree (1964) from Hamline University, St. Paul, Minnesota, M.S. degree (1966) from the University of Wyoming, in Laramie, and Ph.D. degree (1970) from the University of Kansas in Lawrence, with postdoctoral work in behavior genetics and psychiatric epidemiology at the University of Minnesota and the University of Iowa.

RALPH W. RICHTER is Clinical Professor of Neurology and Clinical Associate Professor of Psychiatry at the University of Oklahoma Tulsa Medical College. He also serves as Director of the Alzheimer's Disease Research Unit at St. Johns Medical Center in Tulsa, Oklahoma. Dr. Richter previously served as professor of clinical neurology at Columbia University College of Physicians and Surgeons, New York, NY. Dr. Richter has authored or coauthored over 90 articles, abstracts, book chapters and proceedings papers on pertinent areas of research and was appointed to the Task Force on Alzheimer's Disease by the Governor of Oklahoma. He is a Fellow of the American College of Physicians and American Academy of Neurology, and member of the Tulsa County Medical Society, Oklahoma State Medical Society, and American Medical Association. Dr. Richter received the A.B. degree (1952) from Columbia University in New York, and M.D. degree (1956) from the Columbia University College of Physicians & Surgeons.

JOHN P. BLASS is Winifred Masterson Burke Professor in the Departments of Neurology and Medicine for Cornell University Medical College in New York City. He also serves as Staff Physician and Director of the Dementia Research Service for the Burke Rehabilitation Center in White Plains, New York. Dr. Blass has authored or coauthored more than 250 journal articles, book chapters, and abstracts, as well as a pamphlet entitled Alzheimer's Disease. He is a member of the American Federation of Aging Research, American Geriatrics Society, Gerontological Society of America, Alzheimer's and Related Disorders Association, among other professional societies. Dr. Blass received the A.B. degree (1958) from Harvard College in Massachusetts, Ph.D. degree (1960) in biochemistry from the University of London, and M.D. degree (1965) from Columbia University in New York.

JIMMIE L. VALENTINE is Chairman and Professor of Pharmacology at the Oral Roberts University School of Medicine. Dr. Valentine has authored or coauthored numerous articles in refereed journals and several book chapters. He is a member of the American Society for Pharmacology and Experimental Therapeutics, American Pharmaceutical Association, International Society for Immunopharmacology, among other professional societies. Dr. Valentine received the B.S. degree (1962) in biology and (1964) in chemistry from Centenary College of Louisiana, M.S. degree (1966) and Ph.D. degree (1968) in medicinal chemistry from the University of Mississippi.

LINDA A. WINTERS-MINER is Cofounder and Vice President of the Familial Alzheimer's Disease Research Foundation, Tulsa, Oklahoma. She also serves as Coordinator of the Tulsa Alzheimer's Disease Community Resource Center at the University of Tulsa and is working with the Department of Biostatistics and Epidemiology at the University of Oklahoma Health Sciences Center, Oklahoma City, to develop an epidemiological study of Alzheimer's Disease in the Cherokee Indian Nation of Oklahoma. Dr. Miner has coauthored several articles, abstracts, and proceedings papers on Alzheimer's disease and was awarded a post-doctoral fellowship in psychiatric epidemiology from the University of Iowa. She received the B.S. (1967) and M.S. (1971) degrees from the University of Kansas in Lawrence, and Ph.D. degree (1977) from the University of Minnesota in Minneapolis.